Growing Inequality:
Bridging Complex Systems, Health Disparities, and Population Health

GROWING INEQUALITY

BRIDGING COMPLEX SYSTEMS, POPULATION HEALTH, AND HEALTH DISPARITIES

■

**GEORGE A. KAPLAN, ANA V. DIEZ ROUX,
CARL P. SIMON, AND SANDRO GALEA**

EDITORS

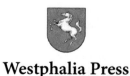

Westphalia Press
An Imprint of the Policy Studies Organization
Washington, DC
2017

GROWING INEQUALITY:
BRIDGING COMPLEX SYSTEMS, HEALTH DISPARITIES, AND POPULATION HEALTH

Westphalia Press
An imprint of Policy Studies Organization
1527 New Hampshire Ave., NW
Washington, D.C. 20036
info@ipsonet.org

ISBN-10: 1-63391-517-4
ISBN-13: 978-1-63391-517-6

Cover and interior design by Jeffrey Barnes
jbarnesbook.design

Daniel Gutierrez-Sandoval, Executive Director
PSO and Westphalia Press

Updated material and comments on this edition
can be found at the Westphalia Press website:
www.westphaliapress.org

CONTENTS

ACKNOWLEDGEMENTS

An edited volume often simply reflects the aggregation of related work by multiple authors. This volume is quite different in that the work included reflects the results of an extended process that brought together scholars from diverse disciplines as part of the Network on Inequality, Complexity, and Health (NICH), who explored the confluence of complex systems simulation methods, and population health and health disparities concerns and research. Above all, we acknowledge the critical contributions of the NICH members whose commitment, ability to transcend disciplinary and methodological boundaries, and depth of knowledge created a fertile and unique environment for pursuing new directions.

Beyond the NICH members, the success of this effort—and the book that showcases its accomplishments—owes much to other people and their institutions. Foremost we acknowledge the leadership and vision of David Abrams, PhD, and Robert Kaplan, PhD, who as Directors of the Office of Behavioral and Social Sciences Research (OBSSR) at the National Institutes of Health (NIH) were critical in providing initial (Abrams) and continuing (Kaplan) support for NICH. The advice, stewardship, creative problem-solving, and commitment to NICH of Helen Meissner, PhD, then Senior Advisor at OBSSR, and G. Stephane Philogene, PhD, Deputy Director of OBSSR, were invaluable. We also thank Patty Mabry, then Senior Advisor at OBSSR, for her support.

The University of Michigan, where all the editors of this book were faculty members at the time that NICH began, contributed in many ways. In particular, the Center for Social Epidemiology and Population Health, and the Center for the Study of Complex Systems provided an environment and colleagues that helped to catalyze this effort. We also recognize financial support from the University of Michigan School of Public Health and the Office of the Vice President for Research. In addition to generous funding for NICH from OBSSR (HHSN276200800013C), work that was integral to the development and conceptualization of NICH was supported by awards from the National Institute of Child Health and Development (NICHD: P50HD038986, R24HD047861) and the Robert Wood Johnson Health and Society Scholars Program. George Kaplan's contributions were also generously supported by the Institute for Integrative Health.

Finally, we would also like to acknowledge the important contributions of Janet Byron and Davis Krauter who have done a wonderful job fine-tuning our words (Byron) and figures (Krauter).

FOREWORD

Robert M. Kaplan, PhD
Director of Research, Clinical Excellence Research Center
Stanford University School of Medicine
Former Director, NIH Office of Behavioral and Social Sciences Research

G. Stephane Philogene, PhD
Deputy Director, NIH Office of Behavioral and Social Sciences Research

David B. Abrams, PhD
Executive Director, The Schroeder Institute for Tobacco Research and Policy Studies,
American Legacy Foundation
Professor, Johns Hopkins Bloomberg School of Public Health
Former Director, NIH Office of Behavioral and Social Sciences Research

The National Institutes of Health (NIH) is the largest supporter of health-relevant research in the world. The NIH provides stewardship for biomedical and sociobehavioral research for the United States and populations throughout the world. The well-known basic science mission of the NIH is to pursue fundamental knowledge about the nature and behavior of living systems. But, perhaps less appreciated is the second clause of the NIH mission statement, which emphasizes the application of knowledge to enhance health, lengthen life, and reduce illness and disability.

It is often assumed that the mechanism for increasing quality of life and life expectancy and reducing the burden of illness and disability is investment in medical care. However, a variety of analyses using several research methodologies have shown that medical care accounts for only a small portion of the variation in health outcomes.[1,2] The United States spends considerably more than any other country on healthcare, but its return on investment in terms of health outcomes has been disappointing. The NIH Office of Behavioral and Social Sciences Research (OBSSR) sponsored a National Research Council/Institute of Medicine study that compared life expectancies and other health indicators of Americans to those of people in other rich countries. Although the life expectancies of Americans are increasing, they are not keeping pace with those in other developed countries. In one comparison of life expectancies in 10 wealthy countries, American women were 3rd out of 10 in 1955, but 9th out of 10 in 2006. Countries with more rapid increases in life expectancy included Japan, France, and Spain. Japan, for example, was considerably below the United

States in 1955 and now is many years ahead. The factors where the United States is number 1 include the prevalence of obesity and overweight youth, adolescent pregnancy, and the number of 15–24 year olds infected with HIV. On measures such as firearm-related homicides, no other wealthy country came close.[3] It was clear that we needed new ways to address the challenge of our relatively poor performance.

In first decade of the twenty-first century, OBSSR realized that new methods were necessary to help us understand a wider range of factors that determine the health of populations. As we learned more about factors associated with longer life, several concerns emerged. First, it was apparent that economic inequality had a profound relationship to life expectancy. Second, most major threats to the public's health were complex; they represent combinations of behavioral and social factors that ultimately have impacts on biological processes, and these influences play out over entire lifetimes. For example, social and environmental influences in prenatal or early childhood can continue to affect health outcomes over the entire human lifespan. Third, it was clear that current research methodologies were inadequate to help us understand the relationship between inequality, complexity, and health. Few behavioral, social, or biological scientists were experienced in the modeling techniques required to pull the pieces together. Perhaps more challenging was that most academic researchers work in intellectually isolated silos. They speak in different technical languages, making it difficult to jointly tackle complex questions. OBSSR recognized that a network of committed experts was needed to develop new synergy and fresh approaches to these problems.

The Network on Complexity, Inequality, and Health

In spring 2007, OBSSR released its second strategic plan, under the leadership of David B. Abrams, PhD. As articulated in the plan, the vision was "to bring together the biomedical, behavioral, social, and public-health science research communities to work more collaboratively to solve the most pressing population health challenges faced by our society."[4] To realize this vision, the office developed a series of initiatives to: (1) facilitate collaborative research across the full range of disciplines and stakeholders; (2) stimulate systems thinking and modeling approaches to research that integrate multiple levels of analysis; and (3) work with other NIH institutes and centers to identify key problems in population health where scientists, practitioners, and decision makers can work together to accelerate the translation, implementation, dissemination, and adoption of behavioral and social sciences research findings. The strategic plan also had a special focus on health disparities, one of the most persistent, policy-resistant, and pressing dilemmas in the United States, and one that we believed demanded new strategies and insights.[5]

Multiple factors may be associated with health disparities, and traditional research methods have not produced enough new insights. Not only do multiple factors contribute to disparities, but the factors also interact with each other in complex and nonlinear ways. On the other hand, colleagues in engineering and computer sciences have been studying complex systems for many years and have developed sophisticated methods for modeling complexity. One of the most important contributions of our project was the importation of systems-science principles from engineering sciences to address an important public health problem. Systems thinking actually expands on traditional biomedical methods because it can incorporate multilevel factors from the biological, psychosocial, and population-level disciplines and professions that can be brought to bear to understand and improve population health and longevity.[4] Various methodologies can be employed, such as system-dynamics simulation, agent-based modeling, network analysis, and Markov modeling to address the heterogeneity of the system, especially when it is not possible or ethical to conduct real-world experiments. This conceptual vision for OBSSR at NIH needed to be translated into concrete blueprints for action using proof-of-concept projects producing practical results.

To begin the process of addressing this problem of how to apply systems science to real-world problems, OBSSR convened a meeting in March 2008 entitled "System Integrative Research to Eliminate Health Disparities." The meeting took place at the Center for Advanced Study in the Behavioral Sciences at Stanford University. About 14 scholars in the population health and health disparities area were invited— including three faculty members from the Center for Social Epidemiology and Population Health at the University of Michigan (George A. Kaplan, Sandro Galea, Ana Diez Roux) and OBSSR staff. The Michigan group was already engaged in the application of systems approaches to understanding health disparities and closely linked areas of population health. The purpose of the meeting was to brainstorm about the best mechanisms and processes required over 1–3 years to develop a "next-generation" research agenda and set of research priorities. We believed that the extraordinary opportunities emerging from integrative systems thinking and transdisciplinary team science should drive this next-generation research agenda. Specifically, we needed a transdisciplinary process that supported and encouraged a meaningful exchange of ideas that could ultimately lead to research with innovative system-based methodologies. The question was how to get there?

We considered a number of ideas. One was Stanford University's "think tank" sabbatical approach, in which the Center for Advanced Study in the Behavioral Sciences brings together scholars from around the world to think, collaborate, and write for a fellowship year in an environment specifically designed to support high-level intellectual work. Likewise, some of the meeting participants had experience working on the MacArthur Foundation's Research Networks. These networks are designed to identify a big problem and bring together researchers, practitioners, and policymakers from multiple disciplines to work collaboratively over an extended period of time. Similarly, the Canadian Institute for Advanced Research's (CIFAR) Population Health Program furthers understanding of the broad and fundamental determinants of health by bringing together multidisciplinary groups of researchers with diverse perspectives. George Kaplan, a member of that program at CIFAR, helped to bridge ideas across different working groups. During the March 2008 meeting at Stanford University, systems-science ideas were considered, but each presented its own set of challenges for implementation as an NIH initiative. By the end of the meeting, the fundamental question remained: What would be the best framework to launch a systems-integrative, transdisciplinary effort that would lead to real breakthroughs in health disparities research?

Following the meeting at Stanford, the first opportunities for implementation of this vision came in March 2008, when the OBSSR received an unsolicited proposal from George Kaplan, Director of the Center for Social Epidemiology and Population Health at University of Michigan. Kaplan proposed a new multidisciplinary approach that would bring together leaders from the biomedical, behavioral, social, and public-health science research communities to work more collaboratively to solve the most pressing population-health challenges faced by our society. The focus of the proposed network was to build bridges between medical, public health, and computer science communities. The new synergy that he proposed would be used to build models of complex systems that serve as the basis for the simulations reported in this volume. Nonetheless, any group that studies complex problems needs a complex name; in this case, we chose the Network on Inequality, Complexity, and Health (NICH), with a primary focus on health disparities and population health.

The Network's Work

The network's progress was slow at first. When we attended the early meetings we wondered whether the network would gain traction. It took time for the investigators to understand one another's methods and to appreciate how hard it is for engineers, system scientists, epidemiologists, physicians, and behavioral scientists to develop a common language to understand the nuances and complexities of one another's disciplines. But within a relatively short time, synergy began to emerge with the group and the work reported in this volume represents one of many exciting projects that emerged from NICH.

The chapters in this book represent innovative, novel, and original contributions that may define a whole new way of examining some of the most challenging problems in population health. As former and current leaders of the OBSSR, we are proud to have been part of this important effort. Ultimately, we hope that it contributes to improving the health-related quality of life not only of the American people but also the people of the world. The rapid emergence of new technologies, tracking systems, digital and social media, and big data and its analysis—while still works in progress—provides powerful new tools to fuel the rapid adoption of systems-integrative approaches to improving the health not only of individuals but critically also of whole populations.

References

1. Murray CJ, Vos T, Lozano R, et al. Disability-adjusted life years (DALYs) for 291 diseases and injuries in 21 regions, 1990–2010: a systematic analysis for the Global Burden of Disease Study 2010. *Lancet.* 2012;380:2197–2223.

2. Schroeder SA. Shattuck Lecture. We can do better—improving the health of the American people. *N Engl J Med.* 2007;357:1221–1228.

3. Woolf SH, Aron LY. The US health disadvantage relative to other high-income countries: findings from a National Research Council/Institute of Medicine report. *JAMA.* 2013;309:771–772.

4. Mabry PL, Olster DH, Morgan GD, Abrams DB. Interdisciplinarity and systems science to improve population health: a view from the NIH Office of Behavioral and Social Sciences Research. *Am J Prev Med.* 2008;35:S211–S224.

5 Abrams DB. Applying transdisciplinary research strategies to understanding and eliminating health disparities. *Health Educ Behav.* 2006;33(4):515–531.

CHAPTER 1

BRIDGING COMPLEX SYSTEMS, HEALTH DISPARITIES, AND POPULATION HEALTH

George A. Kaplan, PhD
Thomas Francis Collegiate Professor Emeritus of Public Health
University of Michigan

Carl P. Simon, PhD
Professor of Mathematics, Complex Systems and Public Policy
University of Michigan

Ana V. Diez Roux, MD, PhD, MPH
Dean and Distinguished University Professor
Dornsife School of Public Health
Drexel University

Sandro Galea, MD, MPH, DrPH
Dean and Robert A Knox Professor
School of Public Health
Boston University

Acknowledgments: Preparation of this chapter was supported, in part, by the NIH Office of Behavioral and Social Sciences Research (Network on Inequality, Complexity and Health; HHSN276200800013, George A. Kaplan, Principal Investigator), the Robert Wood Johnson Foundation Health and Society Scholars Program (George A. Kaplan, Principal Investigator), the University of Michigan Center for Social Epidemiology and Population Health, and The Institute for Integrative Health (George A. Kaplan).

Myra: A Case Study in Growing Inequality

Consider the case of Myra, who is now 12 years old. Her parents have been unemployed on and off for

1

most of her life, including the entire year before she was born. They move from apartment to apartment as one health or job crisis follows another and are evicted because they are unable to pay the rent on time. Sometimes they need to move because heat and hot water are not available enough, or their landlord has lapsed on providing pest control so rats and cockroaches are prevalent. Often they reach the end of the month with little money to spend on food or other necessities, and the little they get in food vouchers has been spent. An occasional treat following a payday for one of her parents is a fast food hamburger, fries, and giant soft drink. They live in a neighborhood bereft of parks but with a surplus of abandoned buildings and crime. Grocery stores with aisles of fresh food are miles away, while stores that feature cigarettes, sugar-filled soft drinks, and chips are around the corner. Myra does not play outside much because it does not feel safe. She did not have any early childhood education classes or informal programs and began school in kindergarten. There are few books but lots television in her home. School is now a refuge for Myra—it is safe and she has friends there, but the teachers are overburdened by too many students, too few books, too little pay, and too little training. She is in 7th grade, but reads at the 4th grade level and is not so sure about simple mathematics. There is no recess, physical or health education, school nurse or counselor, or computer training. Some days she feels pretty low and just does not feel like getting out of bed and going to school, so she just stays home and watches television. Sometimes her friends, also not in school and sometimes older than her, come over.

Her mother has a minimum-wage cleaning job in a mall an hour's ride away by bus, with a work schedule that changes unpredictably from day to day. She is employed on an hourly basis by a subcontractor to the mall and receives no health, retirement, or other benefits. Her father is a non-union carpenter, but works only intermittently due to the poor economy and a previous injury from a fall from unsafe scaffolding. He received unemployment and disability benefits for a while, but they have been discontinued due to time limits on eligibility. Because of the fall and lack of proper medical treatment, he has lost some mobility. Needless to say, even with the Affordable Care Act and expansion of Medicaid in some states (but not theirs), her parents may still not have any health insurance and have to rely on public clinics and emergency rooms for care.

Clearly, the circumstances in which Myra and her family live are difficult and taxing. Many Myras will do fine despite this adversity, but far too many will live out lives of blunted aspirations and achievement. Central to this is poor health, for Myra's circumstances endanger her current and future health, and she is headed for a vicious spiral of poor conditions begetting poor health and poor health leading to worsening conditions.[1,2] We know from the epidemiologic literature that Myra is more likely to develop a large number of health problems in her lifetime, including obesity,[3] asthma and other respiratory diseases,[4] type 2 diabetes,[5] depression,[6] cardiovascular disease,[7] impaired physiological response to stress,[8] neurological changes and dementia, hypertension,[9] hampered resistance to infection,[10] the risks associated with early sexual activity,[11] early substance use,[12] motor vehicle accidents and other injuries,[13] musculoskeletal disorders,[14] and poorer prognosis and faster progression of many of these and more.[15]

The social, environmental, behavioral, and health challenges Myra faces are not independent forces but represent an interconnected ecology of experiences that constrain many aspects of Myra's life over her lifetime, constraints that are likely to be passed on to her children. At the individual level these constraints will exact a toll, but the toll is even greater when we consider the many others like her and how these interconnected challenges result in the collective loss of her and others' contributions to society.

Understanding Myra's Health

But what is to be done about it? The usual approach would be to search for a magic bullet, for example a single factor that would turn Myra's trajectory around such as better food stores, smoking cessation programs, early childhood education, improved access to health care, and a new pharmaceutical agent. Each of these has value, but many of the problems are so intertwined that singling out one remedy might not be effective. For example, if Myra had been fortunate enough to have access to early childhood education, would she have overcome the challenges of attending an under-resourced and overburdened school in a dangerous neighborhood? Or, would the availability of healthier food in her neighborhood help if her parents could not afford it? Or, conversely, would improvement in her parents' economic situation allow her family to move to a better neighborhood, bringing with it higher quality schools, better access to healthy food and recreational facilities, improved air quality, and more positive role models?

Understanding Myra's current and future health and the many other health problems that she faces requires grappling with the multiple, tightly interrelated, and causally tangled determinants of her health, many of which are outside the usual purview of health sciences (figure 1).[16–20] The considerable interconnection and interaction within and across domains that she faces, the multiple levels and scales of the determinants of her health, and the complex dynamics operating over her life course do not easily lend themselves to the conventional tools of the health or social sciences.[21,22]

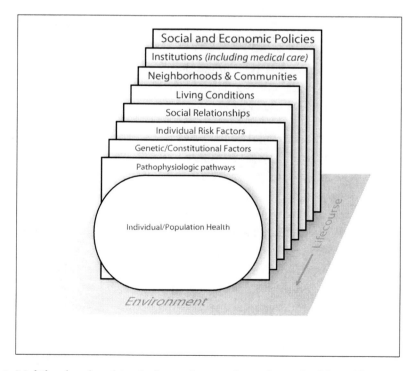

Figure 1. Multilevel and multiscale determinants of population health and health disparities[16]

Many Myras—Populations and Inequality

Myra is one child but she represents many. The interlocking threats to their individual and collective social, economic, and behavioral functioning—biologically embedded over the life course and across generations—create compelling patterns of health inequality that confront our society. These inequalities are all the more dramatic when populations are arrayed by race, ethnicity, or socioeconomic position.[23-27] These threats are not distributed randomly in the population but are burdens reflecting the historical and contemporary social, economic, and political forces that, when bundled together, have a deleterious impact on the health of particular groups.

It is abundantly clear that there are no simple solutions to eliminating these disparities, as they represent the confluence of so many factors that determine levels of health and function.[16] Many of these factors are considerably upstream from the usual focus of the health sciences, and they have a broad footprint on more proximal determinants of health.[27-30] In addition, they do not operate in a vacuum but instead are interacting threads that weave a garment of inequality stretching from conception to death. This dense network of interacting factors—covering multiple domains, extending across multiple levels and scales, and playing out over the life course and across generations—poses major analytic and conceptual challenges to the goal of eliminating, or even reducing, health disparities. The standard approach of looking for single, independent factors and directing interventions at them may not be sufficient to meet the challenges posed by the systematic patterns of disparities in health that we observe between racial, ethnic, and socioeconomic groups. Small steps may be taken, but the level of complexity involved in such an endeavor calls for a new approach.

The Network on Inequality, Complexity and Health (NICH)

On a fall day in 2010, scholars from across the United States and Canada gathered at the University of Michigan to commit themselves to collaborating for the next four and a half years on a new approach to understanding the health of Myra and those like her.

With support from the Office of Behavioral and Social Science Research (OBSSR) at the National Institutes of Health (NIH), they formed the NICH. Representing about 18 academic fields (table 1), their self-described interests cut a broad swath, covering social stratification, neighborhood change, segregation, income inequality, systems thinking, stress, ecology, education and economic development, racial achievement gaps, interventions, stress physiology, neuroscience, health behavior, emotions, socioeconomic position, sex hormones, complexity, dynamic systems, diversity, economic and political systems, genetic and environmental factors in shaping development, bio-behavioral development, social isolation, continuity versus change in development, policy-oriented research on the development of young children focusing on family and community influences, designing and evaluating interventions and policies aimed at enhancing the well-being of children living in poverty, inequalities in communication and health disparities, addressing disparities through communication and dissemination, life events, immunology, social support/networks, life course perspectives, mental health, stress pathways, civil rights, state and local government, state and local finance, land use, regional governance and the legislative process, domestic poverty and federal fiscal policy, social epidemiology, nutrition, minority health and women's health issues

Table 1

NICH Members

Member	Institution	Fields of expertise
George Kaplan, chair	University of Michigan	Social Epidemiology
W. Thomas Boyce	University of California, San Francisco	Developmental Neurosciences
Jeanne Brooks-Gunn	Columbia University	Child Development
Elizabeth Bruch	University of Michigan	Sociology, Complex Systems
Sandro Galea, co-Chair	University of Michigan, Columbia University, Boston University	Epidemiology (Social and Psychiatric)
Ross Hammond	Brookings Institution	Political Science, Complex Systems
Rucker Johnson	University of California, Berkeley	Economics, Public Policy
Shiriki Kumanyika	University of Pennsylvania	Epidemiology, Nutrition
Myron Orfield	University of Minnesota	Law, Inequality
Nathanial Osgood	University of Saskatchewan	Computer Science, Public Health
Sean Reardon	Stanford University	Education, Sociology
Rick Riolo	University of Michigan	Complex Systems
Ana Diez Roux, co-chair	University of Michigan, Drexel University	Social Epidemiology
Carl Simon, co-chair	University of Michigan	Mathematics, Public Policy, Complex Systems
Kurt Stange	Case Western University	Medicine, Epidemiology, Sociology
Steve Suomi	Eunice Kennedy Shriver National Institute of Child Health and Human Development, NIH	Comparative Ethnology, Psychology
Vish Viswanath	Harvard University	Communications
Michael Wolfson	University of Ottawa	Economics, Complex Systems

with a focus on prevention, modeling of population health trends and health policy trade-offs, systems models of disease, development of modeling techniques, clinical research, practice-based research, cancer control, health services research, health policy, minority health, poverty and inequality, neighborhood effects, educational effects, public policy, and the modeling of complex social, economic, and biological systems using agent-based computational models and nonlinear dynamical systems.

Already experts in their fields and likely overcommitted, what would motivate them to commit considerable time and effort to work with colleagues coming from different disciplines, who used different analytic and conceptual tools than they did, and whose professional vocabulary often seemed to require a translator? Their effort, the results of which are reported in this volume, was driven by three considerations. First, there was a critical need to develop a better understanding of the factors contributing to health disparities and population health; second, that the development of such an understanding would be best served by bringing together a broad spectrum of expertise; and finally, that a new approach was needed that embraced and analyzed the complexity of the systems that produce health disparities and population health.

The need to better understand of the determinants of population health and health disparities has been addressed in many places,[16,17,31,32] as has the need for cross- and transdisciplinary approaches.[33] What was unique about this effort was the explicit incorporation of complex systems approaches into the discussion. Starting with the recognition that it is systems that generate health disparities and population health, complex systems approaches allow us to appreciate that the production of health inequalities does not rest only on complicated systems with lots of pieces, but instead on complex systems involving multiple interacting factors with dense, and sometimes nonlinear, feedback. As such, health inequalities, as complex systems, cannot be easily reduced to independent components with analyses of the isolated impacts of single components.

Complex systems approaches provide tools that can accommodate the complex, dynamic, multilevel structures and processes, sometimes nonlinear, that are required for analyzing of many critical problems in health disparities and population health.[22,34] These tools are computational approaches that make use of computer-based algorithms to model dynamic interactions between components, within, and across levels of influence. With the potential for both spatial and temporal dimensions, complex systems analytic approaches allow us to simulate the growth of inequalities across space, time, and generations. While long adopted by many branches of science, complex systems approaches are largely new to population health, and our efforts to understand the complex systems that generate health inequalities and overall patterns of population health remain in their infancy. NICH was the first effort, to our knowledge, to bring together a broad array of health science, social science, and computer science scholars to see what could be added to our understanding of the systems that grow health inequality. The remainder of this volume presents the results of some of our analyses, and ends with thoughts on the strengths and limitations of using complex systems tools and recommendations for moving forward. Our hope is that this work can catalyze the building of further bridges between complex systems, health disparities, and population health researchers.

References

1. Duncan GJ, Brooks-Gunn J, eds. *Consequences of Growing Up Poor*. New York, NY: Russel Sage Foundation; 1999.

2. Lu MC, Halfon N. Racial and ethnic disparities in birth outcomes: a life-course perspective. *Matern Child Health J*. 2003;7(1):13–30.

3. Lee H, Harris KM, Gordon-Larsen P. Life course perspectives on the links between poverty and obesity during the transition to young adulthood. *Popul Res Policy Rev*. 2009;28(4):505–532.

4. Newacheck PW, Halfon N. Prevalence, impact, and trends in childhood disability due to asthma. *Arch Pediatr Adolesc Med*. 2000;154(3):287–293.

5. Maty SA, James SA, Kaplan GA. Life course socioeconomic position and incidence of diabetes mellitus among blacks and whites: the Alameda County Study, 1965–1999. *Am J Public Health*. 2010;100(1):137–145.

6. Everson SA, Sioban C, Lynch JW, Kaplan, GA. Epidemiologic evidence for the relation between socioeconomic status and depression, obesity, and diabetes. *J Psychosom Res*. 2002;53(4):891–895.

7. Johnson-Lawrence V, Galea S, Kaplan G. Cumulative socioeconomic disadvantage and cardiovascular disease mortality in the Alameda County Study 1965 to 2000. *Ann Epidemiol*. 2015;25(2):65–70.

8. McEwen BS. Brain on stress: how the social environment gets under the skin. *Proc Natl Acad Sci USA*. 2012;109(Suppl 2):17180–17185.

9. Morenoff JS, Hansen BB, Williams DR, Kaplan GA, Hunte HE, Jeffrey DH. Understanding social disparities in hypertension prevalence, awareness, treatment, and control: the role of neighborhood context. *Soc Sci Med*. 2007;65(9):1853–1866.

10. Dowd JB, Zajacova A, Aiello A. Early origins of health disparities: burden of infection, health, and socioeconomic status in U.S. children. *Soc Sci Med*. 2009;68(4):699–707.

11. Dupéré V, Lacourse E, Willms JD, Leventhal T, Tremblay RE. Neighborhood poverty and early transition to sexual activity in young adolescents: a developmental ecological approach. *Child Dev*. 2008;79(5):1463–1476.

12. Galea S, Nandi A, Vlahov D. The social epidemiology of substance use. *Epidemiol Rev*. 2004;26(1):36–52.

13. Singh GK. *Child Mortality in the United States, 1935–2007: Large Racial and Socioeconomic Disparities Have Persisted Over Time. A 75th Anniversary Publication*. Rockville, MD: US Department of Health and Human Services, Health Resources and Services Administration; 2010.

14. National Center for Health Statistics. *Health, United States, 2014: With Special Feature on Adults Aged 55–64*. Hyattsville, MD: National Center for Health Statistics; 2015.

15. Hertzman C. The biological embedding of early experience and its effects on health in adulthood. *Ann N Y Acad Sci*. 1999;896(1):85–95.

16. Kaplan GA, Everson S, Lynch JW. The contribution of social and behavioral research to an understanding of the distribution of disease: a multilevel approach. In: Smedley BD, Syme SL, eds. *Promoting Health: Intervention Strategies from Social and Behavioral Research*. Washington, DC: National Academy Press; 2000:31–55.

17. Schoeni RF, House JS, Kaplan GA, Pollack H. *Making Americans Healthier*. New York, NY: Russell Sage Foundation; 2008.

18. Kaplan GA. Economic policy is health policy: findings from the study of income, socioeconomic status, and health. In: Auerbach JA, Krimgold BK, eds. *Income, Socioeconomic Status and Health: Exploring the Relationships*. Washington, DC: National Policy Association; 2001:137–149.

19. Galea S, ed. *Macrosocial Determinants of Population Health*. New York, NY: Springer-Verlag; 2007.

20. Viner RM, Ozer EM, Denny S, et al. Adolescence and the social determinants of health. *Lancet*. 2012;379(9826):1641–1652.

21. Kaplan GA, Galea S. Bridging complexity science and the social determinants of health. *J Policy Complex Syst*. 2014;1(2):88–109.

22. Galea S, Riddle M, Kaplan GA. Causal thinking and complex system approaches in epidemiology. *Int J Epidemiol*. 2010;39(1):97–106.

23. Kaplan GA, Haan MN, Syme SL, Minkler M, Winkelby M. Socioeconomic status and health: closing the gap: the buden of unnecessary illness. *Am J Prev Med*. 1987;3(5):125–129.

24. Centers for Disease Control and Prevention. Health Disparities and Inequalities Report–United States, 2013. *MMWR Morb Mortal Wkly Rep*. 2013;62(Suppl 3):1–186.

25. Krueger PM, Reither EN. Mind the gap: race/ethnic and socioeconomic disparities in obesity. *Curr Diab Rep*. 2015;15(11):95.

26. Kaplan GA. *The Poor Pay More - Poverty's High Cost to Health*. Robert Wood Johnson Foundation; 2009. http://www.rwjf.org/content/dam/farm/reports/reports/2009/rwjf47463.

27. Woolf SH, Braveman P. Where health disparities begin: the role of social and economic determinants—and why current policies may make matters worse. *Health Aff*. 2011;30(10):1852–1859.

28. Shonkoff JP, Phillips DA, eds. *From Neurons to Neighborhoods: The Science of Early Childhood Development*. Washington, DC: National Academies Press; 2000.

29. Williams DR, Sternthal M. Understanding racial-ethnic disparities in health: sociological contributions. *J Health Soc Behav*. 2010;51(Suppl 1):S15–S27.

30. Kaplan GA. Is economic policy healthy policy? *Am J Epidemiol*. 2001;91:351–353.

31. Kaplan GA, Lynch JW. Socioeconomic considerations in the primordial prevention of cardiovascular disease. *Prev Med*. 1999;29(6 pt 2):S30–S35.

32. Glass TA, McAtee MJ. Behavioral science at the crossroads in public health: extending horizons, envisioning the future. *Soc Sci Med*. 2006;62(7):1650–1671.

33. Abrams DB. Applying transdisciplinary research strategies to understanding and eliminating health disparities. *Health Educ Behav*. 2006;33(4):515–531.

34. Diez Roux AV. Complex systems thinking and current impasses in health disparities research. *Am J Public Health*. 2011;101(9):1627–1634.

CHAPTER 2
USING COMPLEX SYSTEMS SIMULATION MODELING TO UNDERSTAND HEALTH INEQUALITY

Ross A. Hammond, PhD
Director, Center on Social Dynamics and Policy
Senior Fellow, Economic Studies
The Brookings Institution

Nathaniel D. Osgood, PhD
Associate Professor, Department of Computer Science
Associate Faculty, Department of Community Health and Epidemiology
University of Saskatchewan

Michael C. Wolfson, PhD
Professor and Canada Research Chair in Population Health Modelling/Populomics
University of Ottawa, Canada

The questions that this book raises about health inequalities represent a significant challenge for analysis. In this chapter we explore these methodological challenges and introduce a powerful set of approaches to address them, known as complex systems modeling, a rapidly growing area of research with wide-ranging literature.[1-10] Although complex systems modeling has been applied to problems in social, biological, and physical sciences, this approach has not yet been widely applied to health inequalities. This book contains a series of illustrative applications of complex systems modeling to health inequalities. To provide context for this effort, the current chapter introduces several kinds of complex systems models, with comparisons to more conventional social and epidemiological approaches to analyzing health inequalities. We then explore agent-based modeling, a commonly used modeling approach, in more detail. We provide an overview of agent-based models, including how they are constructed and used, to aid in reading and synthesizing the case studies that follow.

The Analytical Challenge of Health Inequalities

The story of Myra in the previous chapter illustrates some of the many factors that together influence a person's trajectory of health over the life course. For Myra, these diverse factors combine to lead to health prospects that are likely considerably worse than those of a person growing up in more advantaged circumstances. The story demonstrates how health inequalities—differences in health systematically associated with differences in socioeconomic status (SES), race/ethnicity, or other markers of social position—involve a tangled web of causes and influences, with no simple sequential pathway from a single cause to a single effect.

Myra's story and related evidence from social epidemiology and other fields point to central features of this tangled web of causality; these features form the basis for understanding the analytical challenge posed by health inequalities, and any successful analysis must encompass them. First, health inequality is defined in populations of individuals; it cannot be studied effectively by looking at just one individual, even they are an average or representative person. Next, individuals are heterogeneous along many salient dimensions. In Myra's case, these include health-influencing factors such as diet, schooling, and physical activity. More broadly, they include elements of her context, such as characteristics of her neighborhood, school classroom, and social network. And, of course, they include various aspects of her health status—both in terms of diseases like diabetes as well as learning and physical skills.

Another feature of central importance is time. The characteristics of individuals evolve and co-evolve over time. This poses challenges for designing interventions. For diverse infectious diseases, for example, prevention via vaccination is clearly better than treatment after illness has struck. But when myriad factors interact—for example, parental income and school quality, diet, and physical activity—intervention becomes more challenging: not only are there different times along a person's life course when programs and policies can be applied, but there are also different dimensions or factors that can be targeted. Which timing or intervention target(s) will provide the most benefit may not be obvious. Time also matters because a person's characteristics tomorrow are highly, but not perfectly, correlated with their characteristics today, and the situation now can importantly and persistently shape the situation in the future—a phenomenon sometimes called "path dependence." Some evidence suggests that there may be critical periods of exposure with long-lasting consequences and that effects may extend across long periods of time.

From these features, it follows that understanding health inequalities will require analysis that is *dynamic*; it must allow for interactions among individuals and among contexts and allow for influences between the various characteristics of an individual. For example, physical activity today will probably influence overweight and obesity next year. Such influences are often nonlinear (beyond a certain point, more physical activity will have no further effect on weight) as well as reciprocal (where being overweight may discourage physical activity). These influences also often have a social dimension; for example, the likelihood of engaging in physical activity may depend on the behaviors of one's peers, and one's preferred weight may depend on the weights of people in one's social network. In turn, relevant peer groups may be defined spatially, by neighborhoods, or in terms of social networks, where physical location may be less important. These contributing contextual factors will have varying degrees of influence on the health and SES of population members over the life course, and will themselves change in ways that may be important to capture. Thus, appropriate analysis ideally involves multiple levels and may need to represent dynamic change at each of these levels, beyond the individuals in the population.

Finally, there are many areas where knowledge and evidence are weak or missing. Instead of ignoring questions for which sufficient evidence is lacking, real value may be obtained if analyses can include and critically examine hypotheses that can be characterized qualitatively (if not quantitatively). Even where evidence may seem strong, the explicit consideration of uncertainties in analytical results can also add value.

Therefore, understanding health inequalities and how to best ameliorate them requires:

- Tools with sufficient richness to capture outcomes that are the product of many interacting variables and measures;

- Bridging a population perspective with heterogeneous individuals;

- Consideration of heterogeneities that span a wide range of dimensions or characteristics;

- Consideration of dynamics arising from individuals interacting in various social groupings;

- Analysis encompassing multiple levels, both spatial, such as neighborhoods, and social networks, such as those associated with schools and workplaces;

- Capturing causal influences that are dynamic, nonlinear, and reciprocal, and that may involve positive and negative feedbacks with long lags requiring a life course perspective; and

- Flexibility to consider questions for which empirical foundations are weak or missing, and where even well-established relationships involve a substantial measure of uncertainty; hence, the explicit consideration of randomness or stochasticity.

These requirements have important implications for which methodological approaches are best suited to facilitate progress in understanding health disparities.

Social Epidemiology and Complex Systems Methods

To address these analytic and conceptual challenges, researchers from a wide variety of domains—and increasingly in the health sciences—have turned to complex systems approaches, also sometimes referred to as systems science. The interdisciplinary field of complexity science provides analytic lenses to study systems in which the behavior of the whole cannot easily be determined from consideration of its parts individually. One such lens is provided by dynamic computer simulation modeling, which includes diverse tools such as agent-based models and closely related microsimulation models; system dynamics and mathematically equivalent compartmental models; and workflow process–centric models from the field of discrete event simulation.

While varied, such models share core features, most notably a means of positing a system of causal processes, and a means of mimicking the behavior of the system as it evolves over time from its initial state, driven by these causal processes. Such characterizations allow modelers to capture situations in which system behavior demonstrates properties different from the sum or simple combinations of the behavior of its parts (sometimes called emergent behavior). The results are often surprising, with consequent implications for decision-making.

Dynamic models such as those listed above can readily incorporate features such as feedbacks, delays, heterogeneity, stochastics, and nonlinearity in the relationships between model components. By virtue of capturing both theory (representing processes believed to underlie the system) and empirical data, dynamic models can be used for a wide variety of tasks,[11] including learning more quickly, robustly, and deeply from empirical evidence and gaining insight into the trade-offs between multiple interventions.

While all dynamic modeling techniques share these central features, there are also important differences, reflecting distinct questions emphasized by each technique and differences in the formalisms used to represent processes of interest, making some techniques better suited for specific types of questions or processes. To provide context for the models presented in this book, we briefly describe several of the most prominent dynamic modeling techniques used in health and health-related research and analysis.

Agent-Based and Microsimulation Models

Agent-based models, in their most primitive form, originated in the cellular automata work of von Neumann and Burks[12] and Ulam[13] in the 1940s. While such models were increasingly studied as novel computational mechanisms in the ensuing years, and secured academic interest from an application perspective in the 1970s and 1980s, they became more widely used in the 1990s with the growth of computational power and the proliferation of personal computers. Agent-based models depict one or more populations of individual actors, known as agents, embedded in one or multiple environments (e.g., geographies or networks). Such models provide insights into the co-evolving relationships between individual and system-level behavior, and the interactions of such agents with each other and their environments.

Coming from a parallel tradition with its roots in economics,[14] microsimulation models also depict the evolution of individual agents. In the 1960s and 1970s, microsimulation modeling was employed primarily in the areas of income tax and cash transfer policies. These models generally placed little emphasis on agent–agent interactions beyond those involving members of the same family. Two major groups of microsimulation models developed: cross-sectional and dynamic. For example, the Urban Institute's cross-sectional TRIM model used a large population sample from a Census Bureau survey to estimate income tax revenues and cash transfers, based on the current laws and policy alternatives under discussion.[15] In contrast, dynamic modeling grew out of the vision of Orcutt and colleagues, employing simulation models in which a population of individuals co-evolved in real time.[14,16] In both cases, microsimulation models have traditionally focused on more detailed and empirically observed statistical relationships between variables.

Agent-based models have traditionally focused on relatively simple behavioral rules, sometimes hypothesized and (increasingly) empirically based, and on agent–agent and agent–environment interactions as key drivers of model dynamics. Agent-based models are generally simpler than microsimulation models and have only more recently been applied to policy decisions.[17-23] Agent-based models and microsimulation models can both represent extensive heterogeneity, individual preferences, and decision strategies, and, notably, patterns of individual behavior over time. In a population composed of individuals, the specific trajectories of each individual's characteristics can be tracked over time, generating a synthetic "biography" for each individual. Within both agent-based models and microsimulation models, feedbacks loops can readily characterize the reciprocal causality between factors. To date, agent-based models have been used more extensively to explore such complexity, but this can also be done with microsimulation models in principle.

Both agent-based and microsimulation models have enormous flexibility and representational power. The use of agent-based models to date also demonstrates how very simple models can sometimes uncover important insights; indeed, it has long been recognized that even very simple models of agent behaviors can give rise to unexpected system-wide behavior.

System Dynamics Models

System dynamics modeling harks back to research in control theory and cybernetics in the late 1950s and early 1960s.[24,25] It centers on the principles of feedback—whether regulatory or reinforcing in character—and accumulation. Such feedbacks are found in diverse contexts, including physiologic (for example, when losing weight is recognized to lower metabolic levels, making further weight loss more difficult); behavioral (for example, changes in the mean weight of a population group can affect socially perceived target weights, and thereby physical activity and dietary intake, affecting in turn the weight evolution of that population); or regulatory (for example, imposing a tax on sugar-sweetened beverages can reduce the consumption of such beverages, thereby lowering tax revenues in future years). Since the 1980s, system dynamics has developed with a strong and distinguishing emphasis on both qualitative and quantitative modeling traditions, participatory engagement with communities and stakeholder teams, and visually transparent models that facilitate participatory work.[26-32]

In the health arena, system dynamics models have been most widely used at an aggregate level, e.g. by characterizing one or more populations into distinct categories of "stocks" distinguished from each other by health states or other attributes and "flows" which represent individuals making transitions between those categories. This model structure, represented as differential equations, is also used in compartmental modeling, which has offered exceptional insights in communicable disease epidemiology for a century.[33,34] Both techniques tend to emphasize capturing semi-aggregated or average patterns of behavior (e.g., the rates by which a homogeneous population transitions from prediabetic to diabetic), as compared to the individual-level characterization of these kinds of transitions (a particular person's development of diabetes) as found in agent-based models and microsimulation models.[35] As a result, system dynamics models tend to emphasize deterministic formulations[3] (formulations that lack stochastics), though an important subset of system-dynamics models employs stochastic representations as a central feature.[36]

Along with its many advantages, system dynamics modeling has some limitations. It generally provides only an aggregate or partially disaggregated view of a population over time, making it largely impossible to follow the evolution of an individual within the population over time. The implications that are developed by the models about individual trajectories are obscure,[37] and handling substantial heterogeneity can become unwieldy. Similarly, capturing explicit spatial geometries, or multiple distinct aspects of individual co-evolution (e.g., changes to co-morbidities or multiple behavioral risk factors[38]) can be challenging. System-dynamics models are often used to study populations, but can also be used to study changes over time within an individual or organization. Such models are particularly useful for characterizing regulatory processes, such as in physiology (e.g., weight regulation), psychology (e.g., stress and addiction dynamics), and organizational behavior (e.g., the responses of clinicians to work pressure). Individual-level use of system dynamics models can also be combined with agent-based modeling in powerful hybrid models.

Discrete Event Simulation

The origins of the simulation tradition generally known as "discrete event simulation"[1] lie in the general simulation program work of K.D. Tocher in the late 1950s and 1960s;[39,40] classic examples include simulating ships in a harbor waiting to dock or customers queuing for bank tellers. Discrete event simulation has been applied extensively by operations researchers in manufacturing and industrial processes, as well as in healthcare research—particularly in the health services arena. The approach focuses on characterizing the resource-constrained flow of entities (e.g., patients) along well-defined pathways (e.g., treatments, contact tracing, or process workflows). Within this approach—and in contrast to the other individual-based approaches introduced above—entities are almost universally treated as passive, being operated upon by workflow processes (e.g., undergoing MRI imaging, being triaged by a nurse, or being screened by a community health worker) contingent for their operation on resource availability (e.g., an imaging machine, nurse, procedure room, or vaccine dose).

In contrast to agent-based modeling, there is a sharp dichotomy in discrete event simulation between entities (e.g., patients) and the resources that support the processing of those entities (e.g., MRI machines). In line with their passive role, such entities do not interact directly with each other, but do have indirect interactions. Specifically, the processing of such entities is often constrained by resources, and when a required resource is unavailable (e.g., due to the MRI already being in use or a clinician being previously booked) the entity is placed in a queue awaiting its availability. This provides a form of indirect agent–agent interaction, but falls far short of supporting the more central roles that agent–agent and agent–environment interactions play in agent-based modeling and system dynamics.

Process-centric discrete event simulation models commonly incorporate simple representations of the spatial location of resources and entities, and of the paths over which they travel, together with visualizations of such resources and behavior. The benefits include greater transparency for stakeholders, and thereby greater capacity for elicitation of tacit stakeholder knowledge and building stakeholder confidence. In addition, discrete event simulation provides powerful tools for examining how alternative configurations of resource placement and spatial availability may affect system-level outcomes. Process-centric discrete event simulations excel at the crisp characterization of well-defined, resource-constrained workflows, and economical investigations into the impact of resource availability on system—and particularly service—outcomes. The building blocks of such models are readily understandable, often depicted with easy-to-understand graphics.

---

1   With simulation traditions coming from different backgrounds, the naming of today's traditions is fraught with a confusing cacophony of labels. While the term "discrete event simulation" is used for the specific tradition noted here, several of the other simulation traditions, including some agent-based and microsimulation models, also make use of instantaneous or discrete events (in continuous time) to drive model behavior. It must therefore be recognized that what distinguishes this tradition is not necessarily the presence of discrete events, but the features noted.

However, discrete event simulation models are comparatively poor at representing the more flexible causal pathways and agent–agent and agent–environment interactions often characterized in agent-based and system dynamics models, as well as agent decision-making and the situation of agents in nested contexts (such as membership in multiple overlapping social networks layered on top of physical geography). As a result, it may be profoundly difficult for such models to specify the dynamics seen across even a mid-sized facility such as a hospital. Despite their broad and highly successful use in the health service delivery arena, it is difficult for these models to represent aspects of recognized importance in care pathways, such as the interactions between patients and informal caregivers, patients and other patients, and other types of more flexible patient–provider and provider–provider interactions. The combination of individual-level characterization and heavy use of stochastics in discrete event simulation can also lead to very computationally expensive models.

Hybrid Models

The various simulation modeling techniques just described are not simply competing methods vying to provide the same understanding of complex systems. Rather, their most critical differences reflect both different origins and different goals. The focus of discrete event simulation on service characteristics and the quality of service, resource availability and placement reflects its emergence from the operations research and industrial engineering communities. System dynamics was shaped by its emergence from the field of cybernetics and its use in management science. Important characteristics of agent-based modeling reflect its origins in computer science, physics, and biology, while the roots of microsimulation lie in economics and applied public-policy analysis.

These origins and other historical elements have resulted in important differences in the goals that are best pursued by employing these techniques. For example, the central focus of system dynamics on changing stakeholders' mental models[3,26] has led to investments in modeling processes and representations that foster early and ongoing transparency, and in qualitative and quantitative elements of the modeling process. In contrast, discrete event simulation has focused much of its design and processes on easing the work required to study system-wide impacts on the performance of structured systems (especially service systems) and of changes in resource availability and placement. Agent-based modeling has traditionally placed a strong emphasis on insights gained from understanding the system-wide implications of interactions between multiple such agents, and between agents and the environment. With the increasing availability of multivariate longitudinal data, microsimulation modeling has evolved toward richer characterizations of public policies in a dynamic context (e.g., pensions).[41,42]

While we have described each technique by itself, hybrid systems-science models are becoming increasingly popular and sophisticated. Such hybrid models are found in combinations even more diverse than the approaches themselves. However, a few combinations show promise in cross-leveraging the strengths of multiple techniques. For example, a growing number of models distinguish particular agents as agent-based modeling does, but use system dynamics to characterize continuous elements of agent evolution (e.g., for factors such as the level of immune system activation and immune memory[43,44] or physiology).

A second increasingly common form of hybrid model is one in which agents within an agent-based

17

model also join (e.g., present for care in) service processes simulated using discrete event simulation.45 In another hybrid form, aggregate system-dynamics models can be used to describe populations in which less detail is required while an individual-based model—whether based on agents or simulating discrete events—simultaneously characterizes one or more populations of particular interest.46 Finally, simulated populations of agents can drive or be driven by aggregate dynamics simulated using system dynamics. This type of model can use aggregate modeling to readily capture environmental factors that are not amenable to individual-level characterization (e.g., levels of water and waterborne pathogens in reservoirs). Similar hybrids can be formed between microsimulation models and macroeconomic models or the computable general equilibrium models commonly used in economics.

Hybrid models are used less often than other models, but offer the advantage of balancing the strengths and weakness of the various techniques that they combine. The bridging of individual complex systems models coming from specific methodological traditions and hybrid combinations is an important growth area.

Each of the techniques described above has important strengths for the study of health disparities and inequality. While members of the Network on Inequality Complexity and Health (NICH) had broad familiarity with all these techniques, the models described in this volume made heavy use of agent-based modeling, with one using more of a microsimulation approach (chapter 12) and another making notable use of a hybrid technique that complements traditional agent-based modeling with discrete event simulation to characterize care processes of significance to population health (chapter 11).

Because agent-based modeling predominates in the NICH's work, we now introduce that technique in greater detail, characterize its common characteristics, and describe its particular relevance to the study of in health disparities. Later chapters will build on this understanding to introduce successive models that serve as lenses to investigate particular problems involving health inequalities.

Understanding Agent-based Models

Agent-based modeling is a bottom-up simulation technique for modeling complex dynamics. In an agent-based model, individual actors in a system are represented one by one as autonomous "agents" in a computer program. These agents are given algorithmic rules, which govern their behavior through time, including adaptation, interactions with other agents, and interactions with their environment(s). Given a particular starting configuration, an agent-based model then simulates dynamics, both individual trajectories for each and every agent and population-level or spatial patterns, which arise from the decentralized interactions of the individual agents. Agent-based modeling allows for enormous flexibility in assumptions, and can be used in many different ways as part of a research or policy effort. Agents in an agent-based model can be at any or multiple levels of scale; for example, each agent can correspond to a human person, an immune cell in the body or a multinational corporation. In some models, more than one level of scale is represented simultaneously with agents of different types. The individual-level focus of the technique allows for extensive heterogeneity across agents without requiring prior aggregation into compartments, representative actors, or well-mixed regions.

Although agent-based models can take many forms, depending on the use for which they are designed, almost all share a set of common core elements. The building blocks of an agent-based model can be organized using the PARTE framework: **P**roperties, **A**ctions, and **R**ules (which define the agents), and **T**ime and **E**nvironment (which define the context for the agents and dynamics). The first three elements (P, A, and R) define the agents while the remaining two (T and E) define the context for the agents and dynamics.[47]

Properties are characteristics belonging to individual agents—who they "are." For human agents, these might include sociodemographic variables such as age and SES, contextual variables such as neighborhood or network position, or biological variables such as disease state and body mass index. Such characteristics can be continuous, ordinal, or categorical. Some properties change endogenously in the model while others are held constant, and some properties may be observable by other agents while others may be unobservable.

Actions define the set of specific behaviors available to each agent—what they can "do." Examples of actions include eating food, smoking tobacco, purchasing a house, applying for college, and playing with a friend. Actions often change properties (either an agent's own properties or another agents') and sometimes the environment.

Rules are algorithms that describe formally or mathematically when and how agents choose to perform actions, and how properties are updated or modified. In an agent-based model, rules drive much of the dynamics through time. Rules can be simple ("turn left at every intersection") or complex ("run regression analysis on data points from individual experience to estimate associations as an input to a cost-benefit assessment to choose the optimal action").

Time is important to all dynamic models; in agent-based models, time is often represented in discrete units referred to as iterations or rounds, referring to one pass through the set of instructions given to the computer simulation. These abstract time units can sometimes be calibrated to real-world time analogues (days, months, years). Different "speeds" of action can co-exist within the same agent-based model (e.g., the spread of a virus and the evolutionary mutation of the virus). In other cases, time can be continuous, as illustrated in chapters 9 and 13.

Environment defines the context for the agents and interactions within the model. An important strength of agent-based models is their flexibility and sophistication in representing different types of environments, including social networks and physical-layered geographies. The environment can shape which agents interact with each other, what resources or actions are available to an individual agent, or the timing with which events occur in the model.

The agent-based models described in this book can all be described according to the PARTE framework, although they vary widely in the specific forms that P, A, R, T, or E take.

Agent-based Modeling Inequality and Health Using Agent-based Models

Agent-based models offer a number of features that are well aligned with the characteristics needed to analyze health inequalities. Drawing on the previous sections of the chapter, we briefly summarize three key points here.

Heterogeneity: Agent-based modeling provides for the explicit representation of each individual actor within the model scope. This allows for enormous (and multidimensional) heterogeneity among actors to be captured in the model, without requiring aggregation or averaging, and permits multiple distinct types of actors within the same model. Connecting individual and population levels, and accounting for heterogeneity across a wide range of dimensions or characteristics are important design goals identified at the beginning of this chapter for analysis of health disparities. The capacity to represent and follow particular individuals over time further supports the representation of path dependence in trajectories (such as capturing within the model the long shadows cast by early life insults) and a life-course perspective, also identified earlier as a key consideration.

Spatial representation: Agent-based models are adept at including sophisticated representations of spatial structures, such as physical geography or social networks, which set the context for agent interactions.[47] Interactions between individual agents and their environment can be bidirectional and co-evolutionary— for example, residential location choices by individual homeowners who are both shaped by and (in sum) define patterns of segregation. As argued above, representation of social groupings and spatial contexts can be critical for the sufficiently rich study of health disparities.

Dynamism: Like some other complex systems modeling tools, agent-based models readily represents dynamics that involve long time lags, nonlinearity, feedback across multiple levels, and randomness or stochasticity—all features likely to arise in the study of dynamic causal relationships in health disparities.

Although the other complex systems modeling tools described above, including systems dynamics and discrete event simulation, have potential strengths for the study of health inequality, the combination of these three particular strengths make agent-based models a compelling starting point for initial applications.

Uses of Agent-based Models

This book offers case studies that apply agent-based or microsimulation models to different aspects of the overall problem of health inequality. While these models share a common complex systems approach, they are heterogeneous in important ways.

The models presented vary in their stated purposes and goals. Models can serve a wide array of goals within a research paradigm.[11] Hammond[47] outlines a typology of three uses of agent-based model common within population health, which largely encapsulate the models described.[11,47]

Prospective: Prospective agent-based models inform the design of policies or interventions by using the virtual world of the model to conduct *in silico* experiments, playing out the anticipated impacts of particular interventions. Trade-offs or synergies between interventions can be considered, as well as distributional or unintended long-term outcomes resulting from adaptive response by agents. Prospective modeling can also include the consideration of future trends in the absence of any interventions (see chapters 5 and 6).

Retrospective: Retrospective agent-based models aim to explain the observed success or failure of existing policies, interventions, or natural experiments by uncovering mechanisms that answer "why" and "how" questions).

Etiology: Etiology agent-based models focus on generating or testing (in the model setting) hypotheses about operative mechanisms that may explain observed pattern, outcomes, or distributions. This can also inform the development of empirical indicators or experiments designed to test competing etiological explanations for patterns observed at the population level (see chapters 5 and 7). HealthPaths builds on this idea by combining evidence on multiple etiologies to draw out their joint implications for summary population health indicators (chapter 12). The hybrid model characterizing interacting dynamics associated with trust and oral health also falls into this category (see chapter 11).

Some models address more than one of these goals simultaneously. A good example is the THIM model (see chapter 9), which addresses all three goals, and the Kasman/Klasik model (see chapter 8), which couples explanatory etiologic modeling with prospective policy-oriented modeling.

The development and use of agent-based models generally follows a set of key steps, ranging from design and implementation through testing, calibration, and sensitivity analysis.[47] A second dimension of difference between the models in this book lies in the degree to which they choose to focus on earlier or later stages of the modeling process. In some cases, models aim to engage with data sufficient for extensive calibration, testing, or sensitivity analysis; in others, the aim is to present exploratory models aimed at informing future empirical or experimental research.

This diversity of approaches to using agent-based models reflects the method's flexibility and the many contributions that simulation modeling can make to complement other methodologies in the study of health inequality.

Conclusion

Our partial review of the wide array of distinct and hybrid methods that are part of this interdisciplinary science place the models in this book in a broader context. Complex systems modeling, in general, and agent-based modeling, in particular, offer diverse and compelling opportunities for the analysis of health inequality. The case study applications that follow are a first foray into this rich terrain, providing a sample of the promise and potential that this new field can offer. We hope the framework provided here helps the reader to parse the distinct efforts described in what follows and also to extrapolate from these examples to the broader potential for future work to build on these beginnings.

References

1. Axelrod R. *The Complexity of Cooperation: Agent-based Models of Competition and Collaboration*. Princeton, NJ: Princeton University Press; 1997.

2. Holland JH. *Adaptation in Natural and Artificial Systems*. Cambridge, MA: MIT Press; 1992.

3. Sterman JD. *Business Dynamics: Systems Thinking and Modeling for a Complex World*. Boston: Irwin/McGraw-Hill Education; 2000.

4. Tesfatsion L, Judd KL. eds. *Handbook of Computational Economics: Agent-Based Computational Economics*, Vol. 2. Amsterdam: Elsevier; 2006.

5. Mabry PL, Marcus SE, Clark PI, Leischow SJ, Méndez D. Systems science: a revolution in public health policy research. *Am J Public Health*. 2010;100:1161–1163.

6. Eubank S, Guclu H, Anil Kumar VS, et al. Modeling disease outbreaks in realistic urban social networks. *Nature*. 2004;429:180–184.

7. Gillman MW, Hammond RA. Precision treatment and precision prevention: integrating "below and above the skin." *JAMA Pediatr*. 2016;170(1):9–10.

8. Hammond RA, Dube L. A systems science perspective and transdisciplinary models for food and nutrition security. *Proc Natl Acad Sci USA*. 2012;109(31):12356–12363.

9. Berger T, Birner R, McCarthy N, Díaz J, Wittmer H. Capturing the complexity of water uses and water users within a multi-agent framework. *Water Resour Manage*. 2007;21(1):129–148.

10. Brady M, Sahrbacher C, Kellermann K, Happe K. An agent-based approach to modeling impacts of agricultural policy on land use, biodiversity and ecosystem services. *Landsc Ecol*. 2012;27(9):1363–1381.

11. Epstein JM. Why model? *J Artif Soc Soc Simul*. 2008;11(4):12.

12. Von Neumann J, Burks AW. Theory of self-reproducing automata. *IEEE Trans Neural Netw Learn Syst*. 1966;5(1):3–14.

13. Ulam S. Some ideas and prospects in biomathematics. *Annu Rev Biophys Bioeng*. 1972;1:277–292.

14. Orcutt GH. A new type of socio-economic system. *Rev Econ Stat*. 1957;39:116–123.

15. Beebout H, Sulvetta MB. *Trim, a Microsimulation Model for Evaluating Transfer Income Policies*. Washington, DC: The Urban Institute; 1974.

16. Orcutt, GH, Caldwell S, Wertheimer RF. *Policy Exploration Through Microanalytic Simulation*. Washington, DC: Urban Institute; 1976.

17. Burke DS, Epstein JM, Cummings DA, et al. Individual-based computational modeling of smallpox epidemic control strategies. *Acad Emerg Med*. 2006;13(11):1142–1149.

18. Epstein JM. *Toward a Containment Strategy for Smallpox Bioterror: An Individual-based Computational Approach*. Washington, DC: Brookings Institution Press; 2004.

19. Longini Jr IM, Halloran EM, Nizam A, et al. Containing a large bioterrorist smallpox attack: a computer simulation approach. *Int J Infect Dis*. 2007;11(2):98–108.

20. Heckbert S, Baynes T, Reeson A. Agent-based modeling in ecological economics. *Ann N Y Acad Sci*. 2010;1185:39–53.

21. Schlüter M, Pahl-Wostl C. Mechanisms of resilience in common-pool resource management systems: an agent-based model of water use in a river basin. *Ecol Soc*. 2007;12(2):4.

22. Farmer JD, Foley D. The economy needs agent-based modelling. *Nature*. 2009;460(7256):685–686.

23. Luke DA, Sorg AA, Mack-Crane A, et al. Tobacco Town: Modeling the effects of tobacco retail reduction. State and Community Tobacco Control Initiative, National Cancer Institute; Chicago, IL: 2014. Poster presentation at annual investigators meeting.

24. Forrester JW. Industrial dynamics: a major breakthrough for decision makers. *Harv Bus Rev*. 1958;36(4):37–66.

25. Forrester JW. *Industrial Dynamics*. Cambridge, MA: MIT Press; 1961.

26. Hovmand P. *Community Based System Dynamics*. New York, NY: Springer; 2014.

27. Vennix J. *Group Model Building: Facilitating Team Learning Using System Dynamics*. New York, NY: Wiley; 2014.

28. Beall A, Zeoli L. Participatory modeling of endangered wildlife systems: simulating the sage-grouse and land use in Central Washington. *Ecol Econ*. 2008;68(1):24–33.

29. Langsdale SM, Beall A, Carmichael J, Cohen SJ, Forster CB, Neale T. Exploring the implications of climate change on water resources through participatory modeling: case study of the Okanagan Basin, British Columbia. *J Water Resour Plann Manage*. 2009;135(5):373–381.

30. Langsdale S, Beall A, Bourget E, et al. Collaborative modeling for decision support in water resources: principles and best practices. *J Am Water Resour Assoc*. 2013;49(3):629–638.

31. Stave K. Participatory system dynamics modeling for sustainable environmental management: observations from four cases. *Sustainability*. 2010;2(9):2762–2784.

32. Richmond B, Peterson S, Vescuso P, Maville N. *An Academic User's Guide to Stella Software*. Hanover, NH: High Performance Systems; 1987.

33. Ross R. An application of the theory of probabilities to the study of a priori pathometry. Part I. *Proc R Soc Lond A Math Phys Sci*. 1916;92:204–230.

34. Ross R, Hudson HP. An application of the theory of probabilities to the study of a priori pathometry. Part II. *Proc R Soc Lond A Math Phys Sci*. 1917;93(650):212–225.

35. Richardson GP. *Feedback Thought in Social Science and Systems Theory*. Philadelphia, PA: University of Pennsylvania Press; 1991.

36. Osgood N, Kaufman G. A hybrid model architecture for strategic renewable resource planning. Paper presented at: Proceedings of the 21st International Conference on System Dynamics, July 2003; New York.

37. Meng A, Osgood N. Design of the system dynamics longitudinal analysis system: quantifying the hidden trajectories of system dynamics models. Paper presented at: Proceedings of the 29th International conference of the System Dynamics Society, July 22–25, 2012; St. Gallen, Switzerland.

38. Osgood N. Representing progression and interactions of comorbidities in aggregate and individual-based systems models. Paper presented at: Proceedings of the 27th International Conference of the System Dynamics Society, July 2009; Albuquerque.

39. Tocher KD, Owen DG, Cunningham Green RC. *Handbook of the General Simulation Program*. Report issued by Dept. of Operational Research and Cybernetics, United Steel Companies, England; 1959.

40. Tocher KD. *The Art of Simulation*. London: English Universities Press; 1963.

41. Wolfson MC. *Projecting the Adequacy of Canada's Retirement Income System*. IRPP Study No 17. Montreal: IRPP; 2011.

42. Wolfson MC. *Not So Modest Options for Expanding the CPP/QPP*. IRPP Study No 41. Montreal: IRPP; 2013.

43. Vickers D, Osgood N. 2007. A unified framework of immunological and epidemiological dynamics for the spread of viral infections in a simple network-based population. *Theor Biol Med Model*. 2007;4:49.

44. Vickers D, Osgood ND. The arrested immunity hypothesis in an immunoepidemiological model of chlamydia transmission. *Theor Popul Biol*. 2014;93:52–62.

45. Gao A, Osgood ND, An W, Dyck R. 2014. A tripartite hybrid model architecture for investigating health and cost impacts and intervention tradeoffs for diabetic end-stage renal disease. Oral presentation and full paper presented at: Proceedings of the 2014 Winter Simulation Conference, December 7–10, 2014, Savannah, GA.

46. Flynn T, Tian Y, Masnick K, et al. 2014. Discrete choice, agent-based and system dynamics simulation of health profession career paths. Oral presentation and paper presented at: Proceedings of the 2014 Winter Simulation Conference, December 7–10, 2014, Savannah, GA.

47. Hammond RA. Considerations and best practices in agent-based modeling to inform policy. In: Wallace R, Geller A, Ogawa VA, eds. *Assessing the Use of Agent-Based Models for Tobacco Regulation*. Washington, DC: National Academies Press; 2015.

CHAPTER 3

DOES IMPROVING THE NEIGHBORHOOD FOOD, EXERCISE, AND EDUCATION ENVIRONMENT REDUCE BLACK/WHITE DISPARITIES IN BODY MASS INDEX?

Mark G. Orr, PhD
Research Associate Professor
Virginia Bioinformatics Institute, Virginia Polytechnic Institute and State University

Sandro Galea, MD, MPH, DrPH
Dean and Professor
School of Public Health, Boston University

George A. Kaplan, PhD
Thomas Francis Emeritus Collegiate Professor of Public Health
Center for Social Epidemiology and Population Health, University of Michigan

Acknowledgments: The work reported in this chapter was supported, in part, by the NIH OBSSR (Network on Inequality, Complexity and Health; HHSN276200800013, George A. Kaplan, Principal Investigator), the Robert Wood Johnson Foundation Health and Society Scholars Program (George A. Kaplan, Principal Investigator), the Robert Wood Johnson Foundation Investigator Awards in Health Policy Research (Sandro Galeo, George A. Kaplan) the University of Michigan Center for Social Epidemiology and Population Health, the Institute for Integrative Health (George A. Kaplan), and an Epidemiology Merit Fellowship to Mark G. Orr from the Columbia University Mailman School of Public Health.

We thank Nathaniel Osgood, Ronald Mintz, and Dylan Knowles for technical assistance in the development of the agent-based model, and Andrew Kosenko for aid in manuscript preparation.

The Problem

During the first decade of this century, over one-third of adults in the United States were obese, more than double the rate of the early 1960s.[1,2] The broad footprint of overweight and obesity on health outcomes, quality of life, earnings and productivity, psychological distress, and many other outcomes makes this an alarming trend indeed.[3] Data from the Medical Expenditures Panel Survey suggest that obesity-related conditions may even account for as much as one-fifth of annual healthcare expenditures in the United States.[4]

Like many health conditions and disorders, the prevalence of obesity and overweight is socially patterned, with lower socioeconomic position and racial/ethnic minority status generally associated with higher rates (figure 1).[5]

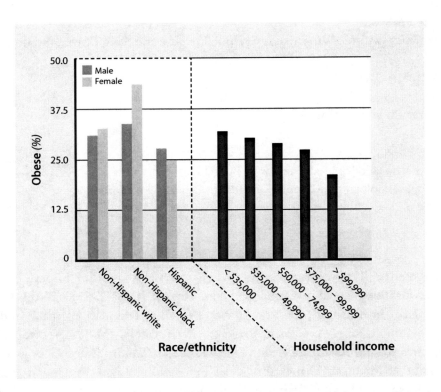

Figure 1. Obesity (percent) by race/ethnicity and household income (US, 2011)[5]

Understanding the determinants of obesity and overweight, how to reduce its prevalence and impacts, and how to eliminate disparities by race/ethnicity and socioeconomic position, is no easy task. Conventionally, obesity and overweight are seen simply as the result of the output of the energy balance equation—input in calories minus energy expenditure in calories. However, many factors contribute to these caloric inputs and energy outputs.[3] For example, the Foresight group's systems map of factors contributing to obesity, and presumably overweight, shows several hundred links between dozens of determinants.[6]

Numerous studies have examined various aspects of the neighborhood food and physical-activity environment and their impacts on body mass index (BMI), obesity, and health outcomes. In recent years, there has been considerable discussion among researchers and policymakers about how these factors can be changed to decrease obesity and overweight.[7] Morland et al.[8] looked at the neighborhood availability of healthy food and found that rates of obesity and overweight were lower where there were more supermarkets versus convenience stores, a proxy indicator of availability. Similarly, Sallis et al.[9] found that higher values on a neighborhood walkability index were associated with lower rates of obesity and overweight. Educational attainment is also considered a contributing factor because of its strong association with obesity, overweight, and BMI, and because it is strongly related to behavioral factors more proximal to BMI, including income and residential mobility.[10]

Racial and socioeconomic segregation is high in the United States, with concurrent impacts on the spatial distribution of food, physical activity, and educational resources, and neighborhood conditions and educational attainment have significant impact on health outcomes. As a result, policies targeting neighborhoods with poor food, physical activity, and educational resources are plausible candidates for lowering racial/ethnic and socioeconomic disparities for many health outcomes and conditions, including overweight and obesity. In this chapter, we build on these research findings to ask whether interventions that aim to improve neighborhood food and physical activity environments and educational attainment may be useful in reducing overall prevalence and black/white and socioeconomic disparities in BMI.

Why Complex Systems?

We report on an agent-based, complex systems model that simulates the effects of various neighborhood-targeted policies and black/white and socioeconomic disparities in BMI. In our analyses, we included individual behaviors, family resources, neighborhood access to healthy food and physical activity infrastructure, high-quality schools, household and neighborhood income, and other factors. Furthermore, we followed agents in the model over the life course as the agents moved between neighborhoods and changed behaviors. Many of these determinants of BMI exhibit feedback, creating a dynamic pattern that further changes with residential mobility. Residential mobility changes neighborhood composition, and these changes in turn alter access to neighborhood resources and in turn individual behaviors, thereby affecting inflows and outflows from the neighborhood, and changing the social influences and norms that may affect diet and physical activity. In short, many characteristics influence this dynamic multilevel system, which exhibits cross-level interdependence and feedback, actors/agents with heterogeneous characteristics, and interdependence between individuals, with change over time. This system is characterized by many positive feedback loops, potentially leading to considerable dynamic, nonlinear behavior—all characteristics that make use of an agent-based model particularly attractive to tackle the problem at hand.[11,12]

Methods

The model. The present analyses use an agent-based model to simulate how neighborhood-targeted policies that affect the availability of healthy food, opportunities for leisure-time physical activity, and educational quality might potentially affect population BMI and black/white and socioeconomic disparities in BMI, as well as the time course of such effects. The neighborhoods targeted for these policies are low in availability of healthy food, opportunities for leisure-time physical activity, or educational quality. We explore the extent to which reducing neighborhood inequality across these dimensions would reduce BMI overall and black/white and socioeconomic disparities in BMI (figure 2).

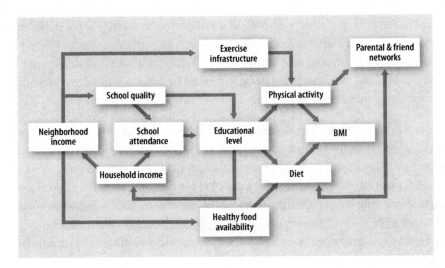

Figure 2. Major domains in model and links between domains

A detailed description of the dynamic, discrete-time, multilevel, agent-based model; the parameters and parameter calculations in the model; and sources for those parameters can be found online (goo.gl/489wgn). To summarize, the simulation starts out with 3,156 agents, with an age and income distribution representative of non-Hispanic whites and blacks in the 100 largest metropolitan areas in the United States. There are 1,280 households, with one to four persons each who live in 64 neighborhoods, each of which has 25 households. Each neighborhood is organized in an 8-by-8 grid, with 80 percent initially occupied, and nine types of neighborhoods based on the race–income distributions in Massey et al.13 The price of housing units varies by median income of the neighborhood. The attributes of each agent include age, race, school attendance, educational attainment, earnings, diet quality, physical activity, smoking, and friends, who are characterized by the same attributes.

Neighborhood characteristics. Neighborhoods were characterized by average income, school quality (SQ), quality of food stores (good food stores; GFS), and neighborhood exercise opportunities (EX). Neighborhood income was the average household income within a neighborhood. We used the student-to-teacher ratio as a measure of school quality[14]; its association with income is modeled on the work of Eide and Showalter.[15] We previously reported that in this model improving educational quality results in improved dietary quality.[16] The number of supermarkets served as a proxy for GFS, with parameters chosen so that its association with income mirrored that found by Moore and Diez Roux.[17] Our measure of EX was based on an environment index that identifies seven neighborhood attributes associated with exercise.[9] For all neighborhood variables, parameters were chosen so that half the neighborhood variation in the index is due to income and half is random.

Agent characteristics. Models are simplifications, and in this initial model agents had no gender. Agents attended school beginning at age 6 and stayed at least until age 13, after which they continued or dropped out, with the timing based on neighborhood school quality, household income, and age with parameters derived from Card and Kreuger[14] and Chapman et al.[18] Parameters were chosen so that at initialization of the model, agents with average school quality and average income attended 13.3 years of school, consistent with national date.[19] Based on the level of attained education, we estimated life-time income and wealth trajectories by education level from national data reported by Day and Newburger[20] and He et al.[21]

Agent levels of exercise, in MET-hours per week (metabolic equivalents), were based on years of education, neighborhood exercise opportunities, friend's activity levels, and parental activity levels. Parameters were adjusted so that an agent with average income and neighborhood exercise opportunities had an average level of exercise activity.[19] Our measure of healthy diet is modeled after the Healthy Eating Index (HEI),[22] and is a function of education,[23] neighborhood availability of good food stores,[24]the availability of healthy foods was directly assessed by using 3 measures: in all food stores within their census tract, in their closest food store, and in all food stores within 1 mile (1.6 km and friend's diets, adjusted so that average input levels result in average level of the HEI.

Friendship networks: Friendship networks were determined by a variant of a probabilistic preferential attachment network.[25] The likelihood of a friendship being formed was a function of the spatial distance between the two agents' households, age, and racial match, and connections were updated each year and with residential mobility. The characteristics of friends figured into the calculation of several mutable agent characteristics.

Residential mobility: In our model, agents could move from one location to another annually. At model initialization, only 80 percent of the housing units were occupied, so there were opportunities to change residential location. Whether or not an agent decided to move was determined by agent characteristics and preferences, and by the availability of housing units that were affordable, based on the agent's income. Households were allowed to spend up to 34 percent of their income on housing[26] and consider all vacant housing units in neighborhoods where housing costs are within 33 percent of the median neighborhood income. Final selection was based on a combination of cost and preferences for neighborhood racial composition.[27]

Births and deaths: When agents reached age 25, they had one child, and that child was added to the pool of agents. Agents died as they aged and accumulated risk throughout model runs, with annual age-specific death rates taken from national tables,[28] supplemented by death rates from coronary heart disease that included the contribution of smoking, BMI, and physical activity.[19,29,30]

Body mass index: Diet and physical activity proximally determined BMI. The association between the HEI and BMI was set to reflect that seen in Gao et al..[22] Data from Miller et al.[31] were used to model the relationship between physical activity and BMI.

A year in the life of an agent: It is useful to consider the "life" of Pat, an agent in the model. Pat is born to a family with certain sociodemographic and behavioral characteristics, enters school at age 6, and leaves between 12 and 25. Pat gets a job after leaving school, has one child at age 25, and retires at age 65. Health behaviors such as smoking, physical activity, and diet quality are updated each year, and reflect individual, social, and neighborhood determinants. Friendships are formed at birth and adjusted annually. Pat may die at some point between age 25 and 100, and pass on any accumulated wealth to his/her child. Pat can move between neighborhoods throughout life depending on various constraints and preferences. Pat's BMI changes over the life course, reflecting the influence of upstream familial, socioeconomic, social, and neighborhood characteristics on Pat's dietary intake and physical activity.

Policy experiments: We calculated the levels of availability of good food (GFS), opportunities for leisure-time physical activity (EX), and school quality (SQ) for each of the 64 neighborhoods. Then we targeted the bottom 20 percent of the neighborhoods on each dimension for policy intervention. The targets and policy interventions were chosen independently for the three dimensions. Five levels of policy intervention were considered: no intervention, and 1–4 standard deviations above the average level at initialization of the model for each dimension. The combination of four levels of policy plus no policy change for each of three dimensions generated 125 separate combinations, each of which was examined in the agent-based model.

Modeling protocol: The ABM was implemented in REPAST (http://repast.sourceforge.net/) an open-source, agent-based modeling and simulation tool. We first examined whether at initialization the model generated bivariate associations on key variables that mirrored what is seen in national data. We then simulated each of the 125 policy conditions separately for blacks and whites. Each condition was simulated 20 times with random starting points and run for 100 time steps (years). Thus, the model generated 250,000 independent BMI estimates. Because of the complexity of this model, it was impossible to predict beforehand the policy impacts, time course of the potential impacts, or differential impacts on black/white or socioeconomic disparities in BMI.

Findings

Calibration of baseline model output: The model was calibrated so that key outputs at baseline, before any policy interventions, were comparable to that observed in national data. For example, model distributions of household income, smoking by age, BMI by age, and percentage of age group in school by grade were all similar to national estimates (figure 3).

Policy effects on black/white disparities in BMI: First, we examined the impact that each of the 125 combinations of policies and policy strengths had on BMI trends for black and whites separately. There was substantial heterogeneity in BMI trends over model time (figure 4), and the policies led to greater changes that were much larger for blacks than whites (figure 5). By 15–20 time steps (years), disparities have been eliminated for some of the policy condition/strength combinations.

We created a BMI disparity index (BDI) as the difference in average BMI between the two groups. Increasing policy strength was associated with decreased BDI (at 20 steps), with the strongest effects for neighborhood physical activity, weak effects for good food stores, and no consistent effects for school quality (figure 6). In other analyses (not shown) that were stratified by age (0–17, 18–24, 25–49, and 50 and older), there was heterogeneity in the effects by policy strength. Policy effects for intervention on the physical activity environment were strongest for those 0–17 and 25–49 years old, and weaker for those 18–24 years old. For those 18–24 years old, the biggest effect was for intervention on school quality, but the other interventions were also effective. Interventions on the availability of good food were strongly effective for those 0–17 years old, but the absolute difference in BDI was quite small in this age group.

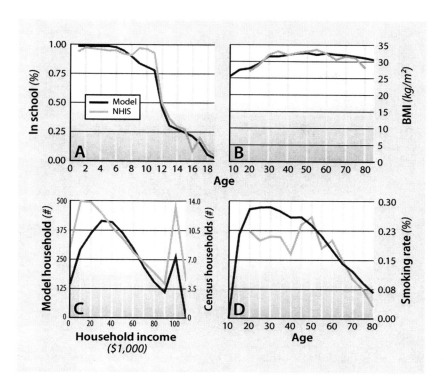

Figure 3. Comparisons between model results at initialization and national data for (A) school attendance by age, (B) BMI by age, (C) household income by age, and (D) rates of current smoking by age

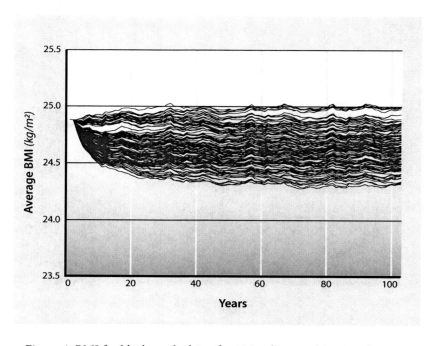

Figure 4. BMI for blacks and whites for 125 policy combinations by time

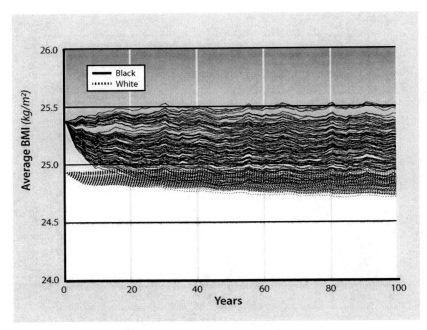

Figure 5. BMI disparity (black BMI—white BMI) by policy strength for each of the policies by time

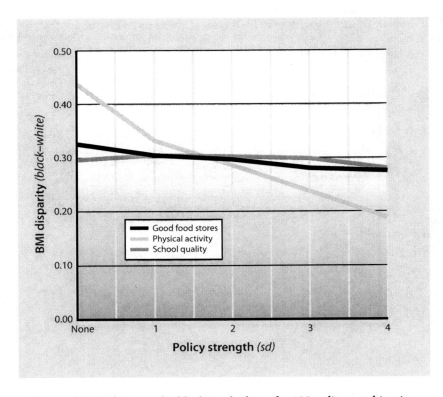

Figure 6. BMI disparity for blacks and whites for 125 policy combinations

Because the pathways by which these three policies might influence BDI are interconnected, it is important to consider their effects simultaneously. While, at first glance, neighborhood physical activity infrastructure seemed to dominate, a different picture appeared when we regressed the BDI on all three policies simultaneously. In such a model, at step 20 (20 years), strength for each of the policies was significantly ($P < 0.05$) associated with a decline in BDI.

We also looked at the results for blacks and whites separately in more detail. Figure 7 shows the impact of each policy separately for black and whites, at the strongest level of intervention (level 4) and the policies combined.

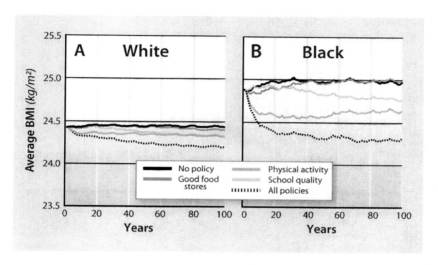

Figure 7. BMI for (A) whites and (B) blacks for maximum policy strength with each policy and all policies combined by time

As suggested by figure 4, the results were considerably different for black and whites. For blacks, the school quality and physical activity infrastructure policies were both associated with reductions in BMI, and there was a strong effect of both policies combined, with the policy effects largely manifested by 20 or so years and little decrease in the BMI after that. Much smaller effects were seen for whites. The picture was similar when the results were examined for different age groups.

Policy effects on socioeconomic disparities in BMI: Similar methods were employed to explore the potential for neighborhood-based interventions to reduce income-associated disparities in BMI. In regression analyses that considered all three policies simultaneously, variations in all policies were significantly ($P < 0.01$) associated with the difference in BMI between those with household incomes of $10,000 to $20,000 and those with incomes greater than $100,000 at 40 years. As seen previously, the effects of policy strength were strongest for the policy that increased neighborhood exercise opportunity and much weaker for the policy that influenced food availability. School quality had a small effect overall, but it was not systematically related to policy strength.

There were considerable differences in the effects of the policies by income level. Figure 8 shows a BMI time series of the effects for the 125 policy and policy strength combinations for those with low incomes and those with high incomes. While there were virtually no effects across the 125 conditions for those with incomes greater than $100,000 per year, there was considerable heterogeneity of effects for those with incomes between $10,000 and $20,000 per year.

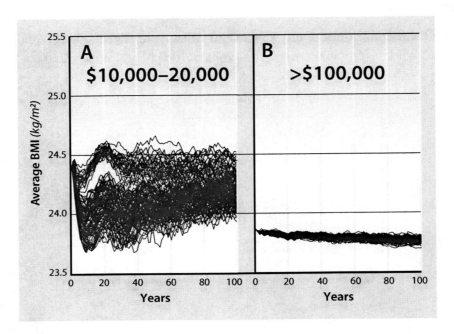

Figure 8. BMI for (A) high-income and (B) low-income groups for 125 policy combinations by time

This pattern was reproduced when we compared the effects of all policies for the strongest interventions (figure 9). Even at the strongest level, the policies had no effect on BMI for those with high incomes. But at low-income levels ($10,000 to $20,000 per year), policies did have an impact on BMI. Neighborhood physical activity infrastructure continued to have the largest effect, but it continuously weakened from around age 15 years. The policies that affected neighborhood food environment and school quality had smaller effects, with somewhat different trends. The intervention to improve school quality took some time to show any effect but remained relatively constant after 30 years or so. Unlike the effects of the combined policies on black–white differences in BMI, which remained fairly constant over time, the combined effects of the three policies on income differences in BMI gradually weakened over time.

Conclusions and Implications

In the chapter, we explored the impact of neighborhood-based policy interventions on black–white and socioeconomic disparities in BMI. We started with an explicitly specified logic model that brings together evidence and speculation about the role of neighborhood physical activity, food environment, and school quality in structuring behavior, contacts with others, socioeconomic trajectories, and other factors that affect individual eating behavior and physical activity. Into this model we inserted a population of individuals that, in some ways, resemble the U.S. population, systematically modified neighborhood

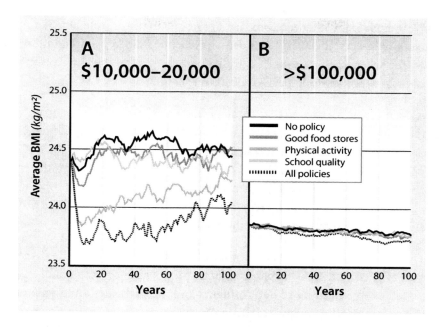

Figure 9. BMI for (A) high-income and (B) low-income groups with maximum policy strength for each policy and all policies combined by time

characteristics, and observed the evolution of BMI over several generations in subgroups that differ by race and socioeconomic position.

When considering the implications of this model, it is helpful to keep in mind the aphorism attributed to the statistician George Box: "Essentially all models are wrong, but some are useful."[32] While Box was principally referring to statistical models, certainly the same can be said of complex systems models.

There are many shortcomings of the agent-based model presented here. It is an idealized representation, and as such cannot be easily generalized to the real world. For example, it is genderless; the characterization of neighborhoods and the spatial distribution of agents and resources are highly schematic; the structure and dynamics of social influences are simplistic; and it leaves out many important pathways. Furthermore, while the overall logic of the model is supported by many studies, it requires the estimation of many parameters, and at the time the model was constructed there were no definitive estimates available for these from systematic reviews or meta-analyses. While that is not an unusual state of affairs in a rapidly changing knowledge environment, even if such reviews and analyses were available, it is not clear how to apply them to the artificial and highly abstracted world represented in this model. Instead we chose parameter estimates from well-known and credible papers that provided the information necessary for the model. In the interest of capturing multiple drivers of BMI, the model contains many parameters, but there are analytical and computational costs associated with such a broad reach. For example, while it would be reassuring to be able to conduct sensitivity analyses for each model parameter, the number of such analyses can increase exponentially with the number of parameters, thereby making such an exploration infeasible.

The model also implements policy interventions that are heroic in magnitude. For example, at the greatest policy strength for school quality, the average student-to-teacher ratio is 7.6! In addition, while it is possible to run the model for several generations, it is unlikely that many of the patterns and parameters built into the model would not vary over long periods of time.

Given all these caveats, it is not surprising that some of the model results deviate from what has been observed in other studies. Indeed, while exact comparisons with national data are difficult given the abstract nature of this model, it does appear to underestimate black–white differences in BMI, with the largest differences on the order of one unit of BMI. On the other hand, the weak results for the effects of the neighborhood food environment reflect increasing uncertainty about such effects, as reported by others.[33] For all these reasons, we view this model and the results that it generated as providing a proof of concept and having heuristic value rather than providing specific policy recommendations.

Nonetheless, we believe that this model has a number of features that fall into Box's category of "useful." While many analyses of BMI and BMI disparities focus on a single or very small number of determinants, we have included a large number of determinants and the pathways and dynamics that link them. Furthermore, given the large and growing literature on the importance of the neighborhood characteristics, this model shows the possible impacts of place-based policy changes and does so with respect to behaviorally relevant and socioeconomic characteristics of neighborhoods. The model also draws upon the growing recognition of the importance of a life-course approach, following individual trajectories over time, and extending across generations. It brings in, albeit in a rudimentary way, social influences; and instead of considering residential mobility as a nuisance, it actually allows residential mobility and tracks its consequences. In doing so, it involves a level of complexity that would be difficult to capture with other analytic methods. Furthermore, the usual problems that stem from unmeasured variables are minimized, because the space that variables are allowed to operate in is explicitly defined. Finally, the specifications of an agent-based model require many decisions, which we were able to fully document.

An important feature of an agent-based model such as ours is that the need to concretely define parameters, linkages, and feedback loops very quickly helps to identify knowledge gaps, which can help to motivate additional data collection and analytic efforts. Finally, our findings hint at some important findings that should be further explored using both agent-based models and conventional techniques. Although we do not believe that these results can be used to choose one neighborhood-based policy over another, they do suggest that some neighborhood-based policies have the potential for reducing or perhaps even eliminating both black–white and socioeconomic disparities in BMI. The analyses further suggest that such reductions can take years, with the time stamps of the policies considered varying between policies and across age groups. Perhaps one of our most interesting findings was that the effects of the neighborhood-based policy interventions that we considered were concentrated on black and poor populations.

The determinants of disparities in BMI and obesity are complex, and no single analysis can capture them all. The work reported here suggests that it is possible to broaden the scope of the analysis, and that agent-based models may prove useful in doing so. The use of such models to approach our understanding of disparities in BMI and obesity is at an early stage, but we posit that the current exercise suggests further steps that can move our understanding forward.

References

1. National Center for Health Statistics. *Health, United States, 2014*. Hyattsville, MD: National Center for Health Statistics; 2015.

2. Ogden C, Carroll M. *Prevalence of Overweight, Obesity, and Extreme Obesity among Adults: United States, Trends 1960–1962 Through 2007–2008*. Hyattsville, MD: Centers for Disease Control and Prevention, National Center for Health Statistics; 2010.

3. Glickman D, Parker L, Sim L, Cook H, Miller E, eds. *Accelerating Progress in Obesity Prevention: Solving the Weight of the Nation*. Washington, DC: Institute of Medicine; 2012.

4. Cawley J, Meyerhoefer C. The medical care costs of obesity: an instrumental variables approach. *J Health Econ.* 2012;31(1):219–230.

5. Schiller, JS, Lucas, JW, Peregoy, JA. Summary health statistics for U.S. adults: National Health Interview Survey, 2011. *Vital Health Stat.* 2005;10(256):1–218.

6. Vandenbroeck P, Goossens J, Clemens M. *Tackling Obesities: Future Choices—building the Obesity System Map*. Foresight Programme. London: UK Government Office for Science; 2007. 80 pp.

7. Krueger PM, Reither EN. Mind the gap: race/ethnic and socioeconomic disparities in obesity. *Curr Diab Rep.* 2015;15(11):95.

8. Morland K, Diez Roux AV, Wing S. Supermarkets, other food stores, and obesity: the Atherosclerosis Risk in Communities Study. *Am J Prev Med.* 2006;30:333–339.

9. Sallis JF, Saelens BE, Frank LD, et al. Neighborhood built environment and income: examining multiple health outcomes. *Soc Sci Med.* 2009;68(7):1285–1293.

10. Ogden C, Carroll M, Flegal K. *Obesity and Socioeconomic Status in Adults: United States 1988–1994 and 2005–2008*. Hyattsville, MD: Centers for Disease Control and Prevention, National Center for Health Statistics; 2010.

11. Kaplan GA, Galea S. Bridging complexity science and the social determinants of health. *J Policy Complex Syst.* 2014;1(2):88–109.

12. Galea S, Riddle M, Kaplan GA. Causal thinking and complex system approaches in epidemiology. *Int J Epidemiol.* 2010;39(1):97–106.

13. Massey DS, Gross AB, Shibuya K. Migration, segregation, and the geographic concentration of poverty. *Am Sociol Rev.* 1994;59(3):425–445.

14. Card D, Kreuger AB. Does School Quality Matter? Returns to Education and the characteristics of public schools in the United States. *J Polit Econ.* 1992;100(1):1–40.

15. Eide E, Showalter MH. Factors affecting the transmission of earnings across generations: a quantile regression approach. *J Hum Resour.* 1997;34(2):253–267.

16. Orr MG, Galea S, Riddle M, Kaplan GA. Reducing racial disparities in obesity: simulating the effects of improved education and social network influence on diet behavior. *Ann Epidemiol.* 2014;24(8):563–569.

17. Moore LV, Diez Roux AV. Associations of neighborhood characteristics with the location and type of food stores. *Am J Public Health.* 2006;96(2):325–331.

18. Chapman C, Laird J, KewalRamani A. *Trends in High School Dropout and Completion Rates in the United States: 1972-2008.* Washington, DC: US Department of Education, National Center Education Statistics. NCES 2011-012; 2010.

19. Centers for Disease Control and Prevention. National Health Interview Survey. 2007 Data Release. http://www.cdc.gov/NCHS/nhis/nhis_2007_data_release.htm.

20. Day J, Newburger E. The big payoff: educational attainment and synthetic estimates of work-life earnings. Current Population Report. . Washington, DC: US Census Bureau; July 2002. p23–210.

21. He W, Sengupta M, Velkoff V, DeBarros K. 65+ in the United States: 2005. Current Population Report. Washington, DC: US Census Bureau; December 2005. p23–209.

22. Gao SK, Beresford SAA, Frank LL, Schreiner PJ, Burke GL, Fitzpatrick AL. Modifications to the Healthy Eating Index and its ability to predict obesity: the multi-ethnic study of atherosclerosis. *Am J Clin Nutr.* 2008;88(1):64–69.

23. Krebs-Smith SM, Cook A, Subar AF, Cleveland L, Friday J. US adults' fruit and vegetable intakes, 1989 to 1991: a revised baseline for the Healthy People 2000 objective. *Am J Public Health.* 1995;85(12):1623–1629.

24. Franco M, Diez Roux AV, Nettleton JA, et al. Availability of healthy foods and dietary patterns: the Multi-Ethnic Study of Atherosclerosis. *Am J Clin Nutr.* 2009;89(3):897–904.

25. Newman M. *Networks: An Introduction.* New York, NY: Oxford University Press; 2009

26. Consumer Expenditures in 2012. US Bureau of Labor Statistics, Report 1046. BLS Reports. March 2014.

27. Bruch EE, Mare RD. Methodological issues in the analysis of residential preferences, residential mobility, and neighborhood change. *Sociol Methodol.* 2012;42(1):103–154.

28. National Center for Health Statistics. *Health, United States, 2009: With Special Feature on Medical Technology.* Hyattsville, MD; National Center for Health Statistics. 2010.

29. Yusuf S, Hawken S, Ounpuu S, et al. Effect of potentially modifiable risk factors associated with myocardial infarction in 52 countries (the INTERHEART study): case–control study. *Lancet.* 2004;364(9438):937–952.

30. National Center for Health Statistics. *Health, United States, 2010.* Hyattsville, MD: National Center for Health Statistics; 2011.

31. Miller W, Koceja D, Hamilton E. A meta-analysis of the past 25 years of weight loss research using diet, exercise or diet plus exercise intervention. *Int J Obes.* 1997;21:941–947.

32. Box GEP; Draper NR. *Empirical Model-Building and Response Surfaces.* New York, NY: Wiley; 1987.

33. Cobb LK, Appel LJ, Franco M, Jones-Smith JC, Nur A, Anderson CAM. The relationship of the local food environment with obesity: a systematic review of methods, study quality, and results. *Obesity (Silver Spring)*. 2015;23(7):1331–1344.

CHAPTER 4

DEVELOPMENTAL COMPLEXITY: MODELING SOCIAL INEQUALITIES IN YOUNG CHILDREN AND MACAQUES

W. Thomas Boyce, MD
Lisa and John Pritzker Distinguished Professor of Developmental and Behavioral Health
Departments of Pediatrics and Psychiatry, School of Medicine, University of California, San Francisco

Rick L. Riolo, PhD
Research Professor Emeritus
Center for the Study of Complex Systems
University of Michigan

Stephen J. Suomi, PhD
Chief of the Laboratory of Comparative Ethology
Eunice Kennedy Shriver National Institute of Child Health and Human Development

Jeanne Brooks-Gunn, PhD
Virginia and Leonard Marx Professor of Child Development
National Center for Children and Families, Columbia University

Kala Groscurth
Center for the Study of Complex Systems
University of Michigan

Sarah T. Cherng, MPH
Department of Epidemiology and Center for the Study of Complex Systems
University of Michigan

Margo Gardner, PhD
Research Scientist
National Center for Children and Families
Columbia University

GROWING INEQUALITY

Bobbi S. Low, PhD
Professor of Resource Ecology
School of Natural Resources and the Environment
University of Michigan

Amanda M. Dettmer-Erard, PhD
Senior Postdoctoral Fellow
National Institute of Child Health and Human Development

Jacob Rosen, MS
Co-founder, CTO
Deftr

Carl P. Simon, PhD
Professor of Mathematics, Complex Systems and Public Policy
University of Michigan

Acknowledgments: This work was supported, in part, by the Division of Intramural Research, *Eunice Kennedy Shriver* National Institute of Child Health and Human Development, National Institutes of Health.

Overview: Social hierarchies and their underlying inequalities have broad implications for health and well-being. These stratifications are usually studied with static models, rarely with dynamic models. In this chapter, we construct and analyze a dynamic agent-based model of the formation of hierarchy and its impact on health and depression. The first section provides a broad background of hierarchies in humans. The second looks at hierarchies among kindergarteners. The third gives a background of hierarchies in a colony of rhesus monkeys. The fourth describes a general agent-based model of hierarchy formation and analyzes the results from a simplified version of that model. The fifth discusses future work, especially extensions of the model for the study of rhesus communities.

Introduction

Human populations such as communities, societies and nations, are often organized into hierarchies through differences in education, income, and job prestige, the defining parameters of SES. These structures produce stable, often heritable and trans-generational, socioeconomic identities with broad implications for population health and well- being. Human societies vary dramatically, however, in levels of income inequality and in the steepness of their socioeconomic gradients of health, and development.[1] They also differ with regard to the overall levels of prosperity. Interestingly, early hominid hunters and gatherers maintained an organizational structure of broad egalitarian cooperation, perhaps suggesting that inequalities and hierarchies are not universal in groups of humans.[2] Although despotic subjugation has characterized the social ordering of many societies in the past and today, a defining attribute of the contemporary, Western industrial era was the rise of egalitarian philosophies[3,4] and welfare laws, such as the Tudor-era English Poor Laws[5] that explicitly undermined the caste and feudal systems of medieval societies. In Western countries today, large differences in socioeconomic gradients exist, but vary dramatically with respect to the differences between those at the top and bottom. The United States, for example, currently has a particularly steep gradient, one that mirrors what existed at the beginning of the Great Depression.

The Network on Complexity, Inequality and Health was formed to consider how such hierarchies and particularly steep gradients influence the health and well-being of individuals and groups of individuals. Our working group focused on how such inequalities influence children in the short- and long-term. We are interested in how hierarchies are formed and how stable they are, how hierarchies are transmitted across generations, and how they are related to health. Our underlying premise is that experiences in childhood influence health and well-being in adulthood (often termed the long reach of childhood).

Just as population-level morbidities are socioeconomically stratified within adult societies, patterns of children's ill health are similarly arrayed along nearly universal gradients of social class.[6] In virtually every human society on Earth, the incidences of biomedical disorders,[7] psychiatric conditions,[8,9] and traumatic injuries[10] within childhood populations increase linearly as SES decreases. The association between SES and child health are graded and monotonic, ubiquitous in a manner irrespective of national development and wealth, and is one of the most powerfully predictive associations in contemporary epidemiology.[11,12]

Social Structure and Health

Socioeconomic status: Children of lower SES encounter multiple sources of chronic adversity and health risk, including food insufficiency and poor diets,[13] exposures to physicochemical toxins,[14] housing instability (including homelessness),[15] dangerous neighborhoods,[16] poor child care and schools,[17] and parents who are disproportionately anxious, depressed, or harsh caregivers.[18] Poorer children sustain higher rates of virtually every form of morbidity, including low birth weight,[19] traumatic injury,[20] infectious diseases,[21] dental problems,[22] psychiatric and developmental–behavioral disorders,[23] and poor academic performance.[24] Growing evidence suggests that socioeconomic inequalities may establish enduring developmental trajectories, leading to lifelong differences in the rates and severities of chronic medical conditions, mental health disorders, and educational and occupational underachievement.[25,26]

Considerable research has focused on children living in impoverished or low-income families. In 2012, about two-fifths of U.S. children aged under 6 lived in low-income families. About one-fifth is living in families with incomes below the U.S. poverty threshold, and another one-fifth is living with families whose income is above the poverty level but under twice the poverty level. Both groups are considered low income, because it is difficult for such families to make ends meet each month.[27] Neuroimaging studies suggest that SES is associated with both brain function and structure, especially in neural regions related to language and self-regulation.[28–30] Physical and psychological adversity may also change the epigenetic markers controlling the expression of stress-responsive genes, leading to differences in responses to environmental events.[31,32]

Despite links between SES and child outcomes, little consensus exists about the mediators of low SES operating at the genesis of health disparities. Some scholars attribute socioeconomic health disparities to material deficits in the lives of poor families: while others regard psychosocial and emotional issues as the major mechanisms through which low-income influences health and behavior problems in poor families.[33] With regard to children, social epidemiologists use the term neo-material to refer to paucities of money or goods money can buy; psychologists consider it an investment problem. Social epidemiologists label the more psychological and interpersonal conditions as social capital, whereas psychologists use the term family stress. Arguments continue about which approach represents reality. Many scholars agree that both of these mechanisms help to explain why children in low-income families are more likely to experience cognitive, emotional, and health problems than those in higher income families. Another version of the same issue is the question of whether absolute deprivation or relative social position within societies with great income inequality is more important for children; we believe that both are important.[34]

Effects of social position: An even more fundamental property may lie beyond the known physical and neuropsychological mediators of socioeconomic influence on child health. Twentieth-century French sociologist Jacques Ellul[35] referred to the preoccupations of modern science with "technique" as deeper ocean currents that "remain the same in spite of the [surface] storm." Similarly, occupying low social status within human societies entails not only the "surface" misfortunes of poor diet, exposure to violence and toxins, and chronic stress, but also the more elemental processes of dominance and subordination, that is, the direct, subjective experiences of subservience, marginalization, and enacted inferiority.[36] Acts of dominance and subordination are universal, prototypical features of the hierarchical social organization that characterizes much of phylogeny, from roundworms[37] and fruit flies[38] to cichlid fish,[39] nonhuman primates,[40,41] and even human children.[42-46] Indeed, Mascaro and Csibra,[47,48] using video-animated agents engaged in dominance-subordination behavior, found that 9-, 12- and 15-month-old infants were progressively capable of inferring stable dominance relations between abstract objects, suggesting that, even in the first year of life, human infants have a rudimentary cognitive schema for understanding and representing asymmetrical and hierarchical human social relationships. The apparent utility of stratification—evolutionary, political, economic, or otherwise—has assured its survival as an enduring, if atavistic, property of both animal and human social organization and behavior.[49]

Thus, across an extraordinary span of evolved species, group organization is shaped by ordered, linearly transitive social relationships, the evolutionary emergence of which has been variously attributed to the adaptive advantages of divisions of labor and social roles,[49] cooperative breeding,[50] leadership provision,[51] checks on aggression,[52] and/or a reduction in the rate or persistence of transmissible disease.[53] Irrespective of its possible adaptive value, exposures to agonistic subordination systematically alter key biological processes, such as cytokine signaling,[54] and stress reactivity pathways,[55,56] modify neurotransmitter and neurotrophin expression patterns in critical brain regions,[57] and undermine disease resistance among subordinate groups.[58]

An association of stress with subordinate social positions is commensurate with prior findings that subjective estimates of social class may be a stronger predictor of health outcomes than objective indicators, such as job status, income, or wealth.[59-61] Dominant status in primate social hierarchies is similarly associated with health, even among captive animals with equal access to food, open environments, and veterinary care.[58,62-64] Individuals occupying subordinate social positions are at greater physical and psychological risk than their higher status peers, even after controlling for the objective socioeconomic conditions of their families and communities. Taken together, these findings suggest that the health disparities associated with SES may be partially attributable—beyond the effects of physical privations, toxic exposures, and experiences to adversity—to differences in an individual's sense of identity, respect, and position within societies marked by nonegalitarian structures and values. Thus, childhood inequalities and their effects on well-being and development may figure prominently in the development of health disparities, acting as antecedents of global SES-linked differences in adult health and morbidity.

Variation in hierarchical structures and effects: The influence of hierarchy within societies on determinants of biology and health shows substantial variability within and across species[65] and plasticity over historical and evolutionary time.[66,67] Such species-typical variation in the "virulence" and consequences of social ordering is comparable with, and perhaps analogous to, the substantially differing slopes of SES/health gradients by nation and state.[68] The origins of this variability[69,70] are obscured, in part, by a lack of consensus regarding what causes health disparities and the debate surrounding the preeminence of material versus psychosocial resource inequalities.[33,71] Such uncertainty has even greater consequences when childhood inequalities are considered, since children vary in their susceptibility[72] to exposures in the material[73,74] and psychosocial[26,75] domains. Furthermore, children are inherently more dependent on adults for the selection and provision of contexts to which they are exposed. Disadvantage within those contexts may have disproportionate and lasting influences on lifelong health.[11] Understanding variation in the health-altering effects of social stratification may assist in discerning the functional core of such stratification.

Largely missing from research in these areas is consideration of how adverse experiences of social subordination[76] may be related to mental disorders, health problems, educational failure, and maladaptive behavior, especially among the young. The works of Strayer,[77] Pellegrini,[78,79] Hawley,[46,80] and their colleagues—describing the developmental emergence, behavioral origins, and social and emotional consequences of childhood dominance relationships—have made notable and important contributions. To further examine linkages between social subordination and maladaptive health outcomes, Boyce et al.[81] studied a socioeconomically and ethnically diverse sample of male and female kindergarten children in Berkeley, California, assessing associations between experiences of dominance-subordination and patterns of prosocial and maladaptive behavior that are known precursors of clinically significant psychopathology.[82]

Dominance Rank and Adaptive Behavior in Kindergartners

Although most studies to date have only documented and described the formation of social-dominance hierarchies within groups of young children, the Berkeley kindergarten work offered a first glimpse into the mental health consequences of occupying subordinate positions in early, novel social groups. Designed as a prospective study of early hierarchical social relationships, the project examined health and development among 338 five-year-old kindergarteners in 29 public school classrooms. Naturalistic behavioral observations in the classroom settings were used to assess dyadic dominance interactions over several weeks. Matrix analysis software was used to ascertain within-classroom dominance positions for each child from nearly 33,000 discrete observations (approximately 28 observations per child). Observations were conducted during structured, semi-structured and free play activities, and social dominance was operationally defined, as first advanced by Schjelderupp-Ebbe[83] and updated by Drews,[84] as a pattern of repeated interactions in which the outcome consistently favored the same dyad member.

Specific interactive behaviors were scored for their levels of dominance and subordination, including winning or losing an object in a struggle; reprimanding or copying a peer; competing for teacher or peer attention; and leading peers or deferring to a peer. Figure 1 shows the decreasing number and proportion of dominant interactions ("wins") and the corresponding increasing subordinate interactions ("losses") among children occupying increasingly subordinate classroom social positions.

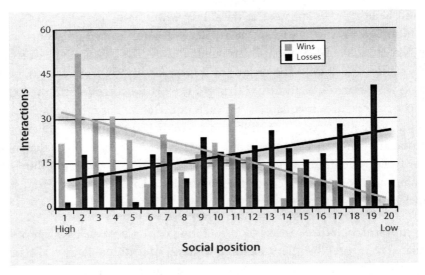

Figure 1. Patterns of winning and losing dyadic interactions by social position for 20 children in a single, representative kindergarten classroom

Adaptive behavior during spring of the kindergarten year was then measured for each child from teacher reports, and the supportiveness and egalitarian character of the classroom climate was estimated from teacher- and child-completed questionnaires. Using multilevel models adjusted for classroom-nested effects, children occupying subordinate positions had significantly more maladaptive behavioral outcomes than their dominant peers, including higher rates of externalizing behavior problems and inattention, poorer academic competence, less-secure peer relationships, fewer prosocial behaviors, and greater depressive symptoms. Although attainment of the children's social positions occurred before their behaviors were monitored, the study took place over only a few months within the kindergarten year. To the extent that social position and maladaptive behavior may be causally associated (an inference beyond the scope of the current data), researchers could not exclude the possibility of reverse causation—that behavior influenced the assignment of social positions or was confounded by child-invariant characteristics.

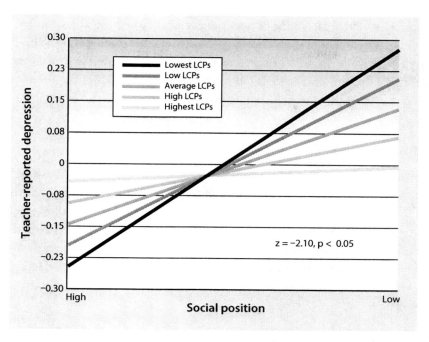

Figure 2. Teacher-reported symptoms of depression in spring by classroom social position. LCPs (learner-centered pedagogical practices), by specific classroom teachers. An interaction between social position and LCPs predicted children's depression, with stronger LCPs diminishing the higher levels of depression identified among subordinate, low-status children

Furthermore, teachers with more egalitarian pedagogical practices diminished the adverse influence of social subordination on depression symptoms (figure 2). In classrooms where teachers had few learner-centered practices (LCPs), the association between children's social position and depression symptoms was high, whereas those classrooms where teachers employed high LCPs showed almost no link between dominance positions and depression. Similar social position–by-teacher LCP interactions were also related to quantifiable behavior problems, less-secure peer relationships, and fewer prosocial behaviors. These results suggest that even within early childhood groups, social stratification occurs promptly and is associated with a partitioning of adaptive behavioral outcomes, such that children occupying subordinate classroom positions show higher levels of problematic, preclinical behavioral difficulties. The results also indicate that the character of larger societal and school structures in which such groups are nested can influence rank–behavior associations.

Observational studies such as the Berkeley kindergarten project suggest that social stratification has developmental and health consequences parallel to those found within larger, socially partitioned adult societies. Although no data currently exist to support the claim, it is possible that the egalitarian versus despotic character of larger societies is developmentally rooted, at least in part, in the early stratification experiences of youth. If formative exposures to dominance and subordination in young lives indeed establish longitudinal trajectories of hierarchical behavior, then early classroom experiences might constitute an ongoing and unplanned natural experiment with profound, unrecognized, and lasting health consequences.

Changing the character of such early school experiences and evaluating the outcomes would be social experiments of potentially enormous cost and magnitude, logistical difficulty, and technical complexity. Nonetheless, it may be critical to conduct experiments that alter structural and pedagogical features such as class size, gender in classrooms and schools (single versus mixed), teacher requirements for educational preparation, and the mainstreaming or sequestration of children with major behavioral challenges.

Social Stratification in Rhesus Monkeys

Insights into fundamental issues regarding social stratification in humans can also be gleaned from extensive studies of social stratification in different animal species, most notably nonhuman primates. Like human children, most primates are inherently social in nature, and virtually all members of virtually all primate species spend their lives residing in social groups that can vary in size, complexity, and permanence. Despite such variation, distinctive social-dominance hierarchies can be readily identified in every group of nonhuman primates, whether naturally occurring or artificially constructed by human investigators.[85] Rhesus monkeys (*Macaca mulatta*, cf.[86]) are among the most clear-cut and most extensively studied over the past 50 years.

Rhesus monkeys are a highly successful species of macaque, arguably more widely distributed geographically and ecologically than any other nonhuman primate species, including all other macaque species and apes.[87] In nature they live in large social groups (troops), ranging in size from several dozen to several hundred individuals, which are typically organized around distinctive, female-headed families (matrilines) spanning multiple generations, with all females remaining in their natal troop for their entire lifetimes and most males leaving around puberty and eventually emigrating to a different social troop. Each troop has several different social-dominance hierarchies. The first is between families, with all members of the highest ranking family dominant over all members of the next highest ranking family, who are dominant over all members of the third-ranking family, and so on. The second is within families; as a general rule, younger daughters outrank older sisters. The third is intergenerational, with an infant's social status mirroring that of its mother, at least initially.[88] These hierarchies, especially those between families, tend to be quite stable from year to year within any given troop, although changes do occasionally occur—and those changes sometimes have dramatic consequences.[89]

Groups of rhesus monkeys maintained in captivity are also characterized by distinctive social hierarchies, basically independent of the relative size of the group and the age range, sex composition, early rearing background, or familiarity of different group members. Indeed, it is essentially impossible to assemble a group of rhesus monkeys and not have a distinctive dominance hierarchy (or multiple hierarchies) rapidly emerge and remain relatively stable in the absence of major changes in group composition. It is clearly in the basic nature of rhesus monkeys to live in socially stratified groups of conspecifics, no matter how those groups were initially put together.[90]

Given the ubiquitous nature of social stratification in rhesus monkey and other nonhuman primate social groups, evolutionary theorists and primate researchers have long speculated about why these hierarchies exist and how individual animals are affected by their social position. Potential hierarchy advantages include access to desirable resources (food, shelter, and potential mates),[85] which are typically identified in behavioral exchanges among male group members.

Some observations have focused on the plight of adult female monkeys that have been low-ranking for extended periods of time. Low-ranking females of all ages have lower levels of play and exploration, are more likely to be physically displaced on a moment-to-moment basis, are more likely to be the targets of physical aggression, are less likely to initiate and to be supported by other group members in agonistic encounters with other group members, are more likely to be physically injured in the course of daily life, and have higher levels of hypothalamic–pituitary–adrenal (HPA) activity (as assessed by hair cortisol concentrations) than their higher ranking counterparts.[64,91,92] Veterinary records on group-living monkeys maintained in captive settings have reported that low-ranking females also require more veterinary treatments for injury and wounds, exhibit different immunologic profiles and have higher rates of infection, and have higher rates of gastrointestinal disorders.[93] In summary, there are major differences in both social opportunities and long-term physical and psychological health outcomes between high- versus low-ranking females in captive rhesus monkey social groups.

Relative social-dominance status appears to be transmitted from mothers to female offspring. For example, high-ranking mothers typically bear and rear daughters who are high-ranking, at least initially, and low-ranking mothers usually have daughters who are low-ranking as well. Elegant cross-fostering studies have demonstrated that such cross-generational transmission of relative dominance status is largely nongenetic, in that infants tend to share the dominance status of their foster mothers rather than that of their biological mothers from their very first days and weeks of life,[94] presumably due to the interactions of each mother and infant with other group members.[95] However, recent data also suggest that biological factors may be involved as well; there appear to be significant genome-wide epigenetic differences between the placentas of fetuses of high-ranking versus low-ranking females, such that cross-generational transmission of relative dominance status may be in part epigenetically mediated through the placenta.[96]

Thus, differences in long-term social status beginning early in life can have profound behavioral, biological, and epigenetic consequences for the development and social status of rhesus monkeys maintained in captive settings, and at least some of these consequences can be transferred to the next generation. These social status-related differences cannot be attributed to differences in food quality or availability, access to veterinary treatment, or differential exposures to toxic and other environmental influences, because all members of these captive groups are maintained with identical rigorous institutional care and use research protocols.[97] Thus, among these rhesus monkeys, the well-documented differences in behavioral and biological functioning and long-term health outcomes can only be attributed to status differences.

Computational Modeling of Early Dominance Relations

Agent-based computational models for classroom experience and behavior provide a plausible and useful alternative to conducting costly educational experiments on a national scale. Simulations of relational dynamics within school classrooms can offer constructed "laboratories" capable of producing valid pedagogical experiments. By manipulating parameters the modeler can shed light on the interactions of personality aspects that observations cannot distinguish, and maybe even suggest which traits play a larger role. In the modeler's toy world, the modeler can test hypotheses that are impossible or unethical to test in the real world and look for and quantify generalities across different social groups and even different species. Models have shed light on important social phenomena, such as disease spread and economic decisions, but little work has focused on education strategies in the classroom. Our models begin that process.

Model Structure

We constructed a model of young children interacting in a play area, employing interactions that affect their status and self-image. Our scenario envisions kindergarten boys or girls during school recess. Since most interactions among kindergarteners are same sex,[81,98,99] we modeled the interactions of boys. Later, we will discuss the modifications that must be made to extend this model to rhesus monkeys interacting in a compound or field site, where intergenerational transfers of status play a critical role.

This model was constructed from two different agent-based modeling programs: NetLogo[100] and a model built on Python. NetLogo models are especially user-friendly; sliders can be moved so that one can watch the effects of changing various parameters. (Our NetLogo model is available by request.) NetLogo is usually used for simpler models than the one constructed for our simulations. It was easier to generate rich output graphs with the Python model, such as graphs of each agent's status over time over multiple runs with differing parameters. Building models in two different platforms allowed us to double check for programming errors. We found no disagreements between the results of these two platforms.

We describe the full model, but when we describe experimental runs we turned off many mechanisms of the general model. We did this because we felt that the model needed substantial verisimilitude to be believable to readers unaccustomed to modeling. For example, the NetLogo versions of the model have a two-dimensional display in which agents can be seen moving around, interacting and reacting to what is happening around them. But this attempt to represent the complexity of the children's behaviors came at a cost: the whole model ended up being quite complex, in both the NetLogo and Python versions. That complexity led to two problems: (1) the program is difficult because it has so many components; and (2) any interesting outcomes could be generated by interactions between two or more components in various combinations making it difficult to isolate proximate causes. By running simplified versions of the model, we built a solid understanding of each mechanism, and then ran models with various combinations of these mechanisms.

Agents and Interactions

For each individual (agent) we track:

- A measure Af-score of their success in play (affiliative resource),
- A measure Ag-score of their success in competitions (agonistic resource), and
- A measure D of their depression level.

Each simulation run has a fixed number N of agents. Each agent initiates a possible interaction once during each round. The initiator of the interaction is called the "focal" agent; the recipient of the interaction is called the "target" agent. A focal agent must do one (and only one) of: (a) play alone, (b) play with a chosen target agent, or (c) compete with a chosen target agent.

In the NetLogo versions, agent locations and movements are represented explicitly. Each agent is given a starting position (x, y) and rules telling them whether they should walk toward another agent to get into the interaction range for competing or playing, walk away from all others to play alone, run away from the victor in a competition, and so on. The agents also have limited vision; they can only choose a target from the agents in sight. These spatial mechanisms and decision rules come at a high complexity cost, so we left the explicit representation of space out of the Python versions to test what differences there were in model outcomes. Interestingly, in the properties we measured for this paper, there was no substantial difference in the outcomes of interest (figure 3).

Results of Interactions

If the focal agent asks a target agent to play with him and the target accepts:

- Both gain affiliative resource (Af),

- Both lose a small amount of depression (D), and

- The lower ranked agent gains agonistic resource (Ag), while

- The higher ranked agent loses a little agonistic resource (Ag).

If the target refuses the offer to play, both lose Af score and Ag score, while the spurned focal agent experiences an increase in D.

If the focal agent challenges his chosen target to a competition,

- The target can accept the challenge or walk away.

- In the case of the accepted challenge, one agent wins and one loses, with the probability of winning depending on the current Ag scores of each player.

- The advantage is always to the player with the higher Ag score. The strength of that advantage is one of the parameters we can vary in our simulations (status advantage).

- The winner's Ag score increases, and the loser's Ag score decreases by the same amount. Both lose Af score. The magnitude of change in Ag scores is modified by a multiplier between 0 and 1 (stake).

- The winner's level of D decreases and the loser's D increases.

- A target agent walking away from a competition challenge is treated as a loss. (A multiplier parameter can be set to make running away more or less costly than fighting and losing.)

GROWING INEQUALITY

As agents interact, the hierarchy determined by the Ag scores changes over time.

We track the distribution of these Ag scores, and how that distribution changes over time. Does it eventually stabilize? Are the Ag scores evenly distributed among the agents, or is the group divided into haves and have-nots? We use a Gini coefficient to shed light on this last question: a Gini coefficient near 1 means that the Ag scores are evenly distributed among agents, and a Gini coefficient near 0 implies a strong inequity among the Ag scores with a small group bunched at the top and another larger group bunched near the bottom of the hierarchy.

Each agent has one turn in a time-step, or round. There are four rounds per recess, 10 recesses per day, and 100 days per simulation run. At the end of each interaction, each agent updates his Ag score, Af score and depression level based on the outcome. In addition, at the end of each day, his depression level (D) moves a bit toward some natural level (D*), assigned to each agent at the beginning of each run.

Following Kahneman's *Fast and Slow Thinking*,[101] we allow focal and target agents to base their choice at all these decision points either via a fast track based solely on recent experiences or a more-complex slow track using preferences over expected outcomes of a myriad of possible interactions. The slow track is forward-looking and represents a deliberative process, while the fast track is a backward-looking, reactive mechanism. For the experiments reported here, the agents use only the deliberative mechanisms.

Adjustable Parameters

This model has a large number of parameters. Choosing base levels for these parameters and learning how to vary them to discover their roles are important parts of these and future simulations (see Appendix).

Key parameters affecting the outcomes of these simulations are:

- Stake: increases the magnitude of the winning and losing amount in any competition.

- Status advantage: increases the probability that the higher ranked Ag score will win the competition.

- The probability that an agent chooses to play alone (for a few agents this probability is very high).

- Distribution of the numbers of agents that will prefer to play alone.

- Size of the class

- The probabilities that agents will use either the fast or the slow track process in their decision processes.

Other parameters that can be adjusted include:

o Each agent's preferred Ag score, a target social position for each individual (aggressiveness), because not everyone wants to be an alpha. The triangular distribution of these values can be adjusted.

o Each agent has a natural level of depression (D*). Their initial distribution is set as a triangle distribution before each run. At the end of each day, each agent's depression level moves back a bit toward their natural level (D*). The strength of the move toward this natural level at the end of each day can also be controlled for each agent.

What We Have Learned So Far

We focused on carrying out a systematic exploration of the key parameters to improve our understanding of how the assumptions and parameter values affected hierarchy outcomes. We performed multiple runs of the model to find interesting relationships among the parameters, so that the model might provide insights on the process of hierarchy formation, elements that empirical studies had not yet found but might look for in the future.

From running the models, we learned that these following inputs and outputs were especially relevant to teachers and those who create educational policy.

Inputs:

- Class size.

- Status advantage.

- Stake (compFracTr, in our computer runs), a parameter between 0 and 1 that captures the benefit in increased Ag score from winning a competition. Stake = 0 means no benefit from winning a competition, and therefore no real competition. A higher stake means that competition losses have a higher impact on the loser.

- Interaction options: (1) Only compete; (2) compete or play, not allowing play refusal; (3) compete or play, allowing play refusal.

Output parameters:

- Average number of rank changes per day in equilibrium (roughly, the stability of the hierarchy).

- Average number of Ag score changes per day in equilibrium (rank based on Ag score).

- Gini coefficient of the hierarchy in the long run.

- The slope of the Ag score versus depression graph.

- Average log run level of depression.

Simplest Models

We began with a very simple model and added to it after reading and discussing relevant literature. We sought to work this simplest model in great detail over all parameter relationships, and then bring in complexities one at a time so that we could better understand the roles of all the assumptions and parameters (figure 3).

For these runs, we summarize how these five outputs are affected by the four inputs. The underlying program is Python, which helped generate illustrative input–output graphs, but we found the same results with NetLogo.

In this preliminary analysis, we looked only at the few inputs and outputs described above, and kept the other parameters fixed. For example, in our reported runs, our agents used only the slow decision process and were not allowed to "play alone." In our unreported work, we did allow these other background parameters to vary widely so that we could be sure that the results reported here hold very generally.

To begin this process, we turned off the play option and limited the agents to competition interactions, for such actions are the heart of the Ag score that determines the hierarchy. In the first column of figure 3A and B, only agents were allowed to compete. In the second column, focal agents could compete or play, but target agents had to accept any offer. In figure 3C, we allow the target of a play offer to reject that offer. The graphs in figure 3C are similar to those in column 2, figure 3A; adding the mechanism of play rejection has minimal effect on the parameter relationships we are considering.

In figure 3A, values of the stake ("compFracTr," in our computer code) are on the horizontal axis, from stake 0 (no gains from competitions, in a sense, no competitions) to stake 1 (losing a competition has a high impact). The curves are color coded by the underlying status advantage from light (low-status player has a high chance of winning) to dark (little chance that the low-status player will win). (Color versions are available at http://bit.ly/2iJ3BQK) The five variables on the vertical axes correspond to our five target outputs.

Figure 3B is a complementary set of graphs in which we have put status advantage ("agonPower" in our computer code) on the horizontal axis and color-coded the curves by the underlying stake from stake <0.1 (lightest) to stake close to 1.0 (darkest). In this dynamic model, all output parameters change over time. Assuming 30 contacts a school day, a complete school year would have 6,000 steps. However, we found that the runs stabilized well before 1,000 steps. We usually carried out a run for about 500 steps. We report the average of each output variable for the last 20 percent of these steps.

Gini coefficient: The Gini coefficient is a number between 0 and 1 that represents the evenness of the distribution of Ag scores across the class. It is usually used to compare income distributions in different countries: 0 means perfectly evenly distributed, the bottom X percent of the population have X percent of the country's wealth; 1 means that the wealthy have a disproportionate amount of the country's wealth. For our virtual classrooms, a high Gini coefficient implied that a few students had very high status and many students had very low status.

In all our runs, the Gini coefficient increased as stake increased and as status advantage increased (row 5 of figure 3A and 3B). The effect of higher stake is especially dramatic (figure 3B). As a function of the underlying stake, there is usually an interval of stake levels in which the Gini coefficient rises rapidly and eventually levels off. This interval of rapid rise is more pronounced for low status advantage values (figure 3A). The value of the Gini coefficient and the shape of its graph appear to be independent of the interaction options.

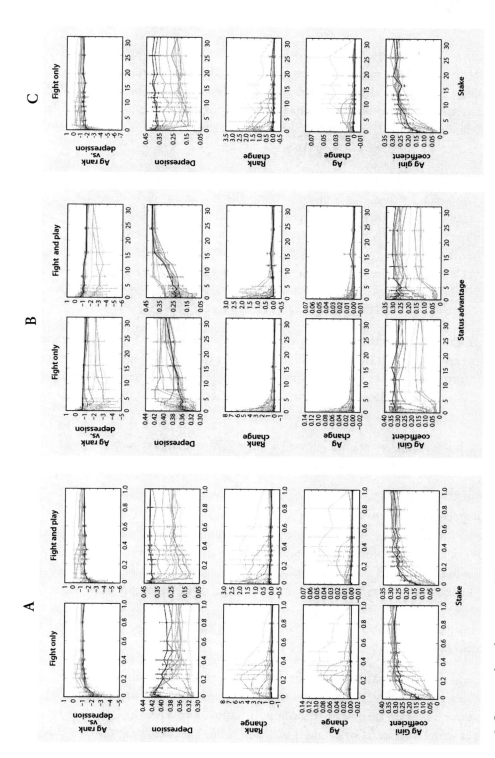

Figure 3. Output values from runs of the model for combinations of stake and status advantage. In (A) and (C), stake is measured along the x-axis and different curves represent different values of status advantage. This is switched in (B). Status advantage varies from its lowest value of 1 (light gray) to its highest value of 32 (black). In "fight only" (column 1 of (A) and (B)), the focal agent chooses which target to have a competition with (fight). "Fight or play" (column 2) has identical parameters, but the focal agent chooses which agent to target and whether to compete or to play with that agent. In (C), the target agent has the option of refusing a play invitation. Principle output measures are: (1) the slope of the depression versus individual Ag rank graph; (2) average depression; (3) average rank change; (4) average Ag score change; and (5) Gini coefficient (G) of population's Ag scores, a measure of how evenly (G = 0) or unevenly (G = 1) Ag scores are distributed across the individuals in the classroom. Measures are calculated at each time step and averaged over the last 20 percent of each run to give an equilibrium value, which is averaged with equilibrium values from eight other runs with identical input parameters (except for random seeds) (http://bit.ly/2iJ3BQK)

There is also a Gini coefficient for the Af scores (not reported). In contrast, its value seems to be independent of stake or status advantage.

In terms of classroom social structure, a teacher who wants to avoid a two-tiered social structure with a few alphas at the top dominating a large number of boys at the bottom would do well to structure competitions so that the stakes of losing a competition are low and lower ranked boys have a decent chance of winning. There is a narrow band of stake values in which the social structure moves from fairly equitable to dramatically two-tiered. Having more play opportunities does not seem to affect this situation.

Long-run changes in the Ag score and Ag score rank: Unlike the uniform character of the Gini coefficient graphs, the graphs of long-run variability of Ag score and Ag score rank have a curious hump shape (rows 3 and 4 in figure 3A). The output variable here is the average number of daily Ag score or Ag rank changes in the last 20 percent of each computer run. A high value implies that the hierarchy is fairly unstable, with many daily changes. A low number suggests that agents are locked into a fairly stable hierarchy. The hump shape in figure 3 indicates that when the stake is small there is little change in the hierarchy over time, but as the stake increases, the social structure becomes more fluid—until the stake reaches a threshold value after which further increasing the stake leads to a less fluid social structure.

These graphs in figure 3 depend strongly on the value of the status advantage setting. The lower the status advantage (so that the lower ranked agent has a reasonable chance of winning a competition) the more pronounced and higher the hump. That makes sense: the smaller the chance of the underdog winning, the less rank change will occur. Alternatively, there is little rank change when the higher ranked agent wins nearly every contest.

In addition, the peak is much higher if agents are not allowed to play (figure 3A). Playing has a smaller effect on an agent's Ag score than competing. On the other hand, there is little difference when play rejection is added to the model (figure 3C).

What leads to this hump-shaped graph of Ag score changes versus stake? When the stake is 0 or close to it, there is nothing to compete for. In particular, Ag scores change very little, if at all, after a competition; so, the order of the Ag scores changes very little too. As stake increases from 0, the wins and losses from competitions begin to make a difference and the graph rises naturally as stake increases. However, during this interval, the long-run Gini coefficient is also rising. Just at the stake value where the Gini coefficient begins its steep slope, the number of rank changes begins to fall. As Ag scores aggregate at the top and at the bottom of their distribution, the number of rank changes dramatically begins to decrease, and the graphs in row 3 of figure 3 decrease toward 0.

Figure 4 shows the connection between peak Ag rank change and the start of the steep portion of the Gini coefficient curve more clearly, for two particularly low values (1.5 and 1.6) of status advantage. Those threshold stakes described above that separate even distributions of status from a two-tiered uneven social structure are also the stakes at which the social structure is the most fluid. These are probably the optimal stake levels from the teacher's perspective.

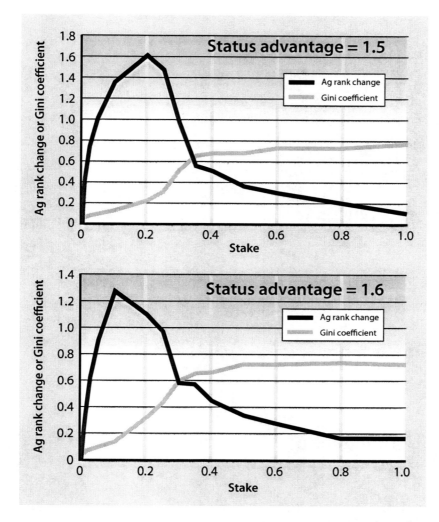

Figure 4. Average Ag rank change and Gini coefficients from single model runs with different values of stake, for status advantage at 1.5 (top) and 1.6 (bottom). The measures are calculated at each time step and those values are averaged over the last 20 percent of each run to give an equilibrium value for that run

For higher values of status advantage, the Gini coefficient begins its steep rise earlier and the rank change graph hits its peak earlier and lower (figure 3A, rows 3, 4, and 5).

This behavior is clearer when one looks at graphs of how individual Ag scores change over time. Figure 5 shows a representative sequence of individual Ag scores over time. In figure 5A, status advantage is fixed at 2 (a level that allows for some lower status victories) while stake is, respectively, 0.1, 0.2, 0.3, 0.4, and 0.5 in the five panels. In the top panel, with stake just above 0, agents' Ag scores take many small steps up and down, and the Ag scores are evenly distributed by step 400 (Gini coefficient = 0.1822). But as stake increases to 0.2, the spread of Ag scores widens, with some agents hitting the max Ag score of 1.0. As the stake increases to 0.3, the Ag scores begin to accumulate at the top (1.0) and at the bottom (0.0) (Gini = 0.5763). The jumps in Ag score are fewer but larger. Finally, when the stake for winning or losing a contest

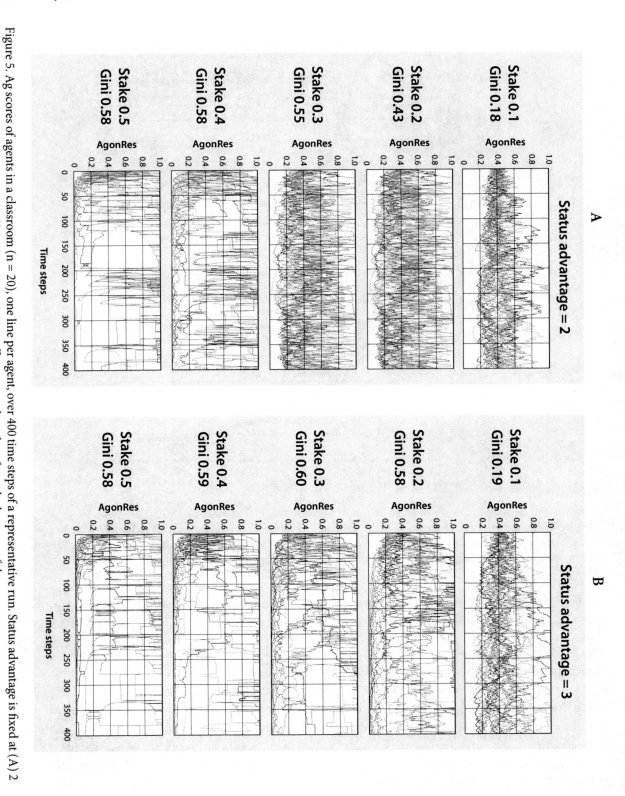

Figure 5. Ag scores of agents in a classroom (n = 20), one line per agent, over 400 time steps of a representative run. Status advantage is fixed at (A) 2 and (B) 3 for all five runs; stake varies from 0.1 to 0.5. Gini coefficients are the values from the last step of the run

is 0.5, we are moving closer to an all or nothing hierarchy, with even fewer and larger jumps in Ag score. Each of these runs started with initial distributions of Ag score around 0.4. We found that as the mean of the initial distribution increases, each of the time graphs moves up a bit too.

Figure 5B shows a similar set of individual Ag scores over time, but with status advantage increased to $p = 3$. This increased advantage to higher status agents leads to a quicker movement to a U-shaped distribution of Ag scores and a correspondingly high Gini coefficient. Figures 3 and 4 give a macro level view of the relative effects of stake and status advantage. Following individuals in figure 5 confirms our earlier interpretation. Increasing the stake beyond some threshold value leads ultimately to a two-tiered social structure. The more certain the competition victory by higher ranked individuals the lower is this threshold.

Just as figure 5 keeps track of the individual Ag scores that lead to the macro-level graphs in row 4 of figure 3A, figure 6 keeps track of the individual Ag ranks that lead to the graphs in row 3 of figure 3A. Figure 6 illustrates how, in a typical run, the number of rank changes increases, peaks, and settles down to 0 over time. As individual Ag scores aggregate near the top and the bottom of the scale, they still preserve their relative positions—ranks—within the social structure. This implies that there is still a hierarchy within the top level and within the bottom level of the social structure.

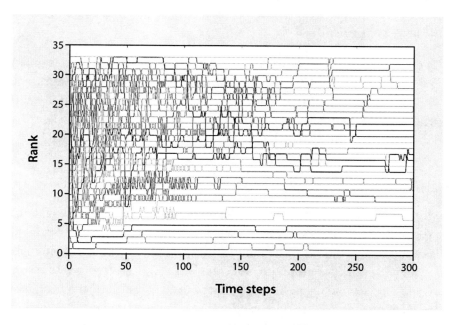

Figure 6. Time-series plot over 300 steps of Ag ranks for 33 children in a classroom, with stake = 0.30, status advantage = 8, and only fighting allowed. Each line shows the Ag rank of an individual child over the whole run

Depression: We care about the Ag score and the resultant rank mostly because of their effects on the self-esteem of agents, or alternatively, their sense of depression. In this model, agents lose self-esteem mostly by losing a competition or by having an offer to play rejected. For every parameter value, there is less depression if the agents are allowed to play (figure 3A). Levels of depression in the first column ("fight only") are higher than those in the other two columns in row 2. Adding the possibility of rejecting play offers has little effect on these graphs.

Furthermore, the average depression level in the group is strongly related to the value of status advantage and is less affected by stake. Average depression level is lower if the underdog has a higher chance of winning (low status advantage) (figure 3B). Conversely, the average level of depression is fairly independent of stake, especially if the stake is greater than 0.3.

The initial distribution of depression level in these runs is a triangle distribution from 0.1 to 0.4, with peak at 0.3. So, the initial values are clustered around 0.33. This level persists over time if there is no stake. However, as stake become positive, the average depression level moves to its stake-independent value, as determined by status advantage. This long-term average is higher than 0.33 if agents can only fight; it is generally lower than 0.33 if agents have the option of choosing play (figure 3A).

In their study of Berkeley kindergarteners, Boyce et al.[81] found that higher Ag scores led to higher self-esteem (lower depression levels). We found the same in our simulations (figure 3A). In our runs, the slopes move to 0 as status advantage decreases. The higher chance that the underdog has of winning competitions, the less the average depression depends on rank or Ag score. In fact, for status advantage near its minimum level of 1, the Ag score/depression curves flatten out. When both play and compete are allowed, the slopes are generally less (figure 3B).

Classroom size: In our models, classroom size did not make a big difference. With status advantage set at the relatively low value of 2.5, the long-run average depression level, Ag score changes, and the Gini coefficients are independent of class size. This independence suggests that whatever number of kids one has to interact with, the effects of the hierarchy depend more upon teacher influences, the intrinsic competitiveness of the other kids, and so on (figure 7).

Model Validation

It would be naïve to presume that the model presented here (and others like it) would enable teachers or administrators to test different policies accurately, such as predicting the effect of reducing classroom size on depression rates and social positions. When modeling a complex adaptive system like a kindergarten, George Box's aphorism is especially appropriate: "Essentially, all models are wrong, but some are useful."[102] It is not a question of the model making perfect predictions of all outputs under all conditions. Rather, it is a matter of deciding whether a model has "face validity": Do experts in the field being modeled judge it to be good enough? These experts can use all the facts from tests of how the various parameters and different mechanisms affect the outputs, all their knowledge about how the mechanisms work, and all the intuition they have developed over time to decide whether the outputs look reasonable over some range of input parameters, and under which conditions do they not.

To establish the face validity of our model, the modelers in our group worked with psychologists in our group and with the psychological literature to choose what to study; in particular, (1) to decide which behaviors, generated by which psychological models of decision-making, operationalize the mechanisms, (2)

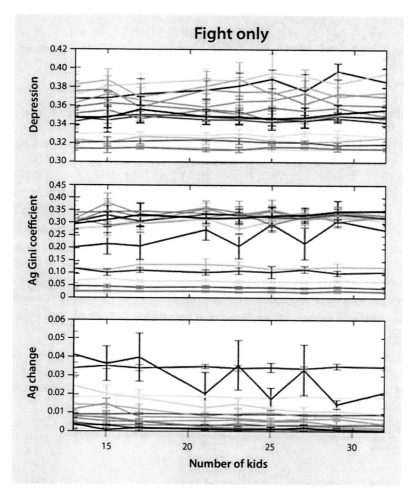

Figure 7. Output values from model runs, with only fighting allowed, for average depression, Gini coefficient, and Ag change. The independent variable on the x-axis is the number of kids. Different curves correspond to different stakes from 0.000 (lightest gray) to 0.999 (black)

to pick values for mechanism parameters, (3) to choose appropriate initial conditions, (4) to define what outputs to measure and, finally, (5) to designate some output measures as "validation targets."

We judge the model's performance as suspect if the numbers and behaviors it produces differ substantially from the chosen validation targets. Of course, which targets to use and how close is good enough is a matter of judgment. We also used the target outcome values to guide our choice of input parameters. Then, we set validation targets so that our choices of model parameters would lead to model results that mirrored the following stylized facts:

1. Ratio of affiliative acts to agonistic acts is 4 to 1.[103,104]

2. Depression falls with higher social position. That is, the slope of D versus Ag score is negative, and the slope of D versus Af score is negative.[81]

3. There is a large fraction of repeat play with the same kids (70–90 percent).

4. Play group size averages 3–4.[104–107]

5. The hierarchy determined by the Ag scores is stable.[45,108]

6. Ten percent of the kids play alone 90 percent of the time.[105,106,109–111]

7. Some agents with high aggressiveness parameters end up near the bottom of the Ag scores hierarchy.[112]

For various versions of our models, we can hit all of the targets considered singly, and some combinations of parameter values and mechanisms that can generate some of targets in combination, but we have not found a set of values that can generate all the targets. Possibly we just have not looked hard enough: The search space is immense and we have only looked in a few corners. Or maybe those targets are incompatible; they come from different classrooms, with kids of different ages, nationalities, and backgrounds.

There is a large body of research on children's behaviors in play groups related to affiliative and aggressive actions, group sizes, playing alone, and hierarchical structures. For example, empirical studies have found that conflicts occur about two to three times per dyad per hour[110]; some children approach others more often[113]; some children have more friends than the others[110,111,114–116]; most friendships are symmetric in terms of dominance[45]; and aggressive children have fewer reciprocated friendships than on-aggressive children.[98,117] An extensive annotated list of such findings is available at http://bit.ly/2im1821. Future extensions of our model will take into consideration more of these empirical observations.

Conclusions

Considering a classroom of younger children,[81] we attempt to shed light on the goals a teacher might have for classroom culture and what might make a difference in achieving those goals. Our simulations relate to goals such as:

- Increasing students' self-esteem, or equivalently lowering their depression and other problem behavior levels.

- Avoiding a ranking in which a small group of students has the highest status, while most of the rest of the cluster at the bottom of the social ladder (high Gini coefficient).

- Avoiding a rigid social structure in which students have little hope or opportunity in improving their relative status.

- Decreasing the strong link between status and depression.

By the way, these goals are the same ones most of us have for the larger society.

Based on our findings, we can suggest abstract strategies that could help a teacher achieve some of these goals:

- Increase the opportunities for play relative to those of fights or competitions.

- Keep the stakes low in competitions that do occur, so that losers do not experience a big drop in social position.

- Encourage rules of competition or types of competitions that give the weaker or less-experienced player a decent chance of winning.

- Lower stakes and status advantage lead to smaller effects of status on self-esteem. Tactics include handicapping favorites, promoting activities in which some low-status children have a better chance of winning, rewarding not just the winner but also to those lower on the list, and keeping prizes reasonably small.

These strategies may be more important considerations than, for example, working hard to reduce class size. But much more work needs to be done to understand how these processes would play out in real-world settings.

Next Steps

A goal of our model is to suggest improvements in how things are done; to that end, real-world tests of the model's conclusions would be instructive. While there may be ethical problems with experimenting in classrooms, some experiments may be possible in prison settings as well as primate field studies.[88,90]

Other next steps include:

- Fine-tune this model, and develop and present more comprehensive lists of the impact of the parameters of this model on the many possible outputs.

- Experiment with advanced search techniques, such as genetic algorithms,[118] to look for combinations of input parameters that can generate outputs closer to all the validation targets in the same run.

- Include inputs that comprehensively mirror the practical actions that teachers can take in classrooms and researchers take in their field studies.

- Extend the model to shed light on the social structures of humans of different ages and, in particular, on the early dominance relations in rhesus monkeys.

Modeling Rhesus Colonies

Is the model we have presented and studied, based on initial observations of interactions among kindergarten children in different classes over time, generalizable to other social situations involving dominance hierarchies in different groups of humans of different ages—or even in a different species, such as rhesus monkeys? Over the past few years, a great deal of observational, biological, and veterinary data have been gathered following the formation of small- to mid-sized groups of juvenile monkeys in standardized laboratory settings, typically beginning at 6–9 months of age (roughly equivalent to 2- to 3-year-old human children) and then followed longitudinally at least until the onset of puberty. In most of these juvenile cohorts, the group members have had different early (first 6–7 months) social experiences, and the groups that have been formed differ from one another with respect to their size, sex composition, presence/absence of adult "foster grandparents," and the relative steepness of the dominance hierarchies established rapidly following group formation.

Data collected on group members include the periodic assessment of social-dominance status,[119] dyadic interaction patterns (including bouts of both play and aggression), social grooming and proximity patterns, activity levels, and biological measures obtained from repeated blood, saliva, and hair sampling. Complete veterinary records have also been maintained for each monkey.

There is considerable overlap between the kindergarten data that provided the basis for our computational model and the data in hand from longitudinal studies of juvenile rhesus monkeys. The agents (individual children versus individual monkeys), actions (play, play alone, compete), and some outcomes have strong behavioral parallels, and some of the biological and health/veterinary records are similar.

One initial question concerns how faithfully the child model represents the actual transactions among the different monkeys. How much do the variables and parameters need to be tweaked to improve the fit between the child model and monkey data, or are such comparisons completely incompatible? Is it possible to modify the existing human model to conform better with what we know empirically about the monkey interactions and the consequences of differences in social dominance among individuals? Next, assuming the model has some comparability across species, do different parameter adjustments yield similar patterns of different outcomes for the two species, and if not, what are the underlying reasons for such discrepancies? Finally, just as one possible goal of developing a model for human kindergarten classes has been to shed light on optimal size, teaching practices, and so on, could the development of a parallel monkey model be useful for making decisions regarding animal husbandry, regarding how factors such as group size, composition, and the advisability of adding or removing group members, influence long-term health and well-being? These questions can now be addressed empirically.

References

1. Keating DP. Developmental health and the wealth of nations. In: Keating DP, Hertzman C, eds. *Developmental Health and the Wealth of Nations: Social, Biological, and Educational Dynamics.* New York, NY: Guilford; 1999:337–347.

2. Erdal D, Whiten A. Egalitarianism and Machiavellian intelligence in human evolution. In: Mellars P, Gibson K, eds. *Modelling the Early Human Mind.* Cambridge, England: MacDonald Institute Monographs; 1996:139–160.

3. Locke J. *Second Treatise of Government.* 1690.

4. Marx K. Critique of the Gotha Program. In: Tucker RC, ed. *The Marx-Engels Reader.* New York, NY: W.W. Norton; 1978:525–541.

5. Leonard EM. *The Early History of English Poor Relief.* Cambridge: Cambridge University Press; 2013.

6. Chen E, Matthews KA, Boyce WT. Socioeconomic differences in children's health: how and why do these relationships change with age? *Psychol Bull.* 2002;128(2):295–329.

7. Chen E, Martin AD, Matthews KA. Socioeconomic status and health: do gradients differ within childhood and adolescence? *Soc Sci Med.* 2006;62(9):2161–2170.

8. McLaughlin KA, Breslau J, Green JG, et al. Childhood socio-economic status and the onset, persistence, and severity of DSM-IV mental disorders in a US national sample. *Soc Sci Med.* 2011;73(7):1088–1096.

9. Reiss F. Socioeconomic inequalities and mental health problems in children and adolescents: a systematic review. *Soc Sci Med.* 2013;90:24–31.

10. Balan B, Lingam L. Unintentional injuries among children in resource poor settings: where do the fingers point? *Arch Dis Child Educ Pract Ed.* 2012;97(1):35–38.

11. Hertzman C, Boyce WT. How experience gets under the skin to create gradients in developmental health. *Annu Rev Public Health.* 2010;31:329–347.

12. Odgers CL, Jaffee SR. Routine versus catastrophic influences on the developing child. *Annu Rev Public Health.* 2013;34:29–48.

13. Chi DL, Dinh MA, da Fonseca MA, Scott JM, Carle AC. Dietary research to reduce children's oral health disparities: an exploratory cross-sectional analysis of socioeconomic status, food insecurity, and fast-food consumption. *J Acad Nutr Diet.* 2015;115(10):1599–1604.

14. Evans GW, Kantrowitz E. Socioeconomic status and health: the potential role of environmental risk exposure. *Annu Rev Public Health.* 2002;23:303–331.

15. Evans GW, Kim P. Childhood poverty and health: cumulative risk exposure and stress dysregulation. *Psychol Sci.* 2007;18(11):953–957.

16. Briggs-Gowan MJ, Carter AS, Ford JD. Parsing the effects violence exposure in early childhood: modeling developmental pathways. *J Pediatr Psychol.* 2012;37(1):11–22.

17. Duncan GJ, Magnuson K, Votruba-Drzal E. Boosting family income to promote child development. *Future Child.* 2014;24(1):99–120.

18. Boe T, Sivertsen B, Heiervang E, Goodman R, Lundervold AJ, Hysing M. Socioeconomic status and child mental health: the role of parental emotional well-being and parenting practices. *J Abnorm Child Psychol.* 2014;42(5):705–715.

19. Blumenshine P, Egerter S, Barclay CJ, Cubbin C, Braveman PA. Socioeconomic disparities in adverse birth outcomes: a systematic review. *Am J Prev Med.* 2010;39(3):263–272.

20. Brown RL. Epidemiology of injury and the impact of health disparities. *Curr Opin Pediatr.* 2010;22(3):321–325.

21. Dowd JB, Zajacova A, Aiello A. Early origins of health disparities: burden of infection, health, and socioeconomic status in U.S. children. *Soc Sci Med.* 2009;68(4):699–707.

22. Boyce WT, Den Besten PK, Stamperdahl J, et al. Social inequalities in childhood dental caries: the convergent roles of stress, bacteria and disadvantage. *Soc Sci Med.* 2010;71(9):1644–1652.

23. US Department of Health and Human Services. *CDC Health Disparities and Inequalities Report—United States, 2011.* Atlanta, GA: Centers for Disease Control and Prevention; 2011.

24. Kawachi I, Adler NE, Dow WH. Money, schooling, and health: mechanisms and causal evidence. *Ann N Y Acad Sci.* 2010;1186:56–68.

25. Keating DP, Hertzman C. *Developmental Health and the Wealth of Nations: Social, Biological, and Educational Dynamics.* New York, NY: Guilford Press; 1999.

26. Shonkoff JP, Boyce WT, McEwen BS. Neuroscience, molecular biology, and the childhood roots of health disparities: building a new framework for health promotion and disease prevention *JAMA.* 2009;301(21):2252–2259.

27. Jiang Y, Ekono M, Skinner C. *Basic Facts about Low-income Children: Children under 6 years.* National Center for Children in Poverty; 2014. http://nccp.org/publications/pub_1088.html.

28. Hackman DA, Farah MJ. Socioeconomic status and the developing brain. *Trends Cogn Sci.* 2009;13(2):65–73.

29. Kishiyama MM, Boyce WT, Jimenez AM, Perry LM, Knight RT. Socioeconomic disparities affect prefrontal function in children. *J Cogn Neurosci.* 2009;21(6):1106–1115.

30. Noble KG, Houston SM, Brito NH, et al. Family income, parental education and brain structure in children and adolescents. *Nat Neurosci.* 2015;18(5):773–778.

31. Olden K, Lin YS, Gruber D, Sonawane B. Epigenome: biosensor of cumulative exposure to chemical and nonchemical stressors related to environmental justice. *Am J Public Health.* 2014;104(10):1816–1821.

32. Boyce WT, Kobor MS. Development and the epigenome: the 'synapse' of gene-environment interplay. *Dev Sci.* 2015;18(1):1–23.

33. Marmot MG, Wilkinson RG. Psychosocial and material pathways in the relation between income and health: a response to Lynch et al. *BMJ.* 2001;322:1233–1236.

34. Odgers CL. Income inequality and the developing child: is it all relative? *Am Psychol.* 2015;70(8):722–731.

35. Ellul J. *Le Bluff Technologique (The Technological Bluff. Trans. Geoffrey W. Bromiley).* Paris (Grand Rapids): Hachette (Eerdmans); 1988 (1990).

36. Hawley PH. The role of competition and cooperation in shaping personality: an evolutionary perspective on social dominance, Machiavellianism, and children's social development. In: Buss DM, Hawley PH, eds. *The Evolution of Personality and Individual Differences.* New York, NY: Oxford University Press; 2011.

37. Ardiel EL, Rankin CH. *C. elegans*: social interactions in a "nonsocial" animal. *Adv Genet.* 2009;68:1–22.

38. Sokolowski MB. Social interactions in "simple" model systems. *Neuron.* 2010;65:780–794.

39. Grosenick L, Clement TS, Fernald RD. Fish can infer social rank by observation alone. *Nature.* 2007;445(7126):429–432.

40. Sapolsky RM. Adrenocortical function, social rank, and personality among wild baboons. *Biol Psychiatry.* 1990;28:862–885.

41. Bastian ML, Sponberg AC, Suomi SJ, Higley JD. Long-term effects of infant rearing condition on the acquisition of dominance rank in juvenile and adult rhesus macaques (*Macaca mulatta*). *Dev Psychobiol.* 2003;42(1):44–51.

42. Strayer FF, Strayer J. An ethological analysis of social agonism and dominance relations among preschool children. *Child Dev.* 1976;47:980–989.

43. Vaughn B, Waters E. Social organization among preschooler peers: dominance, attention and sociometric correlates. In: Omark DR, Strayer FF, Freedman D, eds. *Dominance Relations: An Ethological View of Human Conflict and Social Interaction.* New York, NY: Garland STPM Press; 1978:359–380.

44. Coie JD, Dodge KA, Coppotelli H. Dimensions and types of social status: a cross-age perspective. *Dev Psychol.* 1982;18(4):557–570.

45. La Frenière PJ, Charlesworth WR. Effects of friendship and dominance status on preschooler's resource utilization in a cooperative/competitive situation. *Int J Behav Dev.* 1987;10(3):345–358.

46. Hawley PH. The ontogenesis of social dominance: a strategy-based evolutionary perspective. *Dev Rev.* 1999;19:97–132.

47. Mascaro O, Csibra G. Representation of stable social dominance relations by human infants. *Proc Natl Acad Sci USA.* 2012;109(18):6862–6867.

48. Mascaro O, Csibra G. Human infants' learning of social structures: the case of dominance hierarchy. *Psychol Sci.* 2014;25(1):250–255.

49. Davis K, Moore WE. Some principles of stratification. *Am Sociol Rev.* 1945;10:242–249.

50. Clutton-Brock T. Structure and function in mammalian societies. *Philos Trans R Soc Lond B Biol Sci.* 2009;364(1533):3229–3242.

51. Rowell TE. The concept of social dominance. *Behav Biol.* 1974;11(2):131–154.

52. de Waal FB. The integration of dominance and social bonding in primates. *Q Rev Biol.* 1986;61(4):459–479.

53. Davidson RS, Marion G, Hutchings MR. Effects of host social hierarchy on disease persistence. *J Theor Biol.* 2008;253:424–433.

54. Miller GE, Chen E, Fok AK, et al. Low early-life social class leaves a biological residue manifested by decreased glucocorticoid and increased proinflammatory signaling. *Proc Natl Acad Sci USA.* 2009;106(34):14716–14721.

55. Sapolsky RM. Hypercortisolism among socially subordinate wild baboons originates at the CNS level. *Arch Gen Psychiatry.* 1989;46:1047–1051.

56. McEwen BS, Gianaros PJ. Central role of the brain in stress and adaptation: links to socioeconomic status, health, and disease. *Ann N Y Acad Sci.* 2010;1186:190–222.

57. Kroes RA, Panksepp J, Burgdorf J, Otto NJ, Moskal JR. Modeling depression: social dominance-submission gene expression patterns in rat neocortex. *Neuroscience.* 2006;137:37–49.

58. Cohen S, Line S, Manuck SB, Rabin BS, Heise ER, Kaplan JR. Chronic social stress, social status, and susceptibility to upper respiratory infections in non-human primates. *Psychosom Med.* 1997;59(3):213–221.

59. Adler NE, Epel ES, Castellazzo G, Ickovics JR. Relationship of subjective and objective social status with psychological and physiological functioning: Preliminary data in healthy, White women. *Health Psychol.* 2000;19(6):586–592.

60. Ostrove JM, Adler NE, Kuppermann M, Washington AE. Objective and subjective assessments of socioeconomic status and their relationship to self-rated health in an ethnically diverse sample of pregnant women. *Health Psychol.* 2000;19(6):613–618.

61. Goodman E, Adler NE, Daniels SR, Morrison JA, Slap GB, Dolan LM. Impact of objective and subjective social status on obesity in a biracial cohort of adolescents. *Obes Res.* 2003;11(8):1018–1026.

62. Kaplan JR, Manuck SB, Clarkson TB, Lusso FM, Taub DM. Social status, environment, and athersclerosis in cynomolgus monkeys. *Arteriosclerosis.* 1982;2:359–368.

63. Abbott DH, Keverne EB, Bercovitch FB, et al. Are subordinates always stressed? A comparative analysis of rank differences in cortisol levels among primates. *Horm Behav.* 2003;43(1):67–82.

64. Sapolsky RM. The influence of social hierarchy on primate health. *Science.* 2005;308(5722):648–652.

65. Boehm C. *Hierarchy in the Forest: The Evolution of Egalitarian Behavior.* Cambridge, MA: Harvard University Press; 1999.

66. Knauft BB. Violence and sociality in human evolution. *Curr Anthropol.* 1991;32:391–428.

67. Sapolsky RM, Share LJ. A pacific culture among wild baboons: its emergence and transmission. *PLoS Biol.* 2004;2(4):E106.

68. Ross NA, Wolfson MC, Dunn JR, Berthelot JM, Kaplan GA, Lynch JW. Relation between income inequality and mortality in Canada and in the United States: cross sectional assessment using census data and vital statistics. *BMJ.* 2000;320(7239):898–902.

69. Mackenbach JP, Stirbu I, Roskam AJ, et al. Socioeconomic inequalities in health in 22 European countries. *N Engl J Med.* 2008;358(23):2468–2481.

70. Friel S, Marmot MG. Action on the social determinants of health and health inequities goes global. *Annu Rev Public Health.* 2011;32:225–236.

71. Lynch JW, Smith GD, Kaplan GA, House JS. Income inequality and mortality: importance to health of individual income, psychosocial environment, or material conditions. *BMJ.* 2000;320(7243):1200–1204.

72. Boyce WT, Shonkoff JP. The course of life and life, of course: a commentary on Ben-Shlomo, Cooper and Kuh. *Int J Epidemiol.* 2016;45(4):1000–1002.

73. Schwenk M, Gundert-Remy U, Heinemeyer G, et al. Children as a sensitive subgroup and their role in regulatory toxicology: DGPT workshop report. *Arch Toxicol.* 2003;77(1):2–6.

74. Wild CP, Kleinjans J. Children and increased susceptibility to environmental carcinogens: evidence or empathy? *Cancer Epidemiol Biomarkers Prev.* 2003;12(12):1389–1394.

75. Shonkoff JP, Garner AS, Siegel BS, et al. The lifelong effects of early childhood adversity and toxic stress. *Pediatrics.* 2012;129(1):e232–e246.

76. Keltner D, Gruenfeld D, Anderson C. Power, approach, and inhibition. *Psychol Rev.* 2003;110(2):265–284.

77. Strayer FF, Trudel M. Developmental changes in the nature and function of social dominance among young children. *Ethol Sociobiol.* 1984;5:279–295.

78. Pellegrini AD, Roseth CJ, Mliner S, et al. Social dominance in preschool classrooms. *J Comp Psychol.* 2007;121(1):54–64.

79. Pellegrini AD, Van Ryzin MJ, Roseth C, et al. Behavioral and social cognitive processes in preschool children's social dominance. *Aggress Behav.* 2010;37(3):248–257.

80. Hawley PH, Little TD. On winning some and losing some: a social relations approach to social dominance in toddlers. *Merrill Palmer Q.* 1999;45(2):185–214.

81. Boyce WT, Obradović J, Bush N, Stamperdahl J, Kim YS, Adler N. Social stratification, classroom 'climate' and the behavioral adaptation of kindergarten children. *Proc Natl Acad Sci USA.* 2012;109(Suppl 2):17168–17173.

82. Luby JL, Heffelfinger A, Measelle JR, et al. Differential performance of the macarthur HBQ and DISC-IV in identifying DSM-IV internalizing psychopathology in young children. *J Am Acad Child Adolesc Psychiatry.* 2002;41(4):458–466.

83. Schjelderupp-Ebbe T. Beiträge zur sozialpsychologie des haushuhns. *Z Psychol.* 1922;88:226–252.

84. Drews C. The concept and definition of dominance in animal behaviour. *Behaviour.* 1993;125:283–313.

85. Bernstein IS. Primate status hierarchies. In: Rosenblum LA, ed. *Primate Behavior: Developments in Field and Laboratory Research*, Vol. 1. New York, NY: Academic Press; 1970:71–111.

86. Sade DS. Determinants of dominance in a group of free-ranging rhesus monkeys. In: Altmann SA, ed. *Social Communication among Primates*. Chicago, IL: University of Chicago Press 1967:99–114.

87. Thierry B. Unity in diversity: lessons from macaque societies. *Evol Anthropol*. 2007;16:224–238.

88. Suomi SJ. Conflict and cohesion in rhesus monkey family life. In: Cox MJ, Brooks-Gunn J, eds. *Conflict and Cohesion in Families*. Mahwah, NJ: Erlbaum; 1999:283–299.

89. Dettmer AM, Woodward RA, Suomi SJ. Reproductive consequences of a matrilineal overthrow in rhesus monkeys. *Am J Primatol*. 2015;77:347–352.

90. Novak MA, Suomi SJ. Social interaction in non-human primates: an underlying theme for primate research? *Lab Anim Sci*. 1991;41:308–314.

91. Stevens H, Leckman J, Coplan JD, Suomi SJ. Risk, resilience, and recovery: early manipulations of macaque social experience result in persistent behavioral and neurophysiological sequelae. *J Am Acad Child Adolesc Psychiatry*. 2009;48:114–127.

92. Dettmer AM, Wooddell L, Rosenberg K, et al. Associations between early life experience, chronic HPA axis activity, and adult social rank in rhesus monkeys. *Soc Neurosci*. 2016(in press).

93. Conti G, Hansman C, Heckman JJ, Novak MFX, Ruggiero AM, Suomi SJ. Primate evidence on the late health effects on early life adversity. *Proc Natl Acad Sci USA*. 2012;109:8066–8071.

94. Suomi SJ. Attachment in rhesus monkeys. In: Cassidy J, Shaver PR, eds. *Handbook of Attachment*, 3rd ed. New York, NY: Guilford; 2016:133–154.

95. Berman CM. Immature siblings and mother–infant relationships among free-ranging rhesus monkeys on Cayo Santiago. *Anim Behav*. 1992;44:247–258.

96. Massart R, Sunderman MJ, Nemoda Z, et al. The signature of maternal social rank in offspring placenta DNA methylation profiles in rhesus monkeys. *Child Dev*. 2012:32(44):15626–15642.

97. National Research Council. *Guide for the Care and use of Laboratory Animals*. Washington, DC: National Academy Press; 2011.

98. Hektner JM, August GJ, Realmuto GM. Patterns and temporal changes in peer affiliation among aggressive and nonaggressive children participating in a summer school program. *J Clin Child Psychol*. 2000;29(4):603–614.

99. Maccoby EE. Gender and group process: a developmental perspective. *Curr Dir Psychol Sci*. 2002;11(2):54–58.

100. Wilensky U. 1999. NetLogo. http://ccl.northwestern.edu/netlogo/. Center for Connected Learning and Computer-Based Modeling, Northwestern University. Evanston, IL.

101. Kahneman D. *Thinking Fast and Slow*. New York, NY: Farrar, Strauss & Giroux; 2011.

102. Box GEP, Draper NR. *Empirical Model-Building and Response Surfaces*. New York, NY: Wiley; 1987

103. Howes C, Rubin KH, Ross HS, French DC. Peer interaction of young children. *Monogr Soc Res Child Dev.* 1988;53(1):i–92.

104. Fujisawa KK, Kutsukake N, Hasegawa T. Social network analyses of positive and negative relationships among Japanese preschool classmates. *Int J Behav Dev.* 2009;33(3):193–201.

105. Estell DB. Aggression, social status, and affiliation in kindergarten children: a preliminary study. *Educ Treat Children.* 2007;30(2):53–72.

106. Strayer FF, Santos AJ. Affiliative structures in preschool peer groups. *Soc Dev.* 1996;5(2):117–130.

107. Henzi SP, de Sousa Pereira LF, Hawker-Bond D, Stiller J, Dunbar RI, Barrett L. Look who's talking: developmental trends in the size of conversational cliques. *Evol Hum Behav.* 2007;28(1):66–74.

108. Frankel DG, Arbel T. Group formation by two-year olds. *Int J Behav Dev.* 1980;3(3):287–298.

109. Biehler RF. Companion choice behavior in the kindergarten. *Child Dev.* 1954;25:45–50.

110. Hartup WW, Laursen B, Stewart MI, Eastenson A. Conflict and the friendship relations of young children. *Child Dev.* 1988;59:1590–1600.

111. Howes C. Social status and friendship from kindergarten to third grade. *J Appl Dev Psychol.* 1990;11(3):321–330.

112. Cillessen AH, IJzendoorn HW, Lieshout CF, Hartup WW. Heterogeneity among peer-rejected boys: subtypes and stabilities. *Child Dev.* 1992;63(4):893–905.

113. Dodge KA. Behavioral antecedents of peer social status. *Child Dev.* 1983;54:1386–1399.

114. Cassidy J, Asher SR. Loneliness and peer relations in young children. *Child Dev.* 1992;63:350–365.

115. Ladd GW, Kochenderfer BJ, Coleman CC. Classroom peer acceptance, friendship, and victimization: distinct relation systems that contribute uniquely to children's school adjustment? *Child Dev.* 1997;68(6):1181–1197.

116. Santos AJ, Vaughn BE, Bost KK. Specifying social structures in preschool classrooms: descriptive and functional distinctions between affiliative subgroups. *Acta Ethol.* 2008;11(2):101–113.

117. Snyder J, Horsch E, Childs J. Peer relationships of young children: affiliative choices and the shaping of aggressive behavior. *J Clin Child Psychol.* 1997;26(2):145–156.

118. Mitchell M. *Introduction to Genetic Algorithms.* Cambridge, MA: MIT Press; 1986.

119. Wooddell LJ, Kaburu SK, Dettmer AM, Suomi SJ. Elo ratings as a tool to measure rank changes and dominance stability in semi free-ranging rhesus macaques. *Am J Primatol.* 2015;77:80.

APPENDIX: DETAILED DESCRIPTION OF THE PROGRAM

I.   OVERVIEW

This is a general model of interactions of youngsters in a play area—interactions that affect their status and self-image. Interactions include: "play," "compete," "walk away," and "play alone." As a result of these interactions, the youngsters gain or lose status in the play area hierarchy, with impacts on their levels of stress (depression).

II.   BACKGROUND DETAILS (starred items (*) are user-defined parameters)

1)   * N = Number of agents in the play area (default N = 33, sometimes 20)

2)   * M × M = Size of the play area (default M = 50)

3) (x_j, y_j) = location of agent j in play area, with $0 \leq x_j, y_j < M$.

4)   ** A fixed percentage of the agents are loners (default = 10 percent); a high percentage of the time (default = 90 percent) loners choose to "play alone."

5)   Each agent in turn will decide whether or not to play alone, and if not, to seek an interaction and someone to interact with.

6)   * Each agent j will search only in their **field of vision** FV, a disk of radius R_v about (x_j, y_j). (Default $R_v = 10$).

7)   We will call the chooser/searcher the focal agent or foCus C and the agent he chooses the target agent T.

8)   * When focal agent C chooses target T, C moves into their target's **"interaction zone,"** a ring of outer radius R_+ and inner radius R_- about the target's position. (default $R_+ = 5$; $R_- = .05$).

9)   In each round each agent gets to be the focal agent exactly once, with the order of choice determined randomly at the beginning of each round.

10)   * There is a limit on the number of times that a given agent can be the target agent in any single round, but that limit has rarely been required.

11) * There are 10 rounds per recess.

12) * There are 4 recesses per day.

13) * Currently, there are 100 days per simulation run; eventually this will be the number of school-days per year.

III.   ACTION SUMMARY

1) The focal agent can choose to "play alone," or to offer to "play" or "compete" with some target agent. The offer and the target are, in a sense, chosen at the same time.

2) The agents pre-designated as "loners" have a 90 percent probability of "playing alone" when it's their turn.

3) If the focal agent offers "play," the target can respond with "play" or with "walk away."

4) If the focal agent offers "compete," the target must compete too.

5) After the interactions, various status and stress variables change for both the focal and the target agent.

IV.   PROPERTIES OF EACH AGENT J (Starred items are user-defined)

1) Location in play area (x_j, y_j).

2) Amount of **aFFiliative resource** f_j. This is a measure of agent j's Friendliness. f_j lies in $[0,1]$ and changes over time. It increases with play and decreases with a) competitive acts, b) playing alone, c) walking away.

3) Amount of **aGonistic resource** g_j. This is a measure of the agent's touGhness. It is the primary index of status or rank in the hierarchy in the population. g_j lies in $[0,1]$ and changes over time. It increases with victories in competitions and decreases with losses in competitions. It is zero-sum in that a focal agent's gains or losses in an interaction are the negative of the target agent's losses or gains.

4) * Agent j's target level F_j of f_j. (Default = 1).

5) * Agent j's target level G_j of g_j, called agent j's **competitiveness**.

6) * Agent j's **aggressiveness**, a parameter in $[0,1]$, related to the agent's expectation of winning a competition.

7) * The competitiveness and aggression numbers indicate how much an agent values g over f in interactions. In fact, the weight **D** with which an agent values g over f in his utility function over

outcomes has been assigned in a number of ways in simulations:

  i. a user-defined convex combination of his competitiveness and aggression (to relate to empirical data),

  ii. as a random number chosen from some triangular distribution (so that we could see the role of variance in g_j),

  iii. as the same number for all agents (so we could see the effects of different weights on status g).

8) We consider (f_j, g_j) agent j's **state** at any time.

9) Amount P_j of agent j's **depression** (or stress level). $0 \leq P_j < \infty$. P_j varies over time. It decreases with successful interactions and increases with unsuccessful interactions (like losing a competition or being ignored).

10) * An intrinsic base level of depression P_j^* for each agent j.

11) ** Whether or not agent j is designated as a "**loner.**" A loner decides to "play alone" 90 percent (user-defined) of the times it is his turn. If a loner is chosen as a play target, the loner will choose to walk away. Roughly 10 percent (user-defined) of the agents are randomly chosen as loners at the beginning of the simulation.

12) * There are two decision processes, a fast one and a slower more deliberate one (after Kahneman). Each agent has an a priori probability (user-defined) of choosing the fast process over the slow one at each decision node.

13) * Each agent has a **friendship threshold** FT_j, though it could be the same for all agents. FT is a number that determines "how many more" positive interactions then negative interactions with another agent k does agent j require in order to call agent k his **friend**.

14) Each agent has a memory of past interactions with each agent k. This memory includes:

  a. The round in which interaction with agent k as agent j's target occurred.

  b. Whether or not agent j offered "play" in that interaction.

  c. Whether agent k's response was positive ("play too") or negative ("walk away") to each of these offers.

  d. If the number of positive interactions minus the number of negative interactions is $\geq$ agent j's friendship threshold FT_j, then agent j lists agent k as his **friend**.

V.   RESULTS OF INTERACTIONS (sizes of changes Δ are user-defined)

1) If focal agent C offers target T to play, T can play or walk away.

   a) If both play,

       i. $\Delta p < 0$ for both (both are less depressed)

       ii. $\Delta f > 0$ for both (both increase affiliative resource). Maybe more for C.

       iii. $\Delta g < 0$ for higher g (higher status agent loses a little status)

       iv. $\Delta g > 0$ for lower g (lower status agent gains a little status).

   b) If T walks away,

       i. $\Delta p < 0$ for T, and $\Delta p > 0$ for C. (The spurned are more depressed; the spurner less depressed.)

       ii. $\Delta f < 0$ for both. (Both lose affiliative resource.)

       iii. $\Delta g < 0$ for both. (Both lose status.) Bigger loss for C than for T.

       iv.   [In some runs, no change in f,g,p for T.]

2) If focal agent C offers "compete," T must compete.

   a) Suppose initial states are $(f_C(0), g_C(0))$ for C and $(f_T(0), g_T(0))$ for T. The probability of C winning the competition should be related to $\pi_C \cong g_C(0) / [g_C(0) + g_T(0)]$,

   and similarly the probability of T winning the competition should be related to

   $$\pi_T \cong g_T(0) / [g_C(0) + g_T(0)],.$$

   b) * In our runs, we have chosen to use the expressions

   $$\Pi_C(\text{win} \mid \text{compete}) = (\pi_C)^\rho / [(\pi_C)^\rho + (\pi_T)^\rho] \text{ and } \Pi_C(\text{lose} \mid \text{compete}) = (\pi_T)^\rho / [(\pi_C)^\rho + (\pi_T)^\rho].$$

   for the probabilities of C winning or losing the competition respectively.

   The parameter ρ is user-determined, and is the parameter we call **status advantage** in the text. In 2b) above, $\rho=1$ gives the lower status competitor a reasonable chance of winning the competition. As ρ increases, the probability of the lower status competitor winning declines toward 0.

   c) The computer chooses a winner based on $\Pi_C(\text{win} \mid \text{compete})$ and $\Pi_C(\text{lose} \mid \text{compete})$.

    d)   The winner gains some g and loses some p. The loser loses some g (the same amount as the winner gains), gains some p, and moves away. The amount of g transferred equals:

        (the loser's probability of winning, as in b above)*(loser's Ag score)*(stake).

        The multiplier "**stake**," called "compFracTr" in the program is our key indicator of the relative size of the winning amount.

    e)   These gains and losses have bigger magnitudes if the less likely agent wins the competition.

    f)   The focal agent loses f. The target loses f but less than the focal agent does.

3)   If the focal agent C chooses to play alone, C loses a little f and g and maybe loses a little p.

VI.   CHOICE OF ACTION: THE UTILITY FUNCTION

1)   For slower, more deliberate decisions, each agent evaluates his new state via a utility function that compares the new state with the ideal state.

2)   Suppose that using the scoring rules of Section V, an agent determines that his choice of "play, compete, move away or play alone" yields a new state $(f(1), g(1))$.

3)   The agent wants to compare this new state to his ideal state (F, G), where the default has been $F=1$, using $|f(1) - F|$ and $|g(1) - G|$.

4)   To turn this into a maximization problem, we consider: $(1-|f(1) - F|)$ and $(1 - |g(1) - G|)$. (#)

5)   To turn this into a scalar maximization problem, we weight these by the weight D on toughness discussed in Section IV.7: $(1 - D)*(1 - |f(1) - F|) + D*(1 - |g(1) - G|)$.

6)   Because this linear structure allows less preferred outcomes to occur too frequently, we add a power 2 to both expressions in (#).

7)   In summary, to evaluate new state $((f(1), g(1))$, an agent uses the utility function

    $U(f(1),g(1)) = (1 - D)*(1 - |f(1) - F|)^2 + D*(1 - |g(1) - G|)^2$.

VII.   CHOICE OF ACTION BY THE FOCAL AGENT C

1)   We first check to see whether or not C is a "loner." If C is a loner, C has a 90 percent probability of not interacting with anyone, and a 10 percent probability of choosing an activity/target and following options below. (User-defined percents.)

2)   We suppose now that either C is not a loner or, if he is a loner, that the random number generator

put him in the 10 percent regular activity mode.

3) The program next determines whether agent C will use the fast or slow decision process, based on C's innate proclivity as described in IV.12.

4) If it is determined that C will use his fast process, C looks for a "friend" in his field of vision FV.

5) If he finds one there, he offers to play with this friend.

6) If there is more than one friend in FV, C chooses (stochastically, of course) the one with the highest friendship rating, as described in Section IV.14.e. (In some runs, we have had C choose the friend in FV with whom he interacted with most recently.)

7) If either C has no friends in FV or it is determined that C use his "slow," i.e., more deliberate, decision process, then C uses his utility function U, as described in Section VI.7, to choose an activity/target as follows.

8) Basically, C is going to use U to compute the expected utility of offering play or compete to each agent in his FV. He also computes his utility of playing alone. He stochastically chooses the action/target-agent that yields the highest utility among these options.

9) The process for each agent T in his FV goes as follows:

10) If C were to offer to play with T, C checks his memory of past interactions with T and estimates that the probability that T will choose play (from C's perspective) is

Prob_C (T play | C play) = (#times T accepted C's offer to play) / (#times that C offered T to play).

11) Otherwise, Prob_C (T walk away | C play) = (#times T rejected C's offer to play) / (#times that C offered T to play).

12) If the initial states are $(f_C(0), g_C(0))$ for C and $(f_T(0), g_T(0))$ for T, and if both play, their states change according to Section V.1.a above.

Write $(f_C^{PP}(1), g_C^{PP}(1))$ and $(f_T^{PP}(1), g_T^{PP}(1))$ be their corresponding states after they both play.

13) If C plays and T walks away, then we use Section V.1.b to compute their new states and we write them as $(f_C^{PW}(1), g_C^{PW}(1))$ and $(f_T^{PW}(1), g_T^{PW}(1))$ respectively.

14) Then, C's utility for the Play-Play outcome is:

$$D_C*(1 - |g_C^{PP}(1) - G_C|)^2 + (1-D_C)*(1 - |f_C^{PP}(1) - F_C|)^2$$

15) Similarly, C's utility for the play-walk outcome as

$$D_C*(1 - |g_C^{PW}(1) - G_C|)^2 + (1 - D_C)*(1 - |f_C^{PW}(1) - F_C|)^2$$

Recall that the D_C is C's relative weigh on agonistic resource f. See Section IV.7.

16) Finally, C's expected utility of offering the play option to T is the probability that T will respond with play times the utility to C of the play-play outcome plus the probability that T will respond by walking away times the utility to C of the play-walk outcome:

$Prob_C$ (T play | C play)*$\{ D_C(1 - |g_C^{PP}(1) - G_C|)^2 + (1 - D_C)^* (1 - |f_C^{PP}(1) - F_C|)^2 \}$ + $Prob_C$ (T walk away | C play) * $\{ D_C^*(1 - |g_C^{PW}(1) - G_C|)^2 + (1 - D_C)^* (1 - |f_C^{PW}(1) - F_C|)^2 \}$.

17) Next, C computes the expected utility of offering to compete with T.

18) If C offers "compete," T must compete too. Now the uncertainty is whether C or T wins the competition.

19) Section V.2.b gives the probabilities of C or T winning the competition. Call these Π_C (win | compete) and Π_C (lose | compete).

20) Sections V.2.d–f give the state changes that occur if the agents compete and C wins or loses. Call the new states $(f_C^+(1), g_C^+(1))$ and $(f_C^-(1), g_C^-(1))$, respectively.

21) Then, C's expected utility for playing "compete" with agent T is:

Π_C (win | compete) * $\{ \mathbf{D_C^*(1 - |g_C^+(1) - G_C|)^2 + (1-D_C)^* (1 - |f_C^+(1) - F_C|)^2} \}$ +

Π_C(lose | compete) * $\{ D_C^*(1 - |g_C^-(1) - G_C|)^2 + (1-D_C)^* (1 - |f_C^-(1) - F_C|)^2 \}$.

22) Focal agent C goes through this calculation with each agent T in his FV. Finally, from Section V.3, C computes his expected utility of "playing alone," which ends up in state $(f_C^{P0}(1), g_C^{P0}(1))$, which C values as: $D_C^*(1 - |g_C^{P0}(1) - G_C|)^2 + (1 - D_C)^*(1 - |f_C^{P0}(1) - F_C|)^2 \}$.

23) C compares all these expected utilities and (stochastically) chooses the action/target that yields the highest expected utility.

VIII. CHOICE OF ACTION BY TARGET AGENT T

1) Once the focal agent C has chosen an action and target, the next step is to compute the target's response.

2) If C has chosen "compete," then T must compete, and the outcomes are as listed in Section V.2.

3) If C has chosen "offer play," then T can accept the offer to play or walk away. We now examine T's choice process.

4) If T is a loner, then T has a 90 percent chance of walking away (user-defined).

5) Otherwise, using the parameter described in Section IV.12, it is determined whether T will use his fast or slow decision process.

6) If T uses his fast process, he checks to see whether or not C is listed as a friend on T's list. If C is so listed, T accepts C's offer to play.

7) If C is not on T's friends list or if T uses his slow decision process, then T computes his expected utility of playing with C or of walking away from C's offer. He chooses the action that generates the highest utility.

IX.   EARLY GAME CHOICES

1) We have slid over one complication in the slow decision process: How to estimate a potential agent's reaction if there have been too few interactions for such an estimate: Of course, if C were to offer "compete," T must respond with "compete." If C were to offer "play" and has had too few encounters with the T under consideration, C assumes that T's probability of choosing play versus walk-away mirrors the choices made in the general population so far that round. If that experience is too small still, C assumes that T has a 2/3 probability of choosing play (the probability supported by the psych literature).

X.   THE FLOW OF THE SIMULATION

1) At the beginning of the simulation, the number of agents, the size of the field of vision, the size of the play area, and the size of the interaction zone, and all the other user-defined parameters discussed in Sections II and IV are determined.

2) Each agent is given a value of F, G, P*, loner/nonloner status, and probability of using fast versus slow decision process.

3) Agents are spaced randomly at locations in the play area.

4) At the beginning of each round, agents are given an ordering to determine when they will be the focal agent.

5) There are four rounds to a recess.

6) At the end of each recess, the agents return to their original locations, as prescribed in 3) above,

7) There are ten recesses per day. At the end of the day, each agent retains his f-score and g-score. However, his depression level p is changed to $0.9*p + 0.1*(P* - p)$, a little closer to his innate level.

8) Currently, there are 100 days per simulation; eventually that number will mirror the length of the school year.

CHAPTER 5

NO LONGER LOOKING JUST UNDER THE LAMP POST: MODELING THE COMPLEXITY OF PRIMARY HEALTH CARE

Kurt C. Stange, MD, PhD
Distinguished University Professor, Gertrude Donnelly Hess, MD, Professor of Oncology Research, Professor of Family Medicine and Community Health, Epidemiology and Biostatistics, Sociology, and Oncology
Department of Family Medicine and Community Health
Case Western Reserve University

Sarah T. Cherng, MPH
PhD candidate
University of Michigan Department of Epidemiology and Center for Social Epidemiology and Population Health
University of Michigan School of Public Health

Rick L. Riolo, PhD
Research Professor Emeritus
Center for the Study of Complex Systems
University of Michigan

Laura Homa, PhD
Research Associate
Department of Family Medicine and Community Health
Case Western Reserve University

Johnie Rose, MD, PhD
Assistant Professor and Preventive Medicine Residency Program Director
Department of Family Medicine and Community Health
Case Western Reserve University

GROWING INEQUALITY

Peter S. Hovmand, PhD, MSW
Director
Social System Design Lab, Associate Professor of Practice, Brown School Brown School of Social Work, Washington University in St. Louis

Alison Kraus, MSW
Research Assistant
Social System Design Lab, Brown School of Social Work
Washington University in St. Louis

Acknowledgments: This line of investigation was supported by a contract from the NIH Office of Behavioral and Social Sciences Research to George A. Kaplan at the University of Michigan, to support the Network on Inequalities, Complexity and Health (NICH). The group model building was supported by Contract Number 1IP2PI000216-01 from the Patient-Centered Outcomes Research Institute (PCORI). NICH members were instrumental at every step of the process. George Kaplan, Ana Diez Roux, Tom Boyce, Nate Osgood, Carl Simon, Michael Wolfson, Sandro Galea, Ross Hammond, and Shiriki Kumanyika put in extra effort. Robert Ferrer, MD, MPH, David Katerndahl, MD, and Carlos Jaén, MD, PhD, were vitally helpful in the NICH pilot, which provided important initial conceptualizations for this work. Dr. Stange's time is supported in part by a Clinical Research Professorship from the American Cancer Society, and as a Scholar of The Institute for Integrative Health. This publication additionally was made possible by support from the Clinical and Translational Science Collaborative of Cleveland, UL1TR000439 from the National Center for Advancing Translational Sciences (NCATS) component of the National Institutes of Health and NIH roadmap for Medical Research. Its contents are solely the responsibility of the authors and do not necessarily represent the official views of the NIH. All statements in this report, including its findings and conclusions, are solely those of the authors and do not necessarily represent the views of the Patient-Centered Outcomes Research Institute (PCORI), its Board of Governors, or Methodology Committee.

"Please look with me under this lamppost."

"What are we looking for?"

"My lost keys."

"Where did you lose them?"

"Over there, in the darkness."

"Why are we looking here, under the lamppost?"

"It is so much simpler to see in the light."

Quality measurement in health and health care has made large strides in recent decades.[1-3] But most commonly, health and health care assessment is focused on the parts (diseases), rather than the whole (the health of people, communities, and populations).[4,5] The National Quality Forum, which attempts to catalyze improvements in health care by endorsing and harmonizing the current cacophony of quality measures, has endorsed some global metrics, but the vast majority of health care quality measures are disease-specific.[6] In contrast, an Institute of Medicine report highlights the need for population health measures to guide health policymaking.[7] Another recent Institute of Medicine report, *Vital Signs: Core Metrics for Health and Health Care Progress*,[8,9] demonstrates the growing recognition of the importance of assessing health and health care from the perspective of whole people and populations.

Focusing on body parts and diseases rather than whole persons and populations matters because how we perceive health care guides our efforts to understand, provide, and improve it.[10-13] When health care delivery, documentation, and payment are dominantly disease-focused, they usually lead to reductionist, linear (A→B→C) interventions that risk (often unintentionally) devaluing and sometimes diminishing the health of whole people and communities.[14]

Guiding resources and attention based on a simplistic, linear reductionist model implies that if we just get all the parts right, the whole will be healthy. This may be a helpful approach for simple health and health care interventions, such as the treatment of single acute illnesses or the prevention of diseases for which there is a single dominant cause and a preventive intervention easily targeted toward that cause. But most problems and opportunities in health care and health are complex; the whole is more than the sum of the parts, context matters, and small inputs sometimes have big effects and vice versa. Health emerges from the co-evolution of multiple factors, from the molecular to the social and ecological.[15-23]

Primary care provides an interesting and important case in point, and a surprising paradox. Multiple studies have found that primary care is associated with poorer quality care for individual diseases than care provided by clinicians focused primarily on those diseases.[24,29] Yet, other evidence shows that systems based on primary care have better quality of care, better population health, greater equity, and lower costs.[30-34] This discrepancy has been called the paradox of primary care.[35] Primary care is thought to be particularly important for disadvantaged populations and people with multiple chronic conditions.[36-38]

The complex features of primary care can interact[39,40] to provide value beyond disease-specific care. These features, called the tenets of primary care,[41-45] include:

- Accessibility as the first contact with the health care system;

- Accountability for addressing a large majority of personal health care needs (comprehensiveness);

- Coordination of care across settings; integration of care for acute and (often multiple) chronic illnesses, mental health, and prevention; and guided access to more narrowly focused care when needed;

- Sustained partnerships and personal relationships over time with patients, in the context of their families and communities.

The management of specific diseases is far easier to conceptualize and measure than is the value added by the complex interaction of primary care's elements.[13] During a time of rapid health system change, it is critical to understand the complex mechanisms of primary care that provide its added value,[14,46-49] so that efforts to provide incentives for improving the quality of disease care do not unintentionally diminish other desired effects of primary care.[13,14,46-49] This chapter uses complex systems concepts and methods to elucidate the possible mechanisms by which primary care influences health and health equity.

Why Complex Systems Methods?

Conceptualizing health, health care, and primary care as co-evolving, complex, adaptive systems[5,40,50,51] is helpful to overcome the pitfalls of simplistic, linear, reductionist approaches that do not take into account the paradox of primary care.[52] Computational simulation modeling is a helpful tool for developing and testing hypotheses about the conjoint mechanisms by which emergent properties happen in complex systems.[53]

Agent-based models begin with specifying the characteristics of heterogeneous individuals with many different types of discrete attributes, and their environment, and then observing the system-level effects of agent–agent and agent–environment interactions over time. Since primary care focuses on personalizing, integrating, and prioritizing care based on the particulars of diverse individuals and communities,[54-56] these types of models are particularly appropriate for understanding primary care and its paradox.[57,58]

Recently, principles from community-based, participatory research[59-61] have been used to engage stakeholders with deep personal knowledge of the phenomenon under study to work with scientists to develop, refine, and use models to test relevant hypotheses. Group model- building[62,63] involves stakeholders in the model-building process. While some view group model-building as referring to the involvement of stakeholders at any stage of the process,[62] others restrict it to taking a group of stakeholders through the entire process, from problem conceptualization to formulation, policy analysis, and the transfer of ownership.[63,64] More recent efforts have extended group model-building to engaging and working directly with communities.[65]

Central to group model-building is the use of diagraming conventions from system dynamics,[66] which function as boundary objects[67] that help modelers and participants to communicate their domain-specific perspectives. Boundary objects can include physical prototypes, design drawings, use scenarios, sketches, or standardized reporting forms.[68] Such objects help to make explicit tacit knowledge and assumptions, and make them accessible for group discussion and subsequent computer programming. Effective boundary objects should convey important dependencies in a system, and they should be understandable with a minimal amount of text and modifiable by all group members.[11,69,70] In system-dynamics modeling and simulation, boundary objects such as causal loop diagrams, behavior-overtime charts, and stock-and-flow diagrams form a bridge between the ideas in participants' heads and how those ideas are represented in formal mathematical simulation models.[70] Special challenges in developing boundary objects for agent-based modeling include depicting heterogeneous agent-level decision-making (different agents, such as people, thinking and acting differently from each other) and multiscale processes (problems that play out over different levels of time and/or space).[71] For this reason, group model-building has mainly been used to develop system-dynamics models[52,72,73] and has not been applied to development of agent-based models.[74]

To increase stakeholder participation in the development of an agent-based model for the paradox of primary care, we extended group model-building methods by developing a new set of boundary objects specific to agent-based modeling. In group model-building, boundary objects help to develop common ground for bridging the world views of diverse participants and connecting the insights developed in group discussions with subsequent programming work to create a computer simulation model.

Thus, we set out to pilot test a model of the paradox of primary care, and then to engage a community sample of patients, caregivers, and primary care clinicians in a participatory process of developing an agent-based model, and using it to test hypotheses about possible mechanisms by which primary care might affect population health and equity. Our purpose was not to compare specialty care and primary care, but to elucidate possible mechanisms for the effects of primary care beyond disease-specific care.

Methods

NICH pilot project: The Network on Inequalities, Complexity and Health (NICH),[75] funded by the NIH Office of Behavioral and Social Science Research, provided the supportive space, shared learning, and intellectual foment to launch this line of inquiry. Conversations at NICH led to a pilot study proposal in collaboration with investigators at the University of Texas Health Science Center at San Antonio, Family and Community Medicine (Robert L. Ferrer, MD, MPH, Carlos R. Jaen, MD, PhD, and David A. Katerndahl, MD, MA). This pilot project aimed to develop simple models of the paradox of primary care. It was actualized collaboratively through hands-on programming work by Rick Riolo, PhD, and Sarah Cherng, MPH, and conceptual work by Johnie Rose, MD, PhD, and Kurt C. Stange, MD, PhD, with periodic input from NICH members and from our University of Texas colleagues.

The resulting agent-based models used stylized facts (simplified depictions of empirical findings) about how people lose and regain health and seek health care to examine the effects of different mechanisms of primary care on the health and health equity of people and populations. This work was primarily accomplished in NetLogo,[76] enhanced by software designed by Dr. Riolo that facilitated data visualization and synthesized findings from multiple model runs.

The resulting models allowed us to begin piecing together possible mechanisms by which aspects of primary care, beyond a disease-specific focus, might affect health and health equity.

PCORI project: Based on our NICH pilot project work, we were fortunate to be funded by the new Patient-Centered Outcomes Research Institute (PCORI)[77] to create a participatory model of the paradox of primary care. This work involved ongoing support from NICH and collaboration among research teams at Case Western Reserve University, the Center for the Study of Complex Systems at the University of Michigan, and the Brown School Social System Design Laboratory at Washington University in St. Louis.

We began this work with a practice-based research network serving disadvantaged populations in Cleveland, Ohio, called the Safety Net Providers' Strategic Alliance.[78] We conducted focus groups and individual interviews with patients, caregivers, and primary care clinicians to begin identifying the features of primary care that might be important in addition to disease-specific care. We oversampled patients with multiple chronic conditions and expanded the initial sampling frame to maximize diversity in age, gender, SES, and experience with primary and specialty care. We sought clinicians from different community practice and health care system settings, and in focus groups and interviews selected a maximum diversity sample to participate in group model-building sessions.

These group model-building participants met approximately monthly for eight 2-hour sessions to develop hypotheses and conceptual models of how people become ill and seek health care, and how health care, particularly primary care, affects health. Before, during, and after each session, we worked to adapt group model-building methods—previously developed for system-dynamics modeling[63,79]—to the participatory development and refinement of an agent-based model.[52]

Between group model-building sessions, the conceptual models developed by participants were operationalized[76] and each model iteration was shared with the group at the following session and interactively refined over time.

We present methodological findings and the output from two different runs using the final model from this process. The presentation of model runs begins with a base model in which primary care features were turned off. Then we show a more fully developed model that simulates what happens when patients receive components of primary care hypothesized by the group model-building participants to provide added value. We examine model outputs of population health, health equity, and number of visits, and examine the effects in advantaged and disadvantaged neighborhoods, and for people with multiple chronic conditions.[80]

The model and its description were published in *Annals of Family Medicine*, with all group model-building participants as authors.[81] That article (www.annfammed.org/content/13/5/456.full) includes appendices (cited below when relevant and available at www.annfammed.org/content/13/5/456/suppl/DC1) with a detailed technical summary of the model (Appendix 2), the computer program (www.annfammed.org/content/13/5/456/suppl/DC2), as well as instructions for downloading the free NetLogo software (Appendix 3, to run it; Appendix 4), and worksheets for performing pre-specified and user-initiated experiments for readers to test their own hypotheses (Appendix 5).

Findings

NICH pilot project: The NICH pilot project allowed us to piece together understanding of mechanisms that could explain the paradox of primary care. One particularly interesting early model led to the surprising finding that over time, access to primary care increased the effectiveness of specialty care in treating individual diseases. This resulted from the ongoing effects of selective referral, as primary care clinicians referred patients based on their knowledge of their patients' specific needs and of specialists' particular expertise, whereas self-referring patients went to specialists whose expertise was not as well tailored to their conditions. Over time, referral minimized the negative effects of specialists' aggressive treatment of diseases for which the ratio of treatment effectiveness to treatment side effects was low, and it allowed specialists to work more closely in their areas of expertise compared to when patients self-referred, bringing a wide variety of complaints only some of which were related to the specialists' particular proficiencies.

Another interesting pilot model paralleled recent Affordable Care Act changes that improved health care access. This model identified mechanisms by which greater access to primary care might improve health equity through earlier disease treatment, health behavior change, and ongoing relationships that reduce high-risk care.

As we added more health care mechanisms and system constraints, the model became increasingly complex. It became more difficult to make sense of emergent findings. In the end, we learned a lot about how to sequentially develop a simple model, testing hypotheses at each step that allowed us to both understand the phenomena under study and the strengths and limitation of each phase of the model's development. We learned how to simply operationalize health loss and health care and the complex mechanisms of primary care. We began to develop an understanding about how the complex interaction of simple aspects of health and health care can lead to sometimes surprising emergent phenomena of health and health equity. We carried these understandings forward into the next phase of the project.

Group model-building process: The participatory group model-building process was successful in engaging eight female and one male patients/caregivers (often with multiple roles) with a variety of medical conditions, and three female and three male clinicians (five family physicians and one nurse practitioner) in working with academicians to develop, refine, and test hypotheses with an agent-based model. In this process, participants shared their experience as patients, caregivers, clinicians, and health care administrators, articulating the simple mechanisms by which primary care operates.

The progression of the group's eight sessions was designed and iteratively refined to increase participant knowledge of the modeling process; engage their diverse experience and expertise in providing relevant information and operationalizations for the model; and increase ownership and understanding of the model as a simple but understandable representation of mechanisms by which primary care might affect the patient-centered outcomes of health and health equity (table 1).

The first two sessions established an initial understanding of the modeling process and elicited group ideas about factors to incorporate into the model. A pivotal moment occurred near the end of the third session. Based on the experience of developing an overly complex and difficult-to-understand model during the NICH pilot, the group facilitator (KCS) had been working hard to simplify the incorporation of the many

Table 1

Group Sessions

Session	Description
1	Problem set up and learning about models by example
2	Develop a simple model
3	Experiment with the initial model, then start over
4	Add complexity to the base case
5	Add more primary care factors
6	Refine and use the model to test hypotheses
7	Review, test more hypotheses and plan next steps
8	Consolidate learning, work on outputs

complex ideas into the model. This kept the model understandable as each small increment was programmed (primarily by LH, but also JR and KCS), and evaluated by the group. However, the group began to feel that their complex ideas were increasingly distant; this disconnect was evidenced by stakeholders talking about "your" model as opposed to "our" model.

Therefore, near the end of the third session, the facilitator summarized another set of small, incremental additions to the model based on the evening's discussion, and then—to the horror of the programming team, which had spent the last three months writing code for the model—he offered the alternative: "We could throw the model out and start over." Two vocal group members endorsed throwing out the model and starting over with a more complex base case. With time running out in the session, the facilitator asked what this new model might look like. A group member who had not said anything during the session proposed one in which people could become ill in three ways: acute illness, chronic illness, and mental illness. One of the vocal members added a fourth option—acute, life-changing illness.

As the meeting disbanded, another participant asked the facilitator: "Why are you doing this? Why are you involving all of us in trying to design this model? Your team knows how to do this. Why don't you just program it and show it to us? Do you really think that all of us can come up with something better than your team?" The facilitator replied: "Yes. I do believe that together, if we consider the diversity of our experience and ideas, we will come up with a better model than a small group of academics would create."

The next morning, once the programming team cooled down, they realized that the participants had come up with an elegant solution—not the oversimplified version in the original model that would have limited the ability of subsequent model versions to be sensitive to changes in how health care is delivered, but not overly-complex, as had been the 20-disease version developed in the NICH pilot study. The result was operationalization of the group's four-disease model as behavior-over-time graphs (figure 1), depicting the average effect of the disease on agents' health, and the average effect of treatment.

The academic team showed the group that they were willing to make themselves vulnerable by throwing out their prior work, as well as their appreciation for the wisdom of the group in developing a simple but elegant base case. This generated loyalty among the entire group, and in subsequent sessions they added

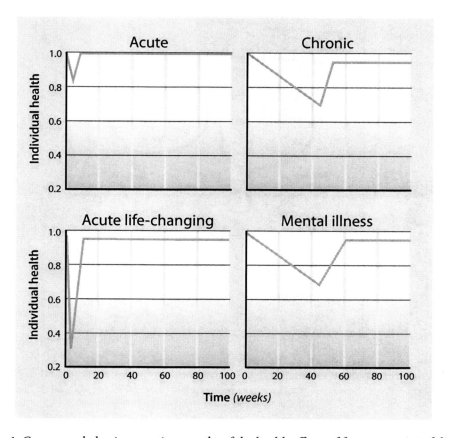

Figure 1. Consensus behavior-overtime graphs of the health effects of four categories of disease

complexity to the base case, operationalized additional features of primary care, ran experiments with the model, and added further refinements.[81] The final session focused on disseminating the work, with each participant leaving with a PowerPoint presentation, worksheets, model description, and an electronic copy of the model program.

Boundary objects: In order to teach participants about agent-based modeling and create a boundary object for synthesizing the group model-building group model-building discussion, we developed drawing conventions for capturing the group discussion in ways that facilitated programming the agent-based computer model. (These conventions are shown in table 2). They were used to some degree by participants, but often the facilitator needed to translate participant words into diagrams that used these conventions. Figure 2 shows the use of these conventions in the boundary object drawn on the white board for the earliest model specified by the group.

In later sessions, participants began specifying characteristics of two kinds of agents: (1) patients from disadvantaged or advantaged neighborhoods and (2) primary and episodic health care providers. In order to easily summarize the characteristics of these agents, and importantly, to facilitate group consideration of possible interactions among these agent characteristics, we used 2 × 2 tables as boundary objects (figure 3).

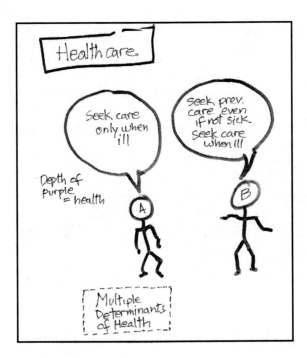

Figure 2. Boundary object that served as the basis for the earliest model specified by the group. Multiple environmental determinants influence the health of individuals, varying from individual to individual. Some patients only seek care when they are ill, while others seek regular preventive care as well as illness care

Over time, as participants worked individually and in smalls groups to test hypotheses hands-on NetLogo model, the graphical user interface began to serve as a boundary object representing the actualization of the group discussions in the figure 4.

Model Elements

In order to be comprehensible and transparent, we created a simple model that operationalized health, illness, health care, and various primary care mechanisms. The model included three types of agents: patients, primary care clinicians, and specialty-care clinicians, whose characteristics are outlined below.

1) Patients

- Health behaviors, which affect the probability of contracting an illness.

- Care-seeking threshold, the decline in health that patients must suffer before seeking care.

- Care preference, either primary or specialty (does not change over time).

- A patient's health, represented as a number between 0 and 1 (with 1 being perfect health and 0 being dead; health changes when patient contracts or recovers from an illness).

Table 2

Recommended Drawing Conventions for Agent Actions and Interactions

ABM Component	Description	Illustration/Symbol
Environment	A blank white board or large piece of paper	
System facts	Statements written on rays of sun	
Agents	Stick figures or buildings representing different types of people or organizations	
Agent states	Coloring/shading of agent figure	
Agent decision rules	Written in caption bubbles (e.g., as if/then statements)	
Agent actions and interactions	Arrows showing impact on another agent or on another relationship (arrow pointing to an arrow)	
Flow of information*	Arrows indicating the decision process(es) that this information affects	
Agent traits*	Indicated in perforated box under agent	

* Not included in original conventions but added based on demonstrated need.

Patients were at risk of acquiring four disease types: acute, acute life changing, chronic, and mental illness (figure 1). Disease burdens differed based on their initial effect on a patient's health and the type of treatment delivered. Patients' probability of contracting each type of disease depended on their health behaviors and other risk factors.

Patients could suffer from multiple diseases at once. They sought care with their chosen clinician once the combined effects of their illnesses caused their health to decrease below their individual care-seeking threshold.

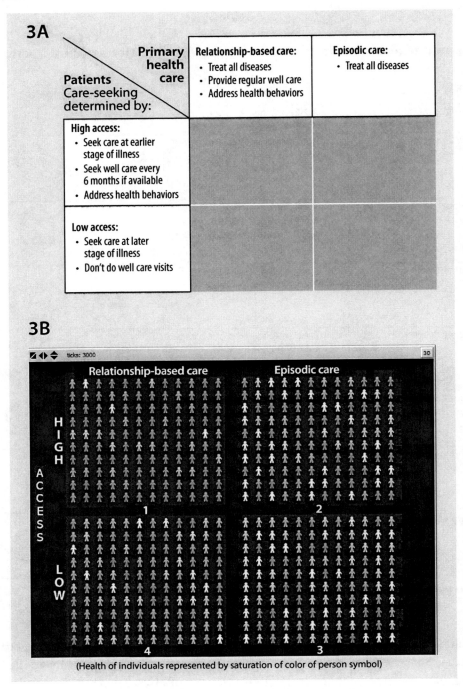

3A

Patients Care-seeking determined by: \ Primary health care	Relationship-based care: • Treat all diseases • Provide regular well care • Address health behaviors	Episodic care: • Treat all diseases
High access: • Seek care at earlier stage of illness • Seek well care every 6 months if available • Address health behaviors		
Low access: • Seek care at later stage of illness • Don't do well care visits		

3B

ticks: 3000   3D

Relationship-based care   Episodic care

HIGH

ACCESS

LOW

1   2   4   3

(Health of individuals represented by saturation of color of person symbol)

Figure 3. (A) 2 × 2 table as a boundary object. This table version shows specified agent characteristics, and the interactions and hypothesized outcomes from these interactions, ready to be filled in during group discussion. (B) Corresponding graphical user interface of 2 × 2 table as a boundary object. Pictorial component of the graphical user interface developed in the NetLogo model, which depicts agents as stick figures placed in two kinds of neighborhoods served by the two kinds of providers

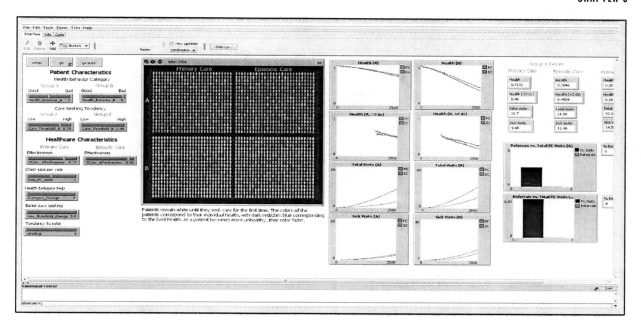

Figure 4. Screenshot of model graphical user interface: user-specified model parameters are on the left, which can be varied with sliders; 2 × 2 pictorial representation is in the middle; and graphical and numerical summaries of model output are on the right

2) Specialty-care clinicians

Specialty-care-seeking patients visit a specialty clinician only when they are ill. Specialty-care clinicians focus their treatment on the disease having the biggest effect on patients' health.

3) Primary care clinicians

Primary care clinicians treated multiple illnesses in a single visit, but in this model they were less effective than specialists in treating any particular disease. Primary care clinicians also potentially had the ability to:

- Help patients improve their health behavior, decreasing their probability of contracting illness.

- Develop a relationship with patients which, over time, caused patients to reduce their care-seeking threshold and seek care earlier in an illness.

- Refer patients to specialty care for treatment, if treatment by a specialist would provide a greater health benefit than treatment by primary care.

Patients visited a primary care clinician when they were ill, but also had the option of making regular check-up visits. At these check-up visits, health problems may be identified and treated even if they have not lowered health below the patient's care-seeking threshold (figure 5).

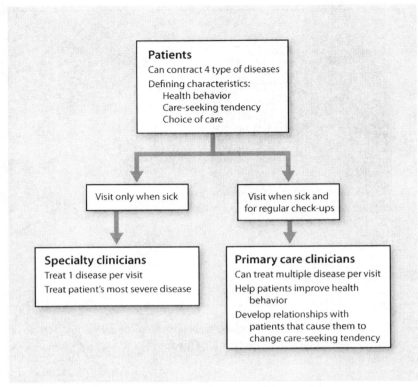

Figure 5. Main mechanisms of the model

NetLogo Model

The model contained 2,000 patients, 1 primary care clinician, and 1 specialty-care clinician (table 3). We split patients evenly into two neighborhoods, labeled A and B. Patients in each neighborhood had their own user-defined health behaviors and care-seeking tendencies. Within these neighborhoods, patients were split evenly between primary-care seekers and specialty-care seekers. Each time step in the model represented 1 week; the model ran for 2,500 time steps, or about 48 years.

As the model ran, we tracked the following averaged outputs for each neighborhood and type of care seeker:

- Health of all patients;

- Health of patients with three or more nonacute diseases;

- Number of total clinician visits per patient;

- Number of sick visits that occurred because patients' health declined below their care-seeking threshold.

For primary care-seeking patients, we also tracked the number of visits that resulted in referrals to specialty care.

Table 3

User-controlled Inputs in the NetLogo Model for Each Type of Agent

Type of Agent	User-controlled Inputs
Patients	Health behavior
	Care-seeking tendency
Specialty-care clinicians	Effectiveness level, which determines the amount of health lost to a single disease that clinician can restore
Primary care clinicians	Effectiveness level (across whatever illnesses the patient has)
	Number of regular check-up visits per year that primary care-seeking patients make
	Extent to which clinicians can help patients improve their health behavior
	Extent to which a primary care-seeking patient will change their care-seeking tendency
	Tendency to refer to specialty care

NetLogo Simulations

We ran a number of different experiments, testing how the average population health and average number of clinician visits per patient were affected when we changed the primary care input variables one at a time. The specific values for each of the input variables for each experiment are included in the worksheets in Appendix 5 of the *Annals* article.[82] Below we describe the results from a simple base model (experiment 1) and a model that includes multiple primary care mechanisms (experiment 6). (Experiments 2–5 added individual primary care mechanisms to the base model.)

In experiment 1, all mechanisms of primary care beyond disease care were turned off, meaning that primary care cannot help patients change their health behaviors or care-seeking tendencies, and cannot refer to specialty care. In addition, patients did not make regular well-care visits to primary care. Furthermore, although primary care can treat multiple diseases per visit, it was less effective than specialty care in treating a single disease.

In experiment 6, all the aforementioned attributes of primary care were turned on.

In each simulation, patients in neighborhood A had low care-seeking thresholds and average health behaviors, while neighborhood B had high care-seeking thresholds (and thus lower access to care) and poorer health behavior (disadvantaged).

In experiment 1, the health of primary-care-seeking patients is worse than that of specialty-care-seeking patients in both neighborhoods for the entire model run (figure 6). This is not surprising, since in this set-up of the model, although primary care treated multiple diseases in a visit, it was less effective than specialty care in treating single diseases and did not offer any additional benefits.

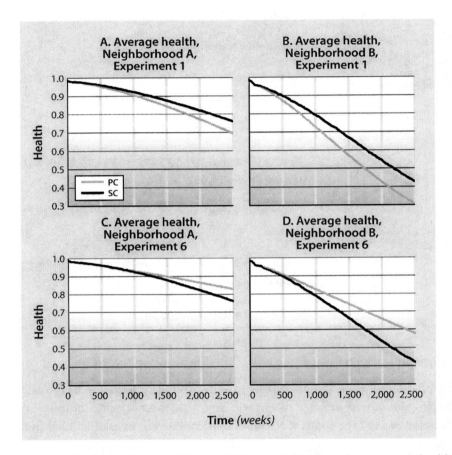

Figure 6. Average health of each neighborhood for base/full models. Top row shows average health of patients in neighborhoods A and B for experiment 1 (no primary care [PC] features turned on), and the bottom row shows the same result for experiment 6 (all primary care features turned on). The dark line shows the average health of specialty-care (SC) seekers in each neighborhood, while the light line shows the health of primary care seekers

In experiment 6, the opposite occurs—primary-care seekers had better average health in both neighborhoods. In this model, we see that the conjoint effect of multiple primary-care features compensates for its lesser disease-specific care.

The health of primary care patients increased more from experiments 1 to 6 for patients in the disadvantaged than the advantaged neighborhood. As a result of their poor health behaviors, patients in neighborhood B were sick more often than those in neighborhood A; additionally, because of their high care-seeking threshold, they tended to wait longer to seek care for an illness.

The primary care effect was greater for people with multiple chronic conditions (figure 7). In experiment 1, the health of primary-care-seeking patients was lower than that of specialty-care-seeking patients, while in experiment 6, the opposite was true. This is similar to what was observed in the overall average health of each neighborhood, but the effect was more pronounced. The difference in health between primary and specialty patients in experiment 6 was greater for patients in neighborhood B (disadvantaged). This difference was greater for patients in neighborhood B with multiple diseases than for the overall neighborhood, suggesting that the primary care benefit in the model was greatest for disadvantaged patients with multiple diseases.

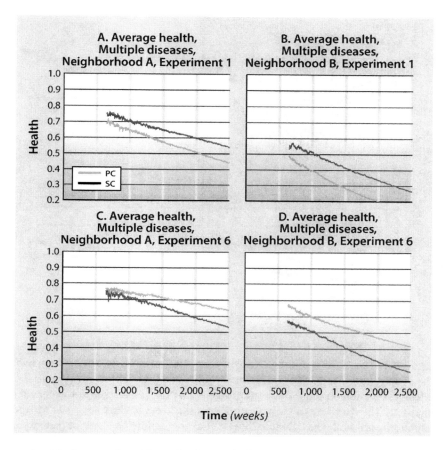

Figure 7. Average health for people with multiple morbidities, receiving primary or specialty care in two neighborhoods. Top row shows average health of patients with three or more non-acute diseases in neighborhoods A and B for experiment 1 (no primary care [PC] features turned on), and the bottom row shows the same result for experiment 6 (all primary care features turned on). The dark line in each graph shows the average health for specialty-care (SC) seekers in each neighborhood, while the light line shows health for primary care (PC) seekers. Note that results are only graphed once the model has run for long enough that enough patients have accumulated multiple diseases

Clinician visits: In experiment 1, primary care and specialtcare seekers had essentially the same number of visits, since in this base model both types of patients sought care only when they are ill, and had similar rates of illness (figure 8). As a result of their poor health behaviors, patients in neighborhood B were more likely to develop illnesses and therefore have more visits than patients in neighborhood A.

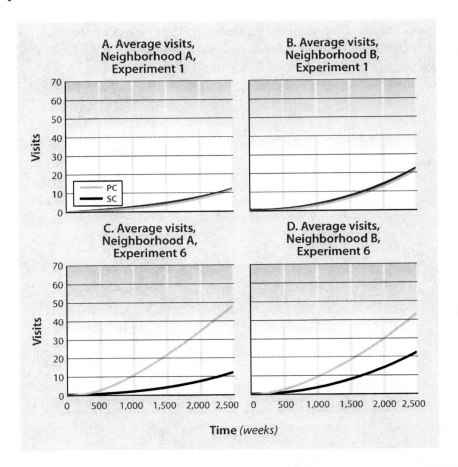

Figure 8. Average number of visits for people receiving primary (PC) or specialty (SC) care in two neighborhoods. Top row shows the average number of clinician visits for patients in neighborhoods A and B for experiment 1 (no primary care features turned on), and the bottom row shows the same result for experiment 6 (all primary care features turned on). The dark line in each graph shows the average clinician visits for specialty-care (SC) seekers in each neighborhood, while the light line shows the average clinician visits for primary care (PC) seekers

In experiment 6, with all the primary care features activated, the number of visits for primary-care seekers increased due to regular preventive visits. Unlike experiment 1, primary care patients in group A have more visits than primary care patients in group B. In experiment 6, primary care patients decrease their care-seeking threshold over time as they develop a relationship with the primary care clinician, which causes their number of visits to increase, particularly for neighborhood A, in which patients initially have a relatively low care-seeking threshold.

Sick visits: In experiment 1, the number of sick visits was the same for primary-care and specialty-care patients (figure 9). The results were more interesting in experiment 6, with the number of sick visits for primary care patients in neighborhood A increasing from experiment 1. This is not because the primary care patients in neighborhood A were sick more often in experiment 6; in fact, they contracted fewer illnesses because their health behaviors were improved from experiment 1. This change is due to patients in neighborhood A decreasing their care-seeking threshold as they developed a relationship with their primary care clinician.

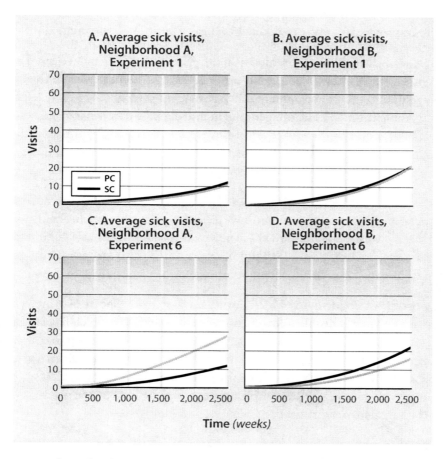

Figure 9. Average number of sick visits for people receiving primary (PC) or specialty care (SC) in two neighborhoods. The top row shows the average number of sick visits for patients in neighborhoods A and B from experiment 1. The bottom row shows the same results for experiment 6. In each graph, the dark line tracks the average sick visits for specialty-care patients, while the light line tracks this number for primary care patients

In contrast, the number of sick visits for primary care patients in neighborhood B decreased from experiments 1 to 6. In experiment 6, primary care patients in group B decreased their care-seeking threshold, which caused their number of sick visits to increase. However, at the same time, they improved their health behavior, causing their number of illnesses, and subsequently their number of sick visits, to decrease. Since primary care patients in group B started with higher care-seeking thresholds than patients in group A, the effect of health behavior change predominated in determining the number of sick visits for patients in group B. The overall effect was a reduction of sick visits in this disadvantaged neighborhood.

Implications

We were able to engage diverse patient, caregiver, clinician, and academic stakeholders in an iterative, participatory process to build an agent-based model. After experiencing the promises and pitfalls of developing an overly complex expert pilot model, grounding the subsequent group-built model in the real experiences of diverse stakeholders helped us to develop a model simple enough to understand, but complex enough to communicate the emerging health care properties that otherwise receive limited attention in current efforts to improve care, advance population health, and eliminate inequalities.[5,13,14,30,38,45,83,84]

In addition, we advanced the field of group model-building by identifying a developmental set of boundary objects by beginning with a teaching set and progressing to graphical conventions that reflected the characteristics of agents and their environment. The subsequent use of a 2 × 2 table fostered participants' ability to identify possible mechanisms for agent-agent and agent-environment interactions, and to consider their possible effects on health, equity, and resource-use outcomes. Ultimately, the computer program's graphical user interface served as an accessible boundary object, allowing users to visualize their collective insights and new discoveries when the computer model ran experiments.

The resulting model operationalizes, in a simple but explicit way, some of the key features of primary care, allowing stakeholders to test hypotheses about how different primary care mechanisms can combine to add value beyond disease treatment and how these mechanisms affect the health of different types of people. The model can be used to improve understanding of primary health care as a complex system in which factors in addition to disease care can affect outcomes such as health, equity, and resource use.

The model shows possible mechanisms by which non-disease-specific aspects of primary care can produce the emergent properties of better health at lower cost and less inequality, which have been observed in epidemiological and ecological studies.[30,32] The resulting understanding could help to overcome reductionist biases[11,85,86] that have resulted in measures of primary-care quality based "one disease at a time" measures, rather than assessing quality in ways that fully consider the complex conjoint effects of multiple mechanisms.[5,11,85,86] Greater understanding of the complexity of primary care could be used to develop systems to support care that is integrated, personalized, preventive, and high value.

This work must be understood in the context of its limitations. The model incorporates the wisdom of diverse health care users and providers, but it is limited to primary care clinicians and patients in a single geographic area and is also limited by the many simplifying assumptions needed to make the model transparent and easy to describe and understand. Primary care involves the complex interaction of many other mechanisms than those proposed here. A group model-building team that included other viewpoints, such as disease specialists, would likely have come up with different parameters and operationalizations of primary care, some of which could equally well represent the mechanisms to explain the paradox of primary care. The model was parameterized to reflect general facts from the health and health care literature, but was limited in not being based on empirical health services and outcome data.

The development of a data-driven model remains an important area for future research. We are currently pursuing funding to support the development of a model in which the base case (how people gain and lose health, and the operationalization of health care and primary care mechanisms) is directly informed by nationally representative data.

In the meantime, the model presented here allows users to explore hypotheses that would be difficult or impossible to test in the real world. We encourage readers to download the model, software, and worksheets, and to do their own experiments by developing hypotheses, varying model parameters, running the model, and tracking results on the worksheets. In order to create an ongoing conversation among model users, we also encourage those doing experiments to report their findings in the *Annals of Family Medicine* online discussion related to the article that first put this model into the public domain.[81] The resulting insights can be used not only to develop more sophisticated models, but also to guide empirical research and advance a more nuanced understanding of what is valuable about primary care and the possible complex interactive mechanisms by which that value emerges over time.

References

1. Agency for Healthcare Research and Quality. The Ambulatory Care Quality Alliance Recommended Starter Set: Clinical Performance Measures for Ambulatory Care. 2005. http://archive.ahrq.gov/professionals/quality-patient-safety/quality-resources/tools/ambulatory-care/starter-set.html.

2. Brook RH. *Redefining Health Care Systems.* Santa Monica, CA: RAND Corporation; 2015.

3. Blumenthal D. The future of quality measurement and management in a transforming health care system. *JAMA.* 1997;278(19):1622–1625.

4. Woolf SH. Patient safety is not enough: targeting quality improvements to optimize the health of the population. *Ann Intern Med.* 2004;140(1):33–36.

5. Heath I, Rubenstein A, Stange KC, van Driel M. Quality in primary health care: a multidimensional approach to complexity. *BMJ.* 2009;338:b1242.

6. National Quality Forum. Quality Positioning System. 2015. http://www.qualityforum.org/QPS/.

7. Institute of Medicine. *For the Public's Health: The Role of Measurement in Action and Accountability.* Washington, DC: National Academies Press; 2011.

8. Blumenthal D, McGinnis JM. Measuring Vital Signs: an IOM report on core metrics for health and health care progress. *JAMA.* 2015;313(19):1901–1902.

9. Institute of Medicine. *Vital Signs: Core Metrics for Health and Health Care Progress.* Washington, DC: National Academies Press; 2015.

10. Cebul RD, Rebitzer JB, Taylor LJ, Votruba M. Organizational fragmentation and care quality in the U.S. health care system. NBER Working Paper. 2008; no. 14212. http://www.nber.org/papers/w14212.

11. Stange KC. The problem of fragmentation and the need for integrative solutions. *Ann Fam Med.* 2009;7(2):100–103.

12. Sweeney SA, Bazemore A, Phillips RL, Jr., Etz RS, Stange KC. A reemerging political space for linking person and community through primary health care. *Am J Public Health.* 2012;102(Suppl 3):S336–S341.

13. Stange KC, Etz RS, Gullett H, et al. Metrics for assessing improvements in primary health care. *Annu Rev Public Health.* 2014;35:423–442.

14. Stange KC. The paradox of the parts and the whole in understanding and improving general practice. *Int J Qual Health Care.* 2002;14(4):267–268.

15. Leykum LK, Lanham HJ, Pugh JA, et al. Manifestations and implications of uncertainty for improving healthcare systems: an analysis of observational and interventional studies grounded in complexity science. *Implement Sci.* 2014;9(1):165.

16. Paley J. The appropriation of complexity theory in health care. *J Health Serv Res Policy.* 2010;15(1):59–61.

17. Greenhalgh T, Plsek P, Wilson T, Fraser S, Holt T. Response to 'The appropriation of complexity theory in health care'. *J Health Serv Res Policy.* 2010;15(2):115–117.

18. Sturmberg JP, Martin CM. Complexity and health—yesterday's traditions, tomorrow's future. *J Eval Clin Pract.* 2009;15(3):543–548.

19. Miles A. Complexity in medicine and healthcare: people and systems, theory and practice. *J Eval Clin Pract.* 2009;15(3):409–410.

20. Kernick D. *Complexity and Healthcare Organization: A View from the Street.* San Francisco: Radcliffe Medical Press; 2004.

21. Sweeney K, Griffiths F, eds. *Complexity and Healthcare: An Introduction.* Abingdon, UK: Radcliffe Medical Press; 2002.

22. Plsek PE, Wilson T. Complexity, leadership, and management in healthcare organisations. *BMJ.* 2001;323(7315):746–749.

23. Plsek PE, Greenhalgh T. Complexity science: the challenge of complexity in health care. *BMJ.* 2001;323(7313):625–628.

24. Harrold LR, Field TS, Gurwitz JH. Knowledge, patterns of care, and outcomes of care for generalists and specialists. *J Gen Intern Med.* 1999;14(8):499–511.

25. Smetana GW, Landon BE, Bindman AB, et al. A comparison of outcomes resulting from generalist vs specialist care for a single discrete medical condition: a systematic review and methodologic critique. *Arch Intern Med.* 2007;167(1):10–20.

26. Shah BR, Hux JE, Laupacis A, Zinman B, Austin PC, van Walraven C. Diabetic patients with prior specialist care have better glycaemic control than those with prior primary care. *J Eval Clin Pract.* 2005;11(6):568–575.

27. McAlister FA, Majumdar SR, Eurich DT, Johnson JA. The effect of specialist care within the first year on subsequent outcomes in 24,232 adults with new-onset diabetes mellitus: population-based cohort study. *Qual Saf Health Care.* 2007;16(1):6–11.

28. Go AS, Rao RK, Dauterman KW, Massie BM. A systematic review of the effects of physician specialty on the treatment of coronary disease and heart failure in the United States. *Am J Med.* 2000;108(3):216–226.

29. Backer V, Nepper-Christensen S, Nolte H. Quality of care in patients with asthma and rhinitis treated by respiratory specialists and primary care physicians: a 3-year randomized and prospective follow-up study. *Ann Allergy Asthma Immunol.* 2006;97(4):490–496.

30. Starfield B, Shi L, Macinko J. Contribution of primary care to health systems and health. *Milbank Q.* 2005;83(3):457–502.

31. Starfield B, Shi L, Grover A, Macinko J. The effects of specialist supply on populations' health: assessing the evidence. *Health Aff (Millwood).* 2005;(Suppl Web Exclusives):W5-97–W95-107.

32. Baicker K, Chandra A. Medicare spending, the physician workforce, and beneficiaries' quality of care. *Health Aff (Millwood).* 2004;(Suppl Web Exclusives):W4-184–W4-197.

33. Donaldson MS, Lohr KN, Vanselow NA, eds. *Primary Care: America's Health in a New Era.* Washington, DC: National Academy Press; 1996.

34. Macinko J, Starfield B, Shi L. Quantifying the health benefits of primary care physician supply in the United States. *Int J Health Serv.* 2007;37(1):111–126.

35. Stange KC, Ferrer RL. The paradox of primary care. *Ann Fam Med.* 2009;7(4):293–299.

36. Lewin S, Lavis JN, Oxman AD, et al. Supporting the delivery of cost-effective interventions in primary health-care systems in low-income and middle-income countries: an overview of systematic reviews. *Lancet.* 2008;372(9642):928–939.

37. Fortin M, Soubhi H, Hudon C, Bayliss EA, van den Akker M. Multimorbidity's many challenges. Time to focus on the needs of this vulnerable and growing population. *BMJ.* 2007;334(7602):1016–1017.

38. Starfield B. Primary care and equity in health: the importance to effectiveness and equity of responsiveness to people's needs. *Humanity Soc.* 2009;33(1/2):56–73.

39. Sturmberg JP, Martin CM, Moes MM. Health at the center of health systems reform: how philosophy can inform policy. *Perspect Biol Med.* 2010;53(3):341–356.

40. Sweeney K. *Complexity in Primary Care.* Oxon, UK: Radcliffe Publishing; 2006.

41. Donaldson MS, Yordy KD, Lohr KN, Vanselow NA, eds. *Primary Care: America's Health in a New Era.* Washington, DC: National Academy Press; 1996.

42. Starfield B. *Primary Care: Balancing Health Needs, Services, and Technology.* Rev. ed. New York, NY: Oxford University Press; 1998.

43. McWhinney IR, Freeman T. *Textbook of Family Medicine.* 3rd ed. New York, NY: Oxford University Press; 2009.

44. Stange KC, Nutting PA, Miller WL, et al. Defining and measuring the patient-centered medical home. *J Gen Intern Med.* 2010;25(6):601–612.

45. Stange KC, Jaén CR, Flocke SA, Miller WL, Crabtree BF, Zyzanski SJ. The value of a family physician. *J Fam Pract.* 1998;46(5):363–368.

46. Marshall MN, Romano PS, Davies HT. How do we maximize the impact of the public reporting of quality of care? *Int J Qual Health Care.* 2004;16(Suppl 1):i57–i63.

47. Casalino LP. The unintended consequences of measuring quality on the quality of medical care. *N Engl J Med.* 1999;341(15):1147–1150.

48. McGlynn EA. Intended and unintended consequences: what should we really worry about? *Med Care.* 2007;45(1):3–5.

49. De Maeseneer J, van Weel C, Egilman D, Mfenyana K, Kaufman A, Sewankambo N. Strengthening primary care: addressing the disparity between vertical and horizontal investment. *Br J Gen Pract.* 2008;58(546):3–4.

50. Sturmberg JP. Systems and complexity thinking in general practice. Part 2: application in primary care research. *Aust Fam Physician.* 2007;36(4):273–275.

51. Sturmberg JP. Systems and complexity thinking in general practice: Part 1: clinical application. *Aust Fam Physician.* 2007;36(3):170–173.

52. Rose J, Riolo R, Hovmand P, et al. Modeling the paradox of primary care. In: Martin C, Sturmberg J, eds. *Handbook on Systems and Complexity in Health.* New York: Springer Press; 2013:815–825.

53. Parunak HVD, Savit R, Riolo RL. Agent-based modeling vs. equation-based modeling: a case study and users' guide. Paper presented at: Proceedings of Multi-agent Systems and Agent-based Simulation. Lecture Notes in Artificial Intelligence, Vol. 1534. Berlin: Springer; 1998: 10–25.

54. McWhinney IR. 'An acquaintance with particulars...'. *Fam Med.* 1989;21(4):296–298.

55. Stange KC. The generalist approach. *Ann Fam Med.* 2009;7(3):198–203.

56. Stange KC. Integrative ways of thinking about generalist practice (Commentary). *Fam Syst Health.* 2001;19(4):375–376.

57. Bankes SC. Agent-based modeling: a revolution? *Proc Natl Acad Sci USA.* 2002;99(Suppl 3):7199–7200.

58. Gilbert N. *Agent-Based Models.* London: Sage Publications; 2007.

59. Israel BA, Eng E, Schulz AJ, Parker EA. *Methods for Community-Based Participatory Research for Health.* 2nd ed. San Francisco, CA: Wiley; 2012.

60. Macaulay AC, Commanda LE, Freeman WL, et al. Participatory research maximises community and lay involvement. North American Primary Care Research Group. *BMJ.* 1999;319(7212):774–778.

61. Macaulay AC, Nutting PA. Moving the frontiers forward: incorporating community-based participatory research into practice-based research networks. *Ann Fam Med.* 2006;4(1):4–7.

62. Vennix J. *Group Model-building.* New York: Wiley; 1996.

63. Richardson GP, Andersen DF. Teamwork in group model-building. *Syst Dyn Rev.* 1995;11(2):113–137.

64. Vennix J. Group model-building: Tackling messy problems. *Syst Dyn Rev.* 1999;15(4):379–401.

65. Hovmand PS. *Community Based System Dynamics.* New York, NY: Springer; 2014.

66. Lane DC. Diagramming conventions in system dynamics. *J Oper Res Soc.* 2000;51(2):241–245.

67. Black LJ, Andersen DF. Using visual representations as boundary objects to resolve conflict in collaborative model-building approaches. *Syst Res Behav Sci.* 2012;29(2):194–208.

68. Levina N, Vaast E. The emergence of boundary spanning competence in practice: implications for information systems' implementation and use. *MIS Q.* 2005;29(2):335–363.

69. Black LJ, Andersen DF. Using visual representations as boundary objects to resolve conflict in collaborative model-building approaches. *Syst Res Behav Sci.* 2012;29(2):194–208.

70. Carlile PR. A pragmatic view of knowledge and boundaries: boundary objects in new product development. *Organ Sci.* 2002;13(4):442–455.

71. Black LJ. When visuals are boundary objects in system dynamics work. *Syst Dyn Rev.* 2013;29(2):70–86.

72. Rose J, Homa L, Hovmand P, et al. Boundary Objects for Participatory group model-building of agent-based models. Paper presented at: System Sciences (HICSS), 48th Hawaii International Conference, January 5–8, 2015.

73. Hovmand PS, Etiënne AJA, Rouwette E, et al. Scriptapedia: a handbook of scripts for developing structured group model-building sessions. Paper presented at: 29th International Conference of the System Dynamics Society, July 25–29, 2011, Washington, DC, USA.

74. Rouwette E, Vennix JAM, Mullekom Tv. Group model-building effectiveness: a review of assessment studies. *Syst Dyn Rev.* 2006;18(1):5–45.

74. Hovmand PS, Etiënne AJAR, Andersen DF, et al. 2011. Scriptapedia 3.04. http://www.systemdynamics.org/other_resources.htm/scriptapedia. Accessed June 17, 2016.

75. Network on Inequality, Complexity & Health. https://obssr-archive.od.nih.gov/scientific_areas/social_culture_factors_in_health/health_disparities/nich.aspx.

76. NetLogo. http://ccl.northwestern.edu/netlogo/. Accessed April 14, 2014.

77. PCORI. Patient-Centered Outcomes Research Institute. www.pcori.org.

78. Practice-Based Research Network Shared Resource. Safety Net Providers' Strategic Alliance. https://sites.google.com/a/case.edu/snpsa/home. Accessed May 15, 2014.

79. Ackermann F, Andersen DF, Eden C, Richardson GP. *ScriptsMap*: a tool for designing multi-method policy-making workshops. *Omega.* 2011;39(4):427–434.

80. Bayliss EA, Bonds DE, Boyd CM, et al. Understanding the context of health for persons with multiple chronic conditions: moving from what is the matter to what matters. *Ann Fam Med.* 2014;12(3):260–269.

81. Homa L, Rose J, Hovmand PS, et al. A participatory model of the paradox of primary care. *Ann Fam Med.* 2015;13(5):456–465.

82. Rose J, Homa L, Kraus A, et al. Boundary objects for participatory group model-building of agent-based models. In: Hawaii International Conference on Systems Sciences, January 5–8, 2015; Kauai, HI.

83. Starfield B. Equity in health. *J Epidemiol Community Health.* 2002;56(7):483–484.

84. Shi L, Starfield B, Kennedy B, Kawachi I. Income inequality, primary care, and health indicators. *J Fam Pract.* 1999;48(4):275–284.

85. Stange KC. A science of connectedness. *Ann Fam Med.* 2009;7(5):387–395.

86. Stange KC. Ways of knowing, learning, and developing. *Ann Fam Med.* 2010;8(1):4–10.

CHAPTER 6

COMPLEX DETERMINANTS OF DISPARITIES IN WALKING WITHIN CITIES

Yong Yang, PhD
Assistant Professor
School of Public Health, University of Memphis

Daniel A. Rodríguez, PhD
Professor
Department of City and Regional Planning
University of North Carolina, Chapel Hill

Daniel G. Brown, PhD
Professor
School of Natural Resources & Environment
University of Michigan

Rick L. Riolo, PhD
Research Professor
Center for the Study of Complex Systems
University of Michigan

Ana V. Diez Roux, PhD, MD, MPH
Dean and Professor
School of Public Health, Drexel University

Acknowledgments: NIH (R24 HD047861), National Heart, Lung and Blood Institute (R21-HL106467 and R01 HL071759), the Robert Wood Johnson Foundation Health and Society Scholars program, and the NIH Office of Behavioral and Social Sciences Research (Network on Inequality, Complexity and Health; HHSN276200800013, George A. Kaplan, Principal Investigator) supported this work.

GROWING INEQUALITY

It is well-established that physical activity is related to numerous health outcomes.[1] Levels of physical activity among U.S. adults are alarmingly low.[2] Because regular participation in moderate activity has been shown to have health benefits similar to those observed for vigorous activity,[1] it has suggested focusing on increasing moderate activities such as walking in daily life. However, only 6 percent and 9 percent of U.S. adults were considered regularly active based on utilitarian walking (e.g., walking to work or the shops) and by walking for leisure (e.g., for exercise or enjoyment), respectively.[3]

During the past two decades, interest in how features of the social and built environment of communities affect the physical activity of residents has exploded.[4-6] Because of the relevance of walking as a component of usual physical activity and the possibility of improving population levels of physical activity by increasing walking in daily life, the study of the environmental determinants of walking has received special attention.

Empirical studies show that walking are related to a number of individual-level characteristics, including age, sex, SES, race/ethnicity, and car ownership.[3,7-11] A large body of work has also documented the association of various features of neighborhood environments and walking behavior,[12-17] including the density of residents, land-use mix, proximity of destinations, street connectivity, presence of sidewalks, features of street design and aesthetics, and social attributes such as safety and violence.[5,7,10,12-21] Areas with higher levels of land-use mix, density of services and residents, greater street connectivity, sidewalks, and interesting or attractive scenery are associated with more walking.[10,5,17-22] Areas with higher levels of safety and lower crime rates are also characterized by more walking among residents.[23-27] Walking can also be influenced by social norms, including support from family and friends and the likelihood of seeing others walking in the neighborhood.[28] In general, different types of walking are associated with different environmental attributes.[29]

The Problem

Despite increasing evidence that features of built and social environments affect levels of walking, the policy implications of this work are uncertain. The majority of existing research has applied statistical models to observational data to estimate associations of environmental characteristics with walking, after controlling for confounding variables. Many studies are cross-sectional and cannot directly address the question of whether changes in environments are associated with changes in walking. To the author's knowledge, virtually all studies are observational and we therefore cannot fully rule out selection effects, such as the possibility that persons with a given propensity to walk (for a variety of individual-level reasons), select, and choose to live in environments that match their walking preferences.[30] In addition, the predominant analytical approach is based on isolating an association between a given factor (e.g., mixed land-use) and an outcome (e.g., walking), while keeping all other factors artificially constant and ignoring feedbacks between individuals, individuals and environments, and various environmental features over time. Not only infectious agents but also behaviors and attitudes may be transmitted through social networks, making individual behaviors highly dependent on that of others.[31,32] Individuals and environments may reciprocally affect each other in complicated ways. Mixed land-use may promote walking and more walking will likely promote greater mixes of land uses as businesses locate to areas with heavy foot traffic.

This in turn may have consequences for automobile traffic, which may increase as a result of greater commercial use, with potentially negative impacts on walking, since more traffic can detract from walkability. Environmental factors may affect each other: for example, greater mix of uses may affect crime, and vice versa.

Why Complex Systems

Systems approaches have great potential for improving our understanding of the environmental determinants of walking. This understanding is critical to identify relevant policies and predict the effect of those policies. Systems-science methodologies including agent-based models[33,34] have received increasing attention as a way to better capture the complex set of relationships inherent in population health problems. Whereas traditional epidemiologic approaches involve manipulating observational data or conducting randomized trials in order to isolate the causal effect of a given factor independent of other factors, systems approaches focus on understanding the functioning of the system as a whole, including feedback loops and network effects, allowing the impact of a given intervention to be evaluated in the context of these dynamic relations.[35] However, few applications to specific research problems exist (outside the transmission of infectious diseases). One area especially amenable to these approaches is the study of environmental or neighborhood effects on health,[36,37] specifically the environmental impacts of walking.[38]

Among available systems approaches, agent-based models [34,39] are particularly well suited to situations involving interactions between heterogeneous agents and between heterogeneous agents and environments, as well as agents and environments that adapt and change over time. The spatial dimensions of the problem, involving interactions in space as well as spatial patterning of individual and environmental characteristics, also make it especially well suited to the use of spatially explicit ABMs.[40,41] They may also be useful for investigating how dynamic processes shape the distribution of health outcomes, and the impacts of policy alternatives when nonlinear relations and feedbacks are present.[36,42] Examples include the transmission of infectious diseases, the determinants of drinking and drug use, and the effects of healthy food availability on diet.[36,43-45]

Agent-based models have been used to study pedestrian movement,[46-49] and researchers have called for their greater use in studying environmental impacts on walking[38,50], but only a few[46-49,51,52] have been applied in this way. In addition, existing models largely focus on how people move around small areas or within buildings, and how features such as the design and layout of buildings and streets influence people's movements. In contrast, the models we developed focus primarily on travel behavior.

Methods

We designed and developed two exploratory, spatial agent-based models to understand how people's walking behavior within a hypothetical city is affected by interactions with their environment and with each other. The first version (V1) was implemented during 2009–2010 as a pilot project.[53,54] Afterward, we developed a second version (V2) during 2011–2012, which was based on V1 with substantial modifications.[55] Because the details of both models have been published elsewhere, we describe the two models in plain language here and avoid the technological details of model implementations (for example, all formulas are excluded).[53-55]

The goal of both models was to enhance scientific understanding of the ways in which environmental factors affect the population levels and socioeconomic factors contributing to walking behavior, utilizing key dimensions and processes judged to be fundamental based on existing empirical works. We asked general questions about basic mechanisms and processes, and the patterns of behavior they generate, rather than questions specific to any given city. We did not attempt to include all possible influences on walking in a real city, but rather those generic dimensions and dynamics likely to operate in a common fashion across cities; we sought to understand general patterns of walking, specifically regarding the impact of mixed land-use and safety—or the effects of policies that alter them—on disparities in walking behavior. We were explicit about the dimensions, dynamics, and assumptions included in our model, so that future iterations can be modified in response to new evidence and empirical observations. Because virtually no prior dynamic modeling of walking behavior exists, we believe that knowledge about the basic dynamics and the impact of changes in land-use and safety in a generic setting is a prerequisite for more sophisticated and realistic future models of specific cities.

Both models represent a city of square shape with 8 km (5 miles) for one side. It is an 800-by-800 grid space, where each cell of size of 10 meters by 10 meters was either occupied by a relevant land use (e.g., a place with a social function) or was empty. The city had 400 equal-sized neighborhoods, each composed of 40-by-40 cells. Model agents included about 100,000 adults (100,800 for V1 and 100,000 for V2, with population density roughly based on Ann Arbor, Michigan), and each household included one or two adults. Income quintiles were assigned to each household randomly from 1 (lowest) to 5 (highest). Every day, individuals could travel to nonresidential locations by a chosen travel mode. We assumed that the travel mode selected was used for both the departing and the returning trips.

For parsimony, the model included only adult travel behaviors on workdays (no weekends). Seasonal variations and weather were ignored. The model assumed that sidewalks were present and walkable. In these time-discrete models, each time step was 1 day.

Key functions in both models included travel-mode choice and feedback mechanisms. Travel-mode choice was defined as the mode selected by a given person for a given trip and how various factors influenced this choice. A person's experience traveling then fed back into their future choices. Feedbacks were implemented through updates to each person's attitude toward each travel mode, which varied with their past experience. Attitude toward a given mode, in turn, affected the likelihood that a person would choose that mode on subsequent days. All attitudes were updated using a similar process. (In V1, a person has an attitude toward walking while in V2, a person has different attitudes toward each travel mode, including walking, public transit, and car.) The key functions were supported by theories and empirical evidence collected from published literature,[56-60] government reports (e.g., Department of Transportation, Bureau of Transportation Statistics, and Bureau of Labor Statistics), and publicly available data sources (e.g., National Health Interview Survey 2005, and National Household Travel Survey 2001 and 2009).

We implemented and ran a series of scenario simulations corresponding to our research questions. For

Table 1

Agent-based Models for Disparities in Walking Behaviors

	V1	V2
Aim	Socioeconomic inequalities in both utilitarian walking and walking for leisure, focusing on neighborhood safety and land-use mix	Socioeconomic inequalities in utilitarian walking and policy, focusing on spatial segregation and travel cost influences
Travel purposes	Work, food shopping, other shopping, social places, and walking for leisure	Work, shops, and all other places
Travel modes and travel-mode choice function	Different functions are used for different travel purposes. Agents selected from: (1) private automobile, and (2) walking. Whether an individual walks is a function of distance to activities, ability, and attitudes. Travel cost is not considered	A general utilities function is used for all travel purposes. Utilities include attitudes toward travel modes and cost. Agents select among three modes: (1) private automobile, (2) public transportation, or (3) walking. Major factors are travel cost and attitudes
Feedback	Four feedbacks that affect attitude toward walking	Nine feedbacks that affect attitude toward walking, public transit, and driving
Personal attributes	1. Attitude toward walking 2. Everyone has a car 3. Social network: each individual has three to five friends who can influence their walking attitude, randomly selected from the people with the same or similar SES (difference no more than 2) 4. Each person has a walking ability, which is assumed not to vary between ages 18 and 37, but decreases linearly starting at age 38. Age and ability remain constant within model time frame 5. Dog ownership	1. Attitude toward three modes 2. Not everyone has a car Households with higher incomes are more likely to own a car 3. A person's social network includes other household members and up to nine friends randomly selected from the same workplace (three), neighborhood (three), and level in the city (three) 4. Walking ability not considered 5. Dog ownership not considered
City level	1. 108,000 individuals (48,000 couples and 12,000 individuals) 2. No public transit 3. Environmental properties: safety and aesthetics	1. 100,000 individuals (50,000 couples) 2. Symmetrical transportation network centered in the city center 3. Environmental properties: safety
Calibration and validation	Parameters such as probabilities and maximum walking distances for different activities were calibrated using data from 2001 National Household Travel Survey. Calibration was performed through an iterative process by which simulation results based on parameter starting values were compared to NHTS characteristics; parameters were adjusted to minimize any differences, simulations run again, and so on until simulated results matched the 2001 NHTS data. For validation, simulated results were consistent with distribution of walking frequency and distance both in general and age-specific from 2001 NHTS data. Model predictions also approximately matched 2003–2005 American Time Use Survey in terms of average trips per day and mean and median distances per trip	We collected reasonable values and ranges for most model parameters, therefore, no calibration was conducted. For validation, we compared the percentage of walking trips by distance and variation of walking by income level with National Health Interview Survey (NHIS) 2005 data [3] and National Household Travel Survey 2001 and 2009 data [62]
Scenarios	1. Variation in spatial distribution of non-household locations and spatial distribution of safety 2. Combinations of strategies (1) improving people's attitudes toward walking; and (2) improving safety	1. Combination of segregation by income, safety, and land use 2. Variable related to travel cost 3. Synergistic effects of combinations of changing attitudes toward travel modes and interventions on travel cost

example, using V1 we varied the spatial distribution of nonhousehold locations and the spatial distribution of safety to investigate the contributions of built and social environments to socioeconomic differences in walking. Using V2, we contrasted the effects of changing travel costs such as gas rates and parking fees to test whether and how various socioeconomic groups status react differently.

Both models were developed in Java (http://java.sun.com) and Repast (http://repast.sourceforge.net/repast_3/). Java is an object-oriented programming language that describes the interactions among these objects; the objects can be understood as pieces of code activated during the simulation. Thus, Java is a suitable language for the implantation of agent-based models. Repast is a family of advanced, free, and open-source agent-based modeling and simulation platforms that have collectively been under continuous development. Repast is one of the most popular tools for agent-based modeling research.[61]

Difference Between Two Models

V1 included all kinds of walking travel while V2 covered utilitarian walking and excluded walking for leisure (table 1). In V1, a person has an attitude toward walking and a binary mode choice, in which individuals chose to walk or travel by car. In V1, travel cost was excluded from the travel-mode choice, and public transit was not included. In contrast, in V2, a person had attitudes toward each travel mode (walking, public transit, and driving), and a more complicated travel-mode choice. V1 had four feedbacks between mode choice and attitude, while V2 had nine feedbacks. V1 and V2 designated different characteristics for describing persons and the city. Different data sources were used for calibration and validation of the two models. In addition, different research questions and scenarios were developed with each model.

In V1, each individual had properties including age, gender, SES, household and workplace locations, and walking ability and attitude, while environmental characteristics included land use, safety, and aesthetics (figure 1). Individuals performed different activities on a regular basis, such as traveling for work, shopping, and recreation. Whether individuals walked and the amount they walked was a function of the distance to different activities, and the individual's walking ability and attitude toward walking, which evolved over time as a function of the attitudes of the other individuals within her/his social network, past experiences, whether others walked along the route, and constraints on distances walked per day.

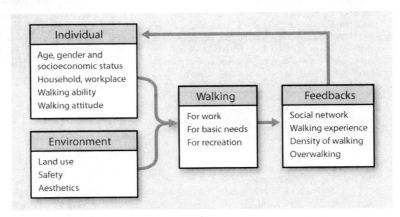

Figure 1. Framework of V1 model

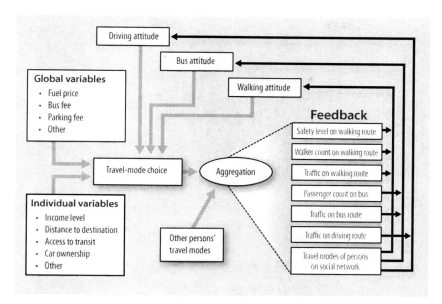

Figure 2. Framework of V2 model

In V2, for each utilitarian trip, a general utility framework is used and the travel modes with higher utility are more likely to be selected (figure 2). The factors affecting utility include attitudes toward and the cost of each travel mode. Agents select among three modes: (1) private automobile, (2) public transportation, or (3) walking. Factors influencing costs of each travel mode include global variables (same value for all persons in the city) such as fuel price, bus fee, and parking fee; and individual variables such as income level (to represent opportunity costs associated with time), distance to destination, access to public transit, and car ownership. Each person's attitude toward each model is updated based on nine feedbacks including the influences of social networks, number of persons using this mode and others, and supporting and experiential factors.

Findings

Variation by SES: In the United States, adults of lower SES tend to walk more for utilitarian purposes and less for leisure than adults of higher SES.[3,11,63] In order to investigate the contributions of built and social environments to socioeconomic differences in walking, we used model V1 to compare different scenarios of socioeconomic segregation and the spatial distribution of land use and safety. We identified one scenario that generated socioeconomic differences in walking which were relatively consistent with those most commonly observed in empirical data.[3,11,63] In this scenario, the city was divided into five concentric zones. There was perfect segregation by SES, such that residents with the lowest SES lived in the core (zone 1), and the SES of residents increased from the core to the periphery (zone 5). The density of nonresidential locations such as worksites or amenities for shopping and recreation declined outward with a ratio of 0.5 from one zone to another. Safety levels increased outwards from zone 1 (lowest safety value of 1) to zone 5 (highest safety value of 5). We believe that this pattern is a stylized representation of a typical U.S. city (figure 3).

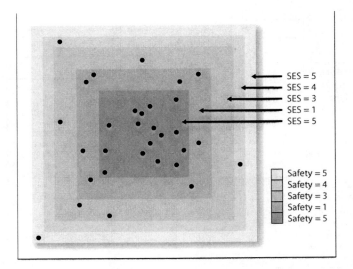

Figure 3. Schematic representation of spatial distribution of land-use and safety for a scenario. Notes: Dots = nonresidential locations. Shading = safety level, with 5 (lightest) most and 1 (darkest) the least safe. Residential segregation increases with further distance from the core, with 1 the lowest and 5 the highest socioeconomic level. In this scenario, more nonhousehold locations cluster in the core, with corresponding lower safety levels

Figure 4 shows walking for different purposes by SES in this scenario. Groups with lower SES walked more for work and less for leisure within the neighborhood than those with higher socioeconomic. This may be explained by the lower safety and closer proximity to work in neighborhoods of lower SES. For basic needs, walking levels were similar across SESs due to the counteracting effects of proximity to destinations and safety. These results help explain the variation in walking by SES observed in empirical data.[53]

Interventions to increase walking: Using model V1 in this scenario, we examined the impact of different combinations of two strategies commonly proposed to increase walking: improving people's attitudes toward walking, for example via individually targeted interventions such as health education campaigns; and improving safety via social environment interventions such as community policing. Also, we examined whether the impacts varied by land-use mix, a feature of the physical environment, implemented in the model by varying the density of nonresidential locations among zones.

Our simulated results indicated that for persons of low SES, increases in walking resulting from improved attitudes toward walking may wear out quickly if other features of the environment such as safety are not conducive. Also, although increasing the safety level of lower SES neighborhoods may in turn increase walking, the magnitude of its effectiveness varies by patterns of land-use mix. Another finding was that safety and land-use mix acted synergistically, such that the effect of one on walking among lower SES groups was magnified in the presence of the other.[54]

Transportation cost policies: Using model V2 and the same scenario again, we examined the contribution of transportation cost policies to income differences in walking, with the rationale that lowering the cost of a desired travel mode (e.g., public transit) and raising the price of an undesired travel mode (e.g., driving) may be an effective strategy for motivating behavior change.

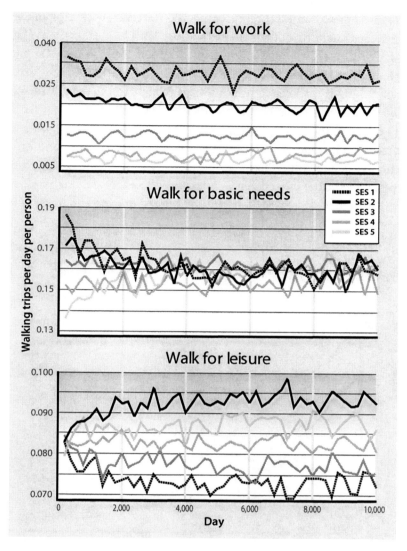

Figure 4. Average walking trips per day per person by purpose and SES group over time in a scenario

We implemented four experiments including driving-optimized, walking-optimized, driving-extreme, and walking-extreme. Under the driving-optimized and driving-extreme optimized scenarios, values of some cost-related parameters were changed to increase the competitive advantage of driving as a travel mode. For example, car speed was increased, and time for parking, parking fee, and fuel price were decreased compared to default values. In addition, the fares and waiting times for public transit were increased, because these changes decrease the competitive advantage of using public transit and thus indirectly increase the competitive advantage of driving. Under the walking-optimized (or driving-constrained) and walking-extreme experiment, the car-related parameters were changed in the opposite direction, and the fares and waiting times for public transit were decreased because the use of public transit involves walking for transit.

In the walking-extreme scenario, walking represented 100 percent of all trips made by those with low incomes but a relatively low share of all trips made by those with higher incomes (figure 5). The income differential was particularly steep where walking trips dropped from nearly 100 percent to 20 percent from the lowest to the highest income. In contrast, in the driving-optimized and driving-extreme experiments, there were only slight differences in walking trips relative to the default scenario. An unexpected result was that for the lowest income level 1, the percentage of walking trips under the driving-extreme experiment was higher than in the driving-optimized and default experiments. This is because under the driving-extreme scenario the number of driving trips increased significantly, and driving trips tended to be concentrated in the city center, which has a higher density of nonresidential locations. Thus, persons with income level 1 who live in the city center were exposed to more driving trips, which, based on the feedbacks encoded in the model, decreases their attitude toward driving and leads to fewer driving trips.

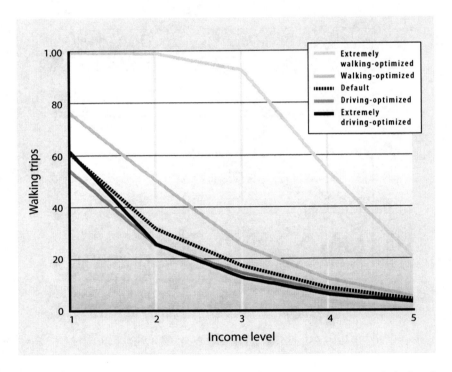

Figure 5. Percentage of walking trips (including for transit) by income level, with default values, driving-optimized experiment, extremely driving-optimized experiment, walking-optimized experiment, and extremely walking-optimized experiment

Compared with the default scenario, strong disincentives placed on driving and a few incentives offered for taking the bus (such as walking-optimized experiment) had the potential to greatly increase walking trips. As expected, the effects of the walking-optimized experiment as a whole, as well as of specific cost-related parameters such as fuel prices and parking, were greater at lower income levels. In contrast, walking by the highest income group was insensitive to fuel price and had relatively low sensitivity to parking costs. Lower income groups were more sensitive to changes in costs of fuel and parking, while higher income groups were unlikely to increase the percentages of walking trips even under the walking-extreme experiment. A key contributor to income differences in walking was encoded in our model because we assumed that the opportunity cost of an hour of local travel was equal to half of an hourly wage.[64] Thus the same time cost more for people with higher hourly wages, that is, those who live outside the city center.

In contrast to walking optimization, the driving optimization scenarios had much smaller impacts on walking, which were approximately similar across income categories. This may reflect the existing orientation toward driving already built into the typical cost structure of transportation options. It may also reflect the relatively high fixed costs associated with driving (e.g., purchasing a vehicle and insurance) relative to lower variable costs (e.g., fuel and parking), which have little effect when altered. For example, national data show that the ownership of even one car dramatically transforms travel behavior: households with no vehicle take 41 percent of trips by walking, compared with 12.5 percent trips by walking for households with one vehicle.[11]

Conclusions and Implications

We used two agent-based models to illustrate the potential and challenges of applying a systems approach to answer policy-relevant questions in population health. Although there have been numerous calls for this approach in public health,[35,65-67] most discussions have been abstract and theoretical. We developed alternative models drawing on existing empirical data, helping to illustrate the data needs required to better understand health-system dynamics and the novel insights that can be gleaned. This work provides a concrete illustration of an innovative way to conduct research and obtain evidence for policy. Although agent-based models have been used in the transportation field to study vehicle flow, traffic congestion, route choice, driving, and travel demand,[68-72] walking itself is rarely investigated. Similarly, studies of pedestrian movement tend to focus on evacuation or crowd behavior within buildings or small areas[46-49] rather than the factors affecting the choice to walk per se. Agent-based models have been proposed as useful tools in the study of walking behavior,[38,50] but few applications exist.

The most noteworthy attribute of both models is that the attitudes of agents toward various travel modes were affected by a number of feedback mechanisms. This is in contrast to most models of travel-mode choice, where attitudes do not vary over time in response to past experiences.[73] By incorporating feedbacks that altered individual walking behaviors in response to social networks, previous experience, and the prevalence of walking they encountered, our relatively simple models were able to generate qualitative patterns of walking behaviors that have been observed in empirical studies. The models allowed for feedbacks over time from features of the built and social environments. In addition, walking for one purpose had effects on walking for other purposes; for example, the models allowed experiences in one realm, such as walking to work, to influence other realms of walking, such as walking to shop.

Another advantage of this work is that it facilitates the examination of interventions using a number of "what-if" scenarios. Using V1 model, we examined the impact of combinations of two strategies and their interactions: improving people's attitudes toward walking and improving safety. Furthermore, we explored whether the effect of these factors was modified by the mix of land-uses. Using the V2 model, we investigated how travel cost can alter the prevalence of walking and income differentials in utilitarian walking and explored the synergistic effects of policies aimed at changing attitudes toward walking and driving with travel cost policies.

Our models and simulations have contributed to understanding the processes driving differences in walking by SES and have indicated that various policy interventions may be needed for different groups. For example, our results show that the co-spatial segregation of SES and safety, such that neighborhoods of low SES have low safety levels, results in less walking among the lower SES groups even when SES is not spatially correlated with land-use mix. Also, as the V2 model showed, lower and higher income groups differed in their sensitivities to the changes in the costs of fuel and parking.

Compared to V1 model, the V2 model is more complicated and has integrated more factors and dynamic processes related to utilitarian walking (for example, the mode of public transit and more types of feedback). V2 may be more advantageous than V1 in terms of practical application, but V1 may better present the decision process of choosing a travel mode at an individual level. Any agent-based model needs an explicit description of the mode-choice process at the individual level. V1 uses a decision-tree or hierarchical structure so that some factors are considered before others. As Alfonzo's hierarchy of walking needs[74] pointed out, some needs are more basic and fundamental than others. An individual must satisfy these more basic needs before they can consider higher order needs. In V1, although the travel-mode choice function is simple, the assumption is that trip distance is a primary factor to be met before the other factors are considered.

Because existing knowledge and data are limited, our ability to justify and calibrate many details of the decision choice—including its hierarchical structure—was as well. We compromised by using knowledge and data at the population level (e.g., on how cost is associated with decisions at the aggregate level) as a substitute for the behavior rules operating at the individual level. This led to the development of V2, which integrated more state-of-the-art knowledge at the population level, but had a more simplified choice structure. Modeling is always a balance between theory and practice; additional research and data collection on individual-level decision-making will allow further refinements of agent-based models.

Our results suggest that interventions at multiple levels may be particularly effective for behavioral change due to possible synergistic effects.[75-78] For example, we identified a synergistic effect between decreasing the attitude toward driving and modifying the cost structure to favor walking. This is just one example of synergies that can affect the complex decision-making that results in the choice of a travel mode. Clearly a diversity of interventions will be required to increase walking. Interventions targeted toward walking (educational campaigns, improved walkability) will be needed along with interventions targeted toward reducing driving (parking policies). Our intent was to assess possible effects of certain types of interventions rather than to make specific predictions. We believe that the assumptions in our two simplified exploratory models were reasonable based on current knowledge, and that the models replicated key patterns observed in the real world. Making reliable predictions about the effects of interventions in a particular setting would require many model refinements and the incorporation of additional data to support the assumptions in and details of the model. Whenever possible, conclusions regarding impacts of interventions should be confirmed with experimental designs.

A major challenge is making these models empirically grounded, given that data to support some parameters may be unavailable or impossible to obtain. For an agent-based model to explicitly and accurately describe the decision process for choosing a travel mode at the individual level, better knowledge and data are needed to justify this type of modeling. Additional research on individual-level decision-making will allow further refinements of agent-based models that are relevant to health policy assessments, which include system-level interactions and responses. For example, in V2, we assume that travel time can be transferred to travel cost with a fixed rate (an hour's travel time equals the individual's half-hour salary).[79] However, evidence shows that uncertainty in time is a key determinant in attitude and travel-mode choice.[79] We need better data and models for incorporating that time uncertainty into the decision choice.

Model validation and calibration of agent-based models is challenging.[80] We performed preliminary calibration by adjusting parameters (for which no empirical data was available) so that summaries of model output were consistent with selected empirical data from the National Household Travel Survey. Discrepancies between model outputs and empirical data may imply the need for further calibration or modification of model assumptions. Also, the replication of existing patterns does not necessarily imply that underlying processes are correctly specified. A valid model requires that relevant agent and environment characteristics are based on existing data whenever possible, but in developing this simple model, it quickly became apparent that there is a dearth of data on which to base model inputs. For example, evidence suggests that dog owners walk more than nonowners, but the magnitude of the difference is not clear.[81] Growing interest in developing these types of models may serve as an impetus to collect these data.

Models cannot include all elements that are likely contributing to the behavior of a complex system. Our models included only a few key elements that allowed us to examine our study questions. For example, we restricted both models to factors directly related to travel-mode choice, which is a short-term choice and does not represent medium-term choices, such as vehicle ownership, and long-term choices, such as residential and work location. Future work may incorporate elements such as traffic safety, urban design, and feedbacks between behaviors and environmental features. For example, walking prevalence may influence land-use mix and safety, and increases in fuel price may result in higher income groups purchasing more fuel-efficient (and costlier) vehicles, which would give them a better cost return on driving. This is a behavioral analog to Jevons paradox, in which greater efficiency has been shown to result in increased consumption. Another potentially important factor the model did not include is habit: daily travel mode may become a habitual behavior after repeating over a period and financial incentives may be insufficient to generate change.[82-84]

The models were developed to be as simple as possible in order to help us to understand model properties before adding more complicated processes, but some of the simplifications may be problematic. One assumption in both models was that all trips always begin and end at the household or workplace, but individuals may combine trips.[85] Residents with limited access to destinations combine more trips, and clusters of destinations serve as activity centers that attract people for multiple reasons.[19,86,87] People may be more likely to walk to an activity center where several errands can be accomplished along the same trip.[88] Different transportation modes may also affect each other in complex ways. For example, those who regularly walk long distances to work may not be inclined to walk in their own neighborhood. Conversely, it is plausible that traveling by car to work or shopping may leave more free time to walk in the neighborhood.

Our models have additional room for refinement. For example, gender differences were not modeled and aesthetic quality was assumed to be constant over space in all scenarios. The feedbacks were based on reasonable guesses and their relative magnitudes need refinement and validation. The social networks were simplistic and the broader roles of social norms (i.e., through media influences) were not considered. Long-term positive feedbacks from habit formation were not considered. The models also did not incorporate feedbacks from walking to environmental features (i.e., endogeneity of environmental features). For example, just as mixed landuse may promote walking, greater walking is likely to promote greater mixes of uses, as businesses locate in areas with heavy foot traffic. In addition, cities may invest more in the aesthetics and safety of neighborhoods where people walk more.

The next step is to implement an agent-based model to a specific real city in order to explore its potential to answer questions relevant to specific conditions in the real world. The data sources should include demographic, land-use, street network, transportation, and crime data, as well as micro-surveys of walking behaviors. After selecting the U.S. city with the best available data, these agent-based models could be modified to include city-specific details.

The ability to capture dynamic processes and incorporate empirical data makes agent-based models powerful tools for exploring the influence of interacting factors on behaviors, and for testing alternative policy interventions. Challenges to building the model algorithms include defining boundaries, accounting for geographic variations, and dealing with variability in human behavior. However, agent-based models can yield insights into basic dynamics that cannot be obtained with other approaches. Together with other methods, including observational studies as well as quasi-experiments and trials, agent-based models may contribute to providing the evidence base necessary to improve population levels of walking and reduce inequalities in walking.

References

1. US Department of Health and Human Services. *Physical Activity and Health: A Report of the Surgeon General.* Atlanta, GA: Centers for Disease Control and Prevention and National Center for Chronic Disease Prevention and Health Promotion; 1996.

2. Macera CA, Ham SA, Yore MM, et al. Prevalence of physical activity in the United States: Behavioral Risk Factor Surveillance System, 2001. *Prev Chronic Dis.* 2005;2(2):A17.

3. Kruger J, Ham SA, Berrigan D, Ballard-Barbash R. Prevalence of transportation and leisure walking among U.S. adults. *Prev Med.* 2008;47(3):329–334.

4. McNeill LH, Kreuter MW, Subramanian SV. Social environment and physical activity: a review of concepts and evidence. *Soc Sci Med.* 2006;63(4):1011–1022.

5. Handy SL, Boarnet MG, Ewing R, Killingsworth RE. How the built environment affects physical activity: views from urban planning. *Am J Prev Med.* 2002;23(2S):64–73.

6. Brownson RC, Hoehner CM, Day K, Forsyth A, Sallis JF. Measuring the built environment for physical activity: state of the science. *Am J Prev Med.* 2009;36(4S):S99–S123.

7. Transportation Research Board. *Does the Built Environment Influence Physical Activity? Examining the Evidence.* TRB Special Report 282; 2005.

8. Cerin E, Leslie E, Owen N. Explaining socio-economic status differences in walking for transport: an ecological analysis of individual, social and environmental factors. *Soc Sci Med.* 2009;68:1013–1020.

9. Cao X, Handy SL, Mokhtarian PL. The influences of the built environment and residential self-selection on pedestrian behavior: evidence from Austin, TX. *Transportation.* 2006;33(1):1–20.

10. Berke EM, Koepsell TD, Moudon AV, Hoskins RE, Larson EB. Association of the built environment with physical activity and obesity in older persons. *Am J Public Health.* 2007;97(3):486–492.

11. Pucher J, Renne JL. Socioeconomics of urban travel: evidence from the 2001 NHTS. *Transport Q.* 2003;57(3):49–77.

12. Owen N, Humpel N, Leslie E, Bauman A, Sallis JF. Understanding environmental influences on walking: review and research agenda. *Am J Prev Med.* 2004;27(1):67–76.

13. Heath GW, Brownson RC, Kruger J, Miles R, Powell K, Ramsey L. The effectiveness of urban design and land use and transport policies and practices to increase physical activity: a systematic review. *J Phys Act Health.* 2006;3(Suppl 1):S55–S76.

14. Humpel N, Owen N, Leslie E. Environmental factors associated with adults' participation in physical activity: a review. *Am J Prev Med.* 2002;22(3):188–199.

15. Lee C, Moudon AV. Physical activity and environment research in the health field: implications for urban and transportation planning practice and research. *J Plan Lit.* 2004;19(147):147–181.

16. Saelens BE, Sallis JF, Frank LD. Environmental correlates of walking and cycling: findings from the transportation, urban design, and planning literatures. *Ann Behav Med.* 2003;25(2):80–91.

17. Saelens BE, Handy SL. Built environment correlates of walking: a review. *Med Sci Sports Exerc.* 2008;40(7 Suppl):S550–S566.

18. Handy S. *Critical Assessment of the Literature on the Relationships Among Transportation, Land Use, and Physical Activity.* Prepared for the Committee on Physical Activity, Health, Transportation, and Land Use. Transportation Safety Board and Institute of Medicine; 2005.

19. Frank LD, Engelke PO, Schmid TL. *Health and Community Design: The Impact of the Built Environment on Physical Activity.* Washington, DC: Island Press; 2003.

20. Frank LD, Kerr J, Sallis JF, Miles R, Chapman J. A hierarchy of sociodemographic and environmental correlates of walking and obesity. *Prev Med.* 2008;47:172–178.

21. Brownson RC, Baker EA, Housemann RA, Brennan LK, Bacak SJ. Environmental and policy determinants of physical activity in the United States. *Am J Public Health.* 2001;91(12):1995–2003.

22. Agrawal AW, Schimek P. Extent and correlates of walking in the USA. *Transp Res Part D Transp Environ.* 2007;12(8):548–563.

23. Suminski RR, Poston WSC, Petosa RL, Stevens E, Katzenmoyer LM. Features of the neighborhood environment and walking by U.S. adults. *Am J Prev Med.* 2005;28(2):149–155.

24. McGinn AP, Evenson KR, Herring AH, Huston SL, Rodriguez DA. The association of perceived and objectively measured crime with physical activity: a cross-sectional analysis. *J Phys Act Health.* 2008;5(1):117–131.

25. Bennett GG, McNeill LH, Wolin KY, Duncan DT, Puleo E, Emmons KM. Safe to walk? Neighborhood safety and physical activity among public housing residents. *PLoS Med.* 2007;4(10):1599–1606.

26. Sallis JF, King AC, Sirard JR, Albright CL. Perceived environmental predictors of physical activity over 6 months in adults: activity counseling trial. *Health Psychol.* 2007;26(6):701–709.

27. McDonald NC. The effect of objectively measured crime on walking in minority adults. *Am J Health Promot.* 2008;22(6):433–436.

28. Eyler AA, Brownson RC, Bacak SJ, Housemann RA. The epidemiology of walking for physical activity in the United States. *Med Sci Sports Exerc.* 2003;35(9):1529–1536.

29. Lee C, Moudon AV. Correlates of walking for transportation or recreation purposes. *J Phys Act Health.* 2006;3(Suppl 1):S77–S98.

30. Handy S, Cao X, Mokhtarian PL. Self-selection in the relationship between the built environment and walking. *J Am Plann Assoc.* 2006;72(1):55–74.

31. Steptoe A, Diez Roux A. Happiness, social networks, and health. *BMJ.* 2008;337:a2781.

32. Christakis NA, Fowler JH. The spread of obesity in a large social network over 32 years. *N Engl J Med.* 2007;357(4):370–379.

33. Axtell R, Epstein JM. Agent-based modeling: understanding our creations. *SFI Bulletin.* 1994;Winter:28–32.

34. Bonabeau E. Agent-based modeling: methods and techniques for simulating human systems. *Proc Natl Acad Sci USA.* 2002;99(Suppl 3):7280–7287.

35. Diez Roux AV. Integrating social and biologic factors in health research: a systems view. *Ann Epidemiol.* 2007;17(7):569–574.

36. Auchincloss AH, Diez Roux AV. A new tool for epidemiology: the usefulness of dynamic-agent models in understanding place effects on health. *Am J Epidemiol.* 2008;168(1):1–8.

37. Giles-Corti B, King AC. Creating active environments across the life course: "Thinking outside the square". *Br J Sports Med.* 2009;43(2):109–113.

38. King AC, Satariano WA, Marti J, Zhu W. Multilevel modeling of walking behavior: advances in understanding the interactions of people, place, and time. *Med Sci Sports Exerc.* 2008;40(7 Suppl):S584–S593.

39. Epstein JM, Axtell RL. *Growing Artificial Societies: Social Science From the Bottom Up.* Cambridge, MA: MIT Press; 1996.

40. Brown DG, Riolo R, Robinson DT, North M, Rand W. Spatial process and data models: toward integration of agent-based models and GIS. *J Geogr Syst.* 2005;7:1–23.

41. Batty M. *Cities and Complexity: Understanding Cities with Cellular Automata, Agent-based Models, and Fractals.* Cambridge, MA: MIT Press; 2005.

42. Galea S, Riddle M, Kaplan GA. Causal thinking and complex system approaches in epidemiology. *Int J Epidemiol.* 2010;39:97–106.

43. Yang Y, Atkinson PM, Ettema D. Simulation of infectious disease transmission within a city: the application of ISTAM to Eemnes by role-based AB simulation. *J R Soc Interface.* 2008;5:759–772.

44. Galea S, Hall C, Kaplan GA. Social epidemiology and complex system dynamic modelling as applied to health behaviour and drug use research. *Int J Drug Policy.* 2009;20(3):209–216.

45. Gorman DM, Mezic J, Mezic I, Gruenewald PJ. Agent-based modeling of drinking behavior: a preliminary model and potential applications to theory and practice. *Am J Public Health.* 2006;96(11):2055–2060.

46. Willis A, Gjersoe N, Havard C, Jon Kerridge RK. Human movement behaviour in urban spaces: implications for the design and modelling of effective pedestrian environments. *Environ Plann B Plann Des.* 2004;31(6):805–828.

47. Turner A, Penn A. Encoding natural movement as an agent-based system: an investigation into human pedestrian behaviour in the built environment. *Environ Plann B: Plann Des.* 2002;29(4):473–490.

48. Batty M. Agent-based pedestrian modeling. In: Longley PA, Batty M, eds. *Advanced Spatial Analysis: The CASA Book of GIS.* Redlands, CA: ESRI Press; 2003.

49. Haklay M, O'Sullivan D, Thurstain-Goodwin M, Schelhorn T. "So go downtown": simulating pedestrian move-ment in town centres. *Environ Plann B: Plann Des.* 2001;28(3):343–359.

50. Saarloos D, Kim J-E, Timmermans H. The built environment and health: introducing individual space-time be-havior. *Int J Environ Res Public Health.* 2009;6:1724–1743.

51. Ronald N, Sterling L, Kirley M. An agent-based approach to modelling pedestrian behaviour. *Int J Simulation: Systems Sci Tech.* 2007;8(1):25–39.

52. Helbing D, Farkas IJ, Molnar P, Vicsek T. Simulation of pedestrian crowds in normal and evacuation situations. In: Schreckenberg M, Sharma SD (eds) *Pedestrian and Evacuation Dynamics.* Berlin: Springer; 2002:21–58.

53. Yang Y, Diez Roux AV, Auchincloss AH, Rodriguez DA, Brown DG. A spatial agent-based model for the simula-tion of adults' daily walking within a city. *Am J Prev Med.* 2011;40(3):353–361.

54. Yang Y, Diez Roux AV, Auchincloss AH, Rodriguez DA, Brown DG. Exploring walking differences by socioeco-nomic status using a spatial agent-based model. *Health Place.* 2012;18(1):96–99.

55. Yang Y, Auchincloss AH, Rodriguez DA, Brown DG, Riolo R, Diez Roux AV. Modeling spatial segregation and travel cost influences on utilitarian walking: toward policy intervention. *Comput Environ Urban Syst.* 2015;51:59–69.

56. Pellegrini PA, Fotheringham AS, Lin G. An empirical evaluation of parameter sensitivity to choice set definition in shopping destination choice models. *Pap Reg Sci.* 1997;76(2):257–284.

57. Barff R, Mackay D, Olshavsky RW. A selective review of travel-mode choice models. *J Consum Res.* 1982;8(4):370–380.

58. Domencich T, McFadden D. *Urban Travel Demand: A Behavioral Analysis.* Amsterdam: North Holland Publishing Company; 1975.

59. Schafer A. Regularities in travel demand: an international perspective. *J Trans Stats.* 2000;3(3):1–32.

60. Miller GA. The magical number seven, plus or minus two: some limits on our capacity for processing informa-tion. *Psychol Rev.* 1956;63(2):81–97.

61. Nikolai C, Madey G. Tools of the trade: a survey of various agent-based modeling platforms. *J Artif Soc Soc Simul.* 2009;12(2):2.

62. Pucher J, Buehler R, Merom D, et al. Walking and cycling in the United States, 2001–2009: evidence from the National Household Travel Surveys. *Am J Public Health.* 2011;101(Suppl 1):S310–S317.

63. Besser LM, Dannenberg AL. Walking to public transit steps to help meet physical activity recommendations. *Am J Prev Med.* 2005;29(4):273–280.

64. US Department of Transportation. Revised Departmental Guidance for the Valuation of Travel Time in Economic Analysis. 2003; http://www.transportation.gov/regulations/revised-value-travel-time-2003.

65. Homer JB, Hirsch GB. System dynamics modeling for public health: background and opportunities. *Am J Public Health.* 2006;96(3):452–458.

66. Mabry PL, Olster DH, Morgan GD, Abrams DB. Interdisciplinarity and systems science to improve population health: a view from the NIH Office of Behavioral and Social Science Research. *Am J Prev Med.* 2008;35(2 Suppl):S211–S224.

67. Sterman JD. Learning from evidence in a complex world. *Am J Public Health.* 2006;96(3):505–514.

68. Dia H. An agent-based approach to modeling driver route choice behavior under the influence of real-time information. *Transp Res Part C Emerg Technol.* 2002;10:331–349.

69. Hidas P. Modeling Lane Changing and merging in microscopic traffic simulation. *Transp Res Part C Emerg Technol.* 2002;10:351–371.

70. Peeta S, Zhou W, Zhang P. Modeling and mitigation of car-truck interactions on freeways. *Trans Res Rec.* 2004;1899:117–126.

71. Wahle J, Bazzan ALC, Klugl F, Schrekenberg M. The impact of real-time information in a two-route scenario using agent-based simulation. *Transp Res Part C Emerg Technol.* 2002;10:399–417.

72. Zhang L, Levinson D. Agent-based approach to travel demand modeling. *Transp Res Rec.* 2004;1898:28–36.

73. Ortúzar JdD, Willumsen LG. *Modeling Transport.* West Sussex, UK: Wiley; 2011.

74. Alfonzo MA. To walk or not to walk? The hierarchy of walking needs. environment and behavior. *Environ Behav.* 2005;37(6):808–836.

75. Weiner BJ, Lewis MA, Clauser SB, Stitzenberg KB. In search of synergy: strategies for combining interventions at multiple levels. *J Natl Cancer Inst Monogr.* 2012;44:34–41.

76. Sallis JF, Owen N, Fisher EB. Ecological models of health behavior. In: Glanz K, Rimer B, Viswanath K, eds. *Health Behavior and Health Education: Theory, Research, and Practice.* San Francisco: Jossey-Bass; 2008:465–482.

77. McLeroy KR, Norton BL, Kegler MC, Burdine JN, Sumaya CV. Community-based interventions. *Am J Public Health.* 2003;93(4):529–533.

78. Stokols D, Allen J, Bellingham RL. The social ecology of health promotion: implications for research and practice. *Am J Health Promot.* 1996;10(4):247–251.

79. Mackie PJ, Jara-Díaz S, Fowkes AS. The value of travel time savings in evaluation. *Transp Res Part E Logist Transp Rev.* 2001;37(2-3):91–106.

80. Cioffi-Revilla C. Invariance and universality in social agent-based simulations. *Proc Natl Acad Sci USA.* 2002;99(Suppl 3):7314–7316.

81. Cutt H, Giles-Corti B, Knuiman M, Burke V. Dog ownership, health and physical activity: a critical review of the literature. *Health Place.* 2007;13(1):261–272.

82. De Bruijn G-J, Gardner B. Active commuting and habit strength: an interactive and discriminant analyses approach. *Am J Health Promot.* 2011;25(3):e27–e36.

83. Murtagh S, Rowe D, Elliott M, McMinn D, Nelson N. Predicting active school travel: the role of planned behavior and habit strength. *Int J Behav Nutr Phys Act.* 2012;9(1):65.

84. Martin A, Suhrcke M, Ogilvie D. Financial incentives to promote active travel: an evidence review and economic framework. *Am J Prev Med.* 2012;43(6):e45–e57.

85. Krizek KJ. Neighborhood services, trip purpose, and tour-based travel. *Transportation.* 2003;30(4):387–410.

86. Sallis JF. Angels in the details: comment on "The relationship between destination proximity, destination mix and physical activity behaviors". *Prev Med.* 2008;46(1):6–7.

87. Moudon AV, Lee C, Cheadle AD, et al. Operational definitions of walkable neighborhood: theoretical and empirical insights. *J Phys Act Health.* 2006;3(Suppl 1):S99–S117.

88. McCormack GR, Giles-Corti B, Bulsara M. The relationship between destination proximity, destination mix and physical activity behaviors. *Prev Med.* 2008;46(1):33–40.

CHAPTER 7

A PROTOTYPE FOR IDENTIFYING POLICY-RELEVANT REASONS FOR GENDER DIFFERENCES IN PHYSICAL ACTIVITY

Shiriki Kumanyika, PhD, MPH
Professor Emerita
Perelman School of Medicine, University of Pennsylvania
Chair, African American Collaborative Obesity Research Network

Matt Kasman, PhD
Research Associate
Center on Social Dynamics and Policy, Brookings Institution

Melicia C. Whitt-Glover, PhD
President and CEO, Gramercy Research Group, Winston-Salem North Carolina and
Physical Activity Lead, African American Collaborative Obesity Research Network

Austen Mack-Crane
Research Assistant
Center on Social Dynamics and Policy, Brookings Institution

George A. Kaplan, PhD
Thomas Francis Collegiate Professor Emeritus of Public Health
Center for Social Epidemiology and Population Health
University of Michigan

Ross A. Hammond, PhD
Senior Fellow in Economic Studies and Director
Center on Social Dynamics and Policy
Brookings Institution

Acknowledgments: This work was supported primarily by the Network on Inequality Complexity and Health (NICH) under contract HHSN27600800013C, Office of Behavioral and Social Sciences Research, National Institutes of Health, awarded to George A. Kaplan at the University of Michigan School of Public Health. The authors acknowledge the contributions of Dr. Helen Meissner at the National Institutes of Health, Dr. Vish Vishnawath at Harvard University, and other members of the NICH for their feedback and suggestions during the development of this project. We also acknowledge the assistance of Caroline Kraus at Gramercy Research Group in the conduct of the literature review for this project.

We developed an agent-based model to evaluate the potential determinants of leisure-time physical activity in black men and women to help inform future physical activity interventions. Effective policies and other new initiatives are needed to prevent or mitigate health risks by increasing regular leisure-time physical activity. The lack of sufficient leisure-time physical activity is a well-established, potentially modifiable risk factor for a range of chronic diseases, including hypertension and type 2 diabetes. Approaches to improve physical activity in population groups at high risk of these diseases are needed in addition to efforts directed to the population at large.

Black men and women have a high burden of chronic diseases, which is disproportionate when compared to that of whites of the same age and gender. Increasing leisure-time physical activity could presumably help to reduce this gap.[1] We focused on gender differences because among diverse racial and ethnic groups, including black Americans, females are less likely than males to achieve physical activity recommendations.

The Problem

Public-Health Significance of Physical Activity

Participation in regular physical activity has been associated with increased longevity and reduced risk of developing myriad metabolic abnormalities and chronic diseases.[1-8] The U.S. government's 2008 Physical Activity Guidelines for Americans documents the beneficial influences of physical activity on health.[9] The Centers for Disease Control and Prevention advises, "Regular physical activity is one of the most important things you can do for your health." Their guidance highlights improved weight control, and reduced risk of heart disease and stroke, type 2 diabetes, and some types of cancer, as well as stronger bones and muscles and improved mental health and mood as direct benefits of engaging in regular physical activity.[10]

Some benefits of regular physical activity are related to its favorable effects on preventing obesity, losing weight, or maintaining weight loss.[9,11] Improving adherence to physical activity guidelines is critical given the high prevalence of obesity in the United States. The National Health and Nutrition Examination Survey (NHANES) data for 2009–2012 show that only about 30 percent of U.S. adults aged 20 years and over were in the healthy weight range, 34 percent were overweight, and 35 percent were obese.[12] In addition, physical activity in those overweight or obese has direct health benefits that are not necessarily related to weight.

Regular physical activity can, therefore, improve the health profiles of people with obesity even if they are not interested in weight loss or are unable to lose weight.[9]

Exercise Levels in the United States

U.S. guidelines recommend that all healthy adults accumulate 150 minutes per week of moderate intensity physical activity or 75 minutes per week of vigorous intensity aerobic activity.[9] These levels of physical activity constitute exercise. For further benefits, adults should aim to increase aerobic physical activity to 300 minutes of moderate intensity or 150 minutes of vigorous intensity activity weekly. Examples of potential ways to engage in leisure-time physical activity include brisk walking, hiking, swimming, water aerobics or aerobic dancing, other types of dancing, bicycling, jogging or running, and playing tennis or active games such as basketball or soccer.[9]

The majority of U.S. adults do not achieve recommended levels of physical activity. Troiano et al.[13] used 2003–2004 NHANES data in which wearable digital devices (accelerometers) were used to estimate the percentage of U.S. adults ages 20–59 years who accumulated at least 30 minutes of moderate- or higher-intensity activity in 10-minute segments on 5 of 7 days per week. Only 3.8 percent of males and 3.2 percent of females met public-health guidelines based on accelerometer data, which would be expected to capture most or all physical activity for the average man or woman.

More commonly, the prevalence of physical activity is based on self-reported data—people's subjective estimates of how active they are. Self-reported data are less accurate than accelerometry and tend to result in overestimates.[13] However, self-reported data may reflect differences in activity levels by gender and age similar to patterns obtained from objective data.[13] One advantage of self-reporting over accelerometry is that it allows for estimations of different types of physical activity. For example, utilitarian activity undertaken as part of a daily transportation routine, or work-related physical activity, can be queried separately from walking or other intentional forms of leisure-time physical activity, which—if low—can then become the focus of exercise interventions.

Even assuming that self-reporting overestimates activity levels, the percentage of U.S. adults who report leisure-time physical activity levels that meet public health recommendations is low. Respondents in the National Health Interview Survey (NHIS) were asked about their frequency and duration of exercise, including vigorous physical activity, moderate physical activity, and muscle-strengthening activities as specified in the 2008 guidelines.[14] Only 26 percent of adults aged 18–44 years and 18 percent of adults aged 45–64 years met both the aerobic activity and muscle-strengthening guidelines; 40 percent and 50 percent, respectively, did not meet either guideline. Lower levels of self-reported leisure-time physical activity in women compared to men and black compared to white adults have been observed consistently (figure 1). Self-reported leisure-time physical activity is higher at higher income levels in both black and white adults (figure 2).

Physical Activity and Health in Black Americans

There are significant disparities between black and white adults in mortality before age 75 from several major causes of death that have been linked to inadequate physical activity, such as the causes shown in figure 3. The data shown in figure 3 are based on years of potential life lost (YPLLs), an indicator of premature mortality that reflects both mortality rate and age at death. In a longitudinal analysis of data from more than 63,000 participants (70 percent black; two-thirds had low income and a high school education or less) in the Southern Community Cohort Study,[15] all-cause, cardiovascular, and cancer mortality risks were significantly reduced after an average of 6-year follow-up among those with the highest versus lowest overall levels of physical activity (i.e., all physical activity rather than only leisure-time physical activity). Similarly, among black Americans included in a longitudinal analysis of pooled data from studies in the National Cancer Institute Cohort Consortium, mortality rates were 20–40 percent lower at higher levels of leisure-time physical activity over a median follow-up period of 14 years.[16]

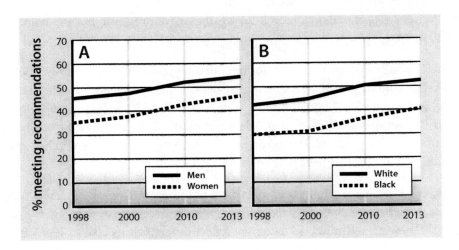

Figure 1. U.S. adults aged 18 years and over meeting federal 2008 physical activity recommendations for aerobic activity, 1998–2013 by gender (A) or race/ethnicity (B). Data are for non-Hispanic whites and non-Hispanic blacks.[12] *Source*: Health United States, 2014, Table 63

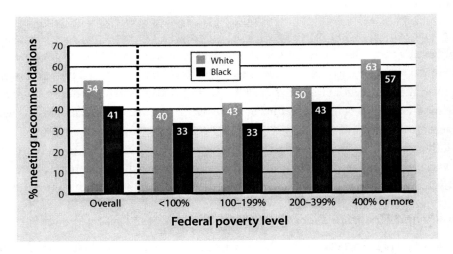

Figure 2. U.S. adults aged 18 years and over meeting recommendations for aerobic activity overall and by income level, as a percentage of federal poverty line (FPL), 2013. Data are for non-Hispanic whites and non-Hispanic blacks.[12] *Source*: National Center for Health Statistics, Health United States, 2014; Table 63

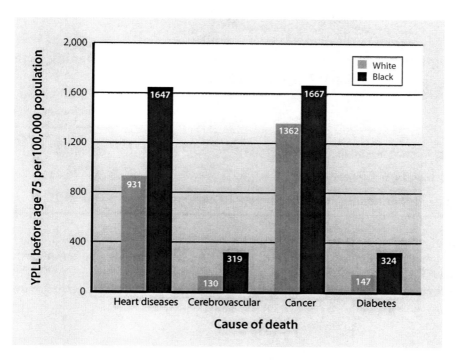

Figure 3. Years of potential life lost (YPLL) for U.S. adults for four major causes of death, 2013, age-adjusted using 2000 standard population. Data are for non-Hispanic whites and for all blacks.[12] *Source*: National Center for Health Statistics, Health United States, 2014; Table 19

The prevalence of obesity, for which physical activity is central to prevention and treatment, is high among Americans in general but is notably higher in black compared to white adults. The 2009–2012 NHANES data indicated that 38 percent of black men compared to 34 percent of non-Hispanic white men had body mass index (BMI) levels in the obese range, and obesity prevalence was 56 percent for black women compared to 32 percent for white women.[12]

Gender Differences in Physical Activity in Black Americans

In three national surveys, the prevalence of self-reported physical activity was 8–10 percentage-points lower for black women compared to black men (table 1).[17] Within these surveys, the percentage of black women who reported leisure-time physical activity levels meeting national recommendations was lowest among those with BMIs of 30 or more; however, this was not observed in black men.

Hypothesis

Our hypothesis was that the gender difference relates to the substantial proportion of leisure-time physical activity ("exercise") that is "socially situated." Specifically, we postulated that black women's lesser likelihood of having built and sociocultural environments that support exercise may explain the lower levels of exercise in black women compared to black men.

This focus on socially situated leisure-time physical activity reflects evidence that exercise behavior is

133

Table 1

Participation in Leisure Time Aerobic and Muscle-Strengthening Activities that Meets Federal Recommendations[17]

	Black men	Black women
	% (95% CI)	
Behavioral Risk Factor Surveillance System (2003)[a]	42 (40,44)	32 (31,34)
National Health Interview Survey (2004)[a]	28 (26,31)	20 (18, 22)
National Health and Nutrition Examination Survey (1999–2004)[b]	30 (28,32)	22 (20,25)

CI = confidence intervals.
[a]Participating in moderate-intensity activity for >30 minutes on >5 days or vigorous intensity activity for >20 minutes on >3 days.
[b]Participating over the past 30 days in moderate-intensity activity for >600 total minutes over >20 days or vigorous intensity activity for >240 minutes on >12 days.

directly or indirectly influenced by the behavior of like-minded peers. Many recommended leisure-time activities require or lend themselves to interactions with others: they are done in teams, classes, group settings, or pairs, or in the presence of others engaging in similar activities, even if there is no direct interaction. In addition, an extensive body of evidence indicates that people need or appreciate companionship and encouragement from others as motivators and supports for exercise.[18-21] "Lack[ing] encouragement, support or companionship from family and friends" is among the 10 most common reasons given by adults for not being more physically active.[10] The principle of homophily indicates that people who share similar characteristics such as age, sex, health-related attitudes, and health status will be perceived as the most influential sources of social support.[22]

Studies of influences on exercise participation in black adults clearly reflect the perceived importance of social engagement as a motivator.[19,23-28] For example, a systematic review of qualitative studies of exercise barriers and facilitators in African Americans concluded that social support, including participation in group activities with peers, played a critical role as a socio-environmental support for the initiation and maintenance of physical activity.[27] These findings applied to both men and women (although studies of only women predominate) and to both younger (18–50 years) and older (over 50 years) respondents. Older adults mentioned the value of dances and exercise programs specifically designed for their age group.

The value of social support may be related to overcoming an intrinsic lack of motivation to exercise, as well as other challenges and disincentives; boosting self-confidence about exercising; providing psychosocial benefits in relationships with partners; or just being in the company of others.[20,26,27] Additional data on sociocultural factors that influence physical activity highlight the importance of collectivism (prioritizing the needs and desires of the group over individuals within a group) as a predictor of physical activity among black men and women.[29]

Research Questions

Following this rationale, the primary research question evaluated in our model was: To what extent might gender differences in socially situated physical activity account for the gender gap in exercise between black men and women? Specifically, we assessed how the gender gap is influenced by differences in: (1) female versus male preferences for the type of social engagement (for example, needing or not needing a specific partner as long as others are exercising); (2) differences in the availability of social partners; (3) one's perception of his or her own availability for exercise given other roles and responsibilities (for example, due to factors that might disproportionately constrain the availability of women); and (4) environmental support for exercise, in terms of neighborhood safety and infrastructure on a continuum of low to high support.

Why Use a Complex Systems Approach?

Our goal was to explore mechanisms that may contribute to differences in physical activity between black men and women, in order to better understand how various factors act, alone or in concert, to generate these differences. Existing observational data do not allow us to easily disentangle these mechanisms using traditional statistical approaches, for three major reasons. First, to our knowledge, no single dataset or appropriate combination of data sources contains observations of socially situated physical activity as well as information related to each of these mechanisms or suitable proxies. Second, even if such a data source did exist it would need to include potentially confounding influences and have sufficient sample size and variation in mechanisms—obviously a steep obstacle to overcome. Finally, socially situated physical activity is an inherently complex phenomenon; individual actions and outcomes will, by definition, influence one another, and assumptions of independence that underlie traditional statistical approaches cannot be met. Therefore, we employed an exploratory, agent-based model to obtain potentially valuable insights. We began by operationalizing decision-making behavior related to socially situated physical activity in an agent-based model framework. We then tested the model's generative sufficiency—which is defined as the ability to reliably reproduce a plausible range of observable outcomes.[30]

This model gave us access to a "virtual laboratory" to conduct experiments exploring our research questions. Using this tool, it was relatively straightforward for us to artificially generate the variation in conditions necessary to thoroughly explore effects on gender differences in physical activity, including nonlinear and interaction effects. However, in order for the results of these analyses to meaningfully reflect the real world, elements of the model such as agent attributes and behavior must be grounded in empirical evidence or theory. The subject of gender differences in physical activity (and the combination of factors that might drive these differences) has received limited scholarly exploration. Therefore, the most appropriate initial agent-based model for this process will be fairly simple, operationalizing current knowledge and theory to map assumptions about the drivers of individual behavior to population-level outcomes.

Our model of physical activity considered three key factors that the literature suggests may generate differences between black men and women in participation in socially situated physical activity, but by necessity it could not incorporate all the related nuances. Specifically, we considered gender differences in exercise engagement, availability for participation (others or self) in exercise, and sensitivity to neighborhood conditions. These broad categories of influences almost certainly comprise multiple components that interact in important ways. We characterized exercise behavior as binary, with individuals always exhibiting either partner- or group-based behavior; in reality, individuals are likely to employ a continuum of strategies under different circumstances. A man or woman's unavailability for exercise is represented as a simple probability in our model rather than a combination of specific influences such as employment obligations, social engagements, physical ailments, work fatigue, and household tasks. When making decisions about participating in physical activity, men and women may respond differently to the infrastructure and safety of neighborhoods; we described these two important factors using a single, simple index score, and for now omit from consideration more complicated ways in which these factors might interact. Despite these limitations, we believe that our relatively stylized (i.e., generalized) modeling approach is an appropriate initial attempt at modeling, sufficient for exploring our research questions.

Methods

Model Assumptions

Our model used socially situated physical activity, a subset of leisure-time physical activity, as the outcome variable. Here, socially situated physical activity refers to physical activity undertaken for recreational or health purposes outside of daily household, occupational, or transportation routines, which is influenced by the supportive or similar behavior of others. In the model, the probability of exercising on any given day for black men and women living in an urban area is a function of (a) peer availability for exercise, (b) decision-making behavior with respect to needing a specific partner from the available pool of same-sex peers, and (c) neighborhood safety and infrastructure.

Constraints on Peer Availability for Exercise

External time demands. Lack of time to exercise is one of the most common reasons cited by adults who do not obtain recommended amounts of physical activity, in the United States as a whole[10] and also among black Americans.[27] From a theoretical perspective, external time demands would individually limit the available time for leisure-time physical activity for both black men and women, varying by circumstance. Women would be expected to have less time available for exercise, on average, because they generally have more household and caregiving responsibilities than men.[31] It is common for women to report that caregiving limits their time to exercise,[32-36] which may be related to the time needed for caregiving (for children or others) as well as the need to arrange for someone else to provide care while they exercise. Time demands are relevant for a significant proportion of black women; of black Americans who are employed, women comprise 54 percent.[37] Twenty-eight percent of black family households are headed by single women,[38] 61 percent of black women have at least one child, and 21 percent have three or more children. These factors may affect black women's perceptions about their own availability to engage in exercise and could also affect the availability of other black women as exercise partners.

Pregnancy. Although pregnancy is not a contraindication for regular leisure-time physical activity, and exercise is recommended during pregnancy for both physical and mental health, women are less likely to exercise when pregnant, particularly in racial/ethnic minority populations.[9,39] Exercise levels during pregnancy are also lower among women who exercised less prior to pregnancy, have more than one child at home, and have less education. In turn, pregnancy can affect the pool of potentially available female exercise partners.

Social norms and expectations. Predispositions to exercise may have their origins in experiences earlier in life for adults in general, including black adults, and evidence suggests that early life experiences may be less supportive of exercising for girls compared to boys. For example, in contrast to men, for whom free play and participation in sports and other forms of exercise may have been strongly encouraged and enjoyable during boyhood, such favorable experiences may have been much less common for girls. Factors that differentially discourage exercise participation in girls, some of which have been cited as more common in black than white Americans, include insensitivity of school physical education curricula to gender differences in exercise preferences; perceptions of adults and children of both genders that certain types of physical activity are more appropriate for boys than girls or that being too active in sports is unfeminine; and girls' greater dislike for the effects of physical activity on personal appearance or hygiene (for example, sweating or messing up their hair).[40,41] In addition, social expectations about female roles may lead girls and women to prioritize caregiving over exercise. When these influences are carried over into adulthood, they could render women less likely than men to have well-established exercise skills, motivations, routines, and self-confidence and more likely to have reservations about the social appropriateness of exercising.

Body image, physical status, or personal appearance. Although many black women want to lose weight and are aware that exercise helps with weight loss, they may also reject society's thin body ideal in favor of wanting to retain the culturally preferred shapely or curvaceous body.[33,42] In some cultural groups, including black Americans, perception of a larger female body size as healthier, more nurturing, or more fertile may exist alongside the less positive attitudes toward overweight and obesity that are typical in American society.[43,44] In terms of physical status, the higher prevalence of obesity and severe obesity in black women also constrains leisure-time physical activity,[17] due to higher levels of musculoskeletal problems and functional limitations associated with larger body size or obesity-related comorbidities.[27]

The impact of exercise on maintaining preferred hairstyles may also be a deterrent to exercise for a substantial proportion of black women[45] compared to black men or to white women. Versey notes that maintaining certain types of hairstyles requiring professional styling may have a particular significance for black women, from a historical and cultural perspective and for personal identity and self-esteem.[45] Popular styles may be achieved by chemical straightening ("relaxers") or by braiding, sewing, or "weaving" synthetic or human hair into one's own hair, which can be time consuming and relatively costly to maintain; they are often not "wash and wear" styles that can be easily restored after a workout.[46] Black females may be socialized from childhood to avoid exercise for this reason[47] and may observe appearance-related avoidance of exercise in their female role models.

Preference for Partnering as an Influence on Exercise Decisions

The positive effect of social support on the leisure-time physical activity of black Americans is well established.[25,27] Much of the evidence describes the role of encouragement from family members and friends or the benefits of social interaction in group exercise settings. A substantial proportion of this evidence is from women-only studies that do not permit direct comparisons of the social support needs of men and women; however, the weight of evidence suggests that social support is important for both. Women may perceive men as needing less support for exercise because of social expectations and circumstances that: favor exercise for males more than for females; socialize men to be more self-motivated and self-confident; or make exercise easier for men to arrange.[48–50]

Although there is substantial uncertainty due to the limited evidence base, it is plausible that black women, or women in general, require more or different (closer) social support compared to black men.[25,42] Disincentives to exercise may predispose black women to require more personalized social support[25]; they may desire direct support from like-minded women who can help them to understand and overcome these disincentives. In a survey of more than 900 black women in South Carolina, encouragement from and accountability to a friend were associated with higher self-reported achievement of physical activity recommendations.[32]

Neighborhood Infrastructure

Many black Americans live in neighborhoods with characteristics that—objectively or as perceived by residents—are not conducive to leisure-time physical activity. In addition to safety, other factors include the availability and accessibility of parks, outdoor recreational facilities, and indoor recreational spaces or centers.[51–53] The cost of using facilities is also a consideration. Cost would presumably be more of a constraint for black women because of the gender gap in wages.[37] Also, where facilities are present, some may be more geared to or used primarily by men, to the potential exclusion of women. A follow-up on physical activity behavior among participants in the longitudinal Coronary Artery Risk in Young Adults (CARDIA) study found that increased access to recreational facilities was associated with lower BMI in men but not women.[54] Men and women may both be concerned about the perceived safety of being outdoors in the evening, but presumably this is of greater concern for women.

Agent-based Model

Data

In order to determine whether our model had the ability to reproduce behaviors and outcomes similar to those in the real world, we first needed to identify data with which the model could be compared. These data needed to be able to provide a basis for agents and environments that could be used in model runs as well as observable behaviors and outcomes analogous to those produced by the model. We used the Chicago Community Adult Health Study (CCAHS) as a foundation for a comparison data source. The dataset contains detailed observations of household demographic characteristics, health behaviors and measurements (including physical activity), and neighborhood and social environments for 3,105 adults living in Chicago between 2001 and 2003.[55] Because of the relatively small sample size of black respondents within specific neighborhoods, we used 2000 census data to determine the black adult population within each neighborhood, disaggregated by gender and age group.

Specifications

The agents in our model represented black adult residents of Chicago, each residing in a specific neighborhood. Agents could be males or females of different ages. During each simulated day, there was a probability that each agent was affected by factors that influenced their availability to exercise (figure 4). Those who did not experience these constraints could potentially engage in exercise. The probability that available male agents would be willing to exercise was proportional to the product of their neighborhood's safety and infrastructure scores. We posited that willing males would actually engage in exercise in a given time period if there were any other similar-aged males who were willing to exercise in their neighborhood, and that female agents would exercise only when they could find a similar-aged female partner in the neighborhood who was not currently exercising with another partner. Female pairs would then exercise with probability proportional to the product of their neighborhood's safety and infrastructure scores. We ran the simulation for a 30-day time period, during which we output exercise rates for men and women both overall and disaggregated by age group.

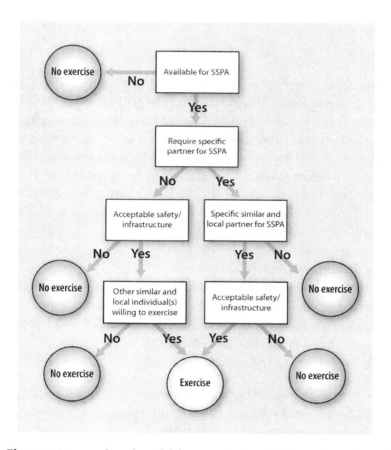

Figure 4. Elements in agent-based model for socially situated leisure-time physical activity

Experimental Variations

In order to explore the role of various mechanisms in generating differences between exercise levels in black men and women, we simulated combinations of the following variations from the baseline model:

1. *Differential availability.* We varied the amount by which female agents were more likely to face constraints on their availability on a given day relative to men.

2. *Differential decision behavior.* We varied the behavior of female agents in the model so that they participated in exercise in the same way as male agents, in terms of partnering.

3. *Differential sensitivity to neighborhood infrastructure and safety.* We allowed for female agents to have either greater or lesser sensitivity to neighborhood infrastructure and safety. We varied this both under baseline conditions—allowing us to explore the role of differential sensitivity in explaining the variation in overall exercise participation rates between men and women—as well as under hypothetical intervention scenarios where infrastructure and safety were improved in particular neighborhoods. This allowed us to explore how such interventions might differentially affect exercise for men and women.

Findings

Before manipulating the model conditions, we first examined how our model output compared to real-world patterns of leisure-time physical activity in a baseline setting analogous to the simulated environment. The CCAHS survey data included responses to several questions about physical activity. The most relevant for our study asked (1) how many days during an average week respondents engaged in light- to moderate-intensity leisure activities for more than 10 minutes and (2) how many days during the average week respondents engaged in vigorous-intensity leisure activities for more than 10 minutes. Both of these measures could be easily translated into daily exercise rates to better correspond to our model's output. Unfortunately, responses to these questions were not completely analogous to the behavior that our model explored. The first question combines light-intensity physical activity (a level that does not contribute to meeting health-related physical activity guidelines) with moderate-intensity physical activity, and responses to these two types of physical activity cannot be separated. Furthermore, we do not know whether gender differences in socially situated physical activity are the same as for overall leisure-time physical activity. However, these responses were useful for comparison to our model output in order to ensure that a minimal validation threshold was reached; if our model output for the gender differences was substantially different from these values, then we should question whether we have correctly operationalized socially situated physical activity for black men and women in Chicago.

Based on mean responses of black men and women aged between 18 and 65 years, reported daily rates of both light- to moderate-intensity and vigorous-intensity physical activity were greater for men than that for women by approximately 4 percent and 8 percent, respectively. Our model produced a range of gender differences in exercise that were generally similar to (and contained) the differences in leisure-time physical activity observed in responses to the two survey questions. Therefore, although we cannot definitively state that our model is an accurate depiction of the processes that it is intended to explore, our evidence suggests that it is a meaningful representation of gender differences in exercise behavior for this set of individuals.

We next explored differences in physical activity between men and women under different conditions. Specifically, we ran simulations using every combination of four differential female availability values, three differential female sensitivities to neighborhood infrastructure and safety, and with differential female exercise behavior both on and off. Figure 5 shows mean gender differences obtained from each of these conditions; it also depicts variations in gender differences across 10 repeated runs per condition. This variation is visible only upon close inspection of the figure, underscoring the overall lack of variation in mean differences in physical activity across the runs; this suggests that the 10 runs we conducted for each condition were sufficient to detect relatively small (one or two percentage points) differences in outcomes between conditions. The female-partner-availability constraint multiplier (x axis) varies within each panel. Male and female availabilities are equivalent when the multiplier is 1, and females are six times more likely to be unavailable when the multiplier is 6. In the top row, men's and women's decisions about exercise partnering are based on equivalent behavior, that is, both men and women did not need to find specific partners, but would exercise if any same-sex, similar-aged peer in the neighborhood was also willing to exercise. In the bottom row, women have different exercise behaviors than men and require specific exercise partners.

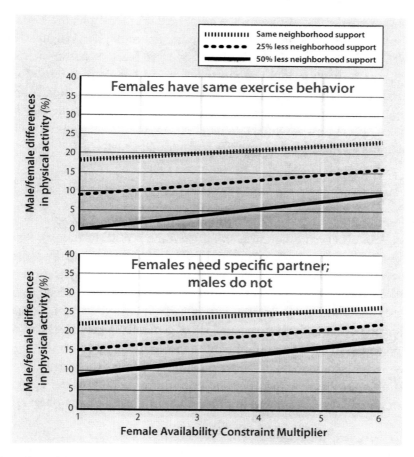

Figure 5. Agent-based model results for socially situated leisure-time physical activity by extent of constraints on female peer availability, varying partnering preferences and supportiveness of neighborhood infrastructure for females and males

Each of the three mechanisms that we explored had an observable and substantial impact on gender differences in exercise, suggesting that they are all potential candidates for interventions to diminish those differences. When none of these mechanisms were present (i.e., when partnering preferences and the effects of neighborhood conditions were the same and the multiplier for female availability constraints is 1, there were also no gender differences in exercise. However, with the addition of each mechanism, gender differences increased.

First, we saw a substantial linear relationship between the female unavailability multiplier and gender differences in physical activity. A change in multiplier from 1 to 6 in figure 5A was associated with the introduction of a 10 percentage-point gender difference in exercise. Next, figure 5B and C shows a gender difference increase of about 10 percent (figure 5B) and 17 percent (figure 5C) relative to figure 5A when neighborhood conditions are, respectively, 25 percent or 50 percent less supportive for women. And finally, figure 5D shows that the effect of females utilizing different behavior than men such that they require specific exercise partners results in an approximately 10 percent increase in gender differences in exercise.

The three mechanisms are generally additive when combined. For example, the slope of the relationship between gender differences and the female availability constraint multiplier in figure 5B and D was roughly the same magnitude as the one in figure 5A. However, we also found negative interaction effects. In the presence of both differential neighborhood supportiveness and female preference for a specific partner (figure 5E and F), the relationship between the female unavailability and gender differences in physical activity decreased slightly relative to that seen in figure 5A. These negative interaction effects can be explained by "floor effects" that appear when certain neighborhoods have no women exercising as a result of either differential neighborhood support or exercise partnering behavior.

Implications

This simple agent-based model supported our hypothesis that socially situated aspects of physical activity can potentially explain observed differences in leisure-time physical activity between black men and women. It offers a novel approach to understanding the dynamics that potentially contribute to lower day-to-day exercise participation in black men and women, and has broader implications for the use of complex systems simulations for the determinants of physical activity. An intentionally simplistic model can provide important insights, especially during the early stages of inquiry into a phenomenon. Although our model is stylized, omitting detail to focus on a small set of generalized behaviors and mechanisms, experiments using this model identified important influences and relationships representing promising avenues for further study. As we better understand gender differences in physical activity, the nuances related to the specific variables of interest can be incorporated into future versions of our agent-based model. This work contributes to a potentially vibrant and important iterative synthesis of observational and complex systems approaches.

Numerous intervention studies have been conducted to understand strategies for successfully increasing and maintaining participation in physical activity among black Americans and other population subgroups that are the least active, both within and outside of the context of weight control studies.[56-61] In general, the intervention strategies show little to no immediate improvements in physical activity, and most show no long-term maintenance of improvements gained during the intervention period. Additional research is needed to understand the factors influencing participation in physical activity and methods to address these factors to successfully increase and maintain physical activity levels and improve related health outcomes.

Our agent-based model generates insights into how key barriers to physical activity, including constraints on women's availability for exercise, combined with neighborhood characteristics that may be more supportive of exercise for men than women, can result in lower levels of exercise in women than in men; this gap widens when women do not have access to social support from specific partners. The model does not address absolute levels of leisure-time physical activity and does not directly simulate or inform policies or programs to increase the percentage of black men and women who achieve recommended levels of physical activity, although we can envision models designed specifically for that purpose. Nonetheless, our results may help to identify strategies for helping black women increase exercise levels to a greater degree than relying only on ongoing initiatives to increase leisure-time physical activity among adults in general. Our results may also offer insights for increasing exercise levels among women in other racial or ethnic groups.

If one assumes that women's preferences for specific partners are not readily modifiable, our model suggests that policies or other initiatives focusing on women's availability for exercise and supportive neighborhood characteristics (both potentially modifiable factors) could improve women's exercise participation relative to that of men. Time demands, exercise during pregnancy, and physical limitations—while not modeled separately—are all potential targets of policies or initiatives in localities or workplaces. For example, providing child care or activities for children in indoor or outdoor home or recreational settings might enable more women to exercise (e.g., in housing developments, gyms, parks, and recreation areas). Similarly, providing activities for parents to do separately or together with their children at child care, school, or after-school settings might be particularly beneficial for black female heads of households (e.g., recreation centers or YMCAs with walking tracks around sports fields, so parents can exercise while children play sports). Increasingly, community-level social networks, such as Black Girls Run! and Girl Trek[62,63], encourage physical activity by engaging black women as leaders to inspire and provide support for other black women and their children to exercise, regardless of weight or fitness level. Girl Trek provides community- and neighborhood-level exercise opportunities in which women are encouraged to bring children in strollers and to involve young children in exercise. A motto of Black Girls Run! is "no woman left behind"; participants are encouraged to cheer on fellow participants until the last ones finish, and faster runners often double back after finishing their workouts to support and encourage slower runners and walkers.

In order to address the reluctance among pregnant women to exercise, health care providers and programs that reach large numbers of pregnant women—such as the federal Supplemental Nutrition Program for Women, Infants, and Children (WIC)—could emphasize the dissemination of exercise recommendations for pregnant women. Other effective strategies may include increasing the availability and visibility of exercise staff trained and certified to address pregnancy-related safety concerns; special classes for pregnant women during prenatal care; and social marketing programs using role models to change norms about appropriate activities for pregnant women. Similar strategies could be applied to enable and encourage exercise among people with physical limitations on the types of exercise they can do. While initiatives directed to women with large body sizes could be perceived as stereotyping or stigmatizing them, initiatives tailored to all levels of functional ability may be useful for reaching heavier women (e.g., Black Girls Run's "Walk Before You Run" program).

Ideally, approaches that improve exercise infrastructure for women would complement initiatives that increase the overall availability of exercise resources in black neighborhoods. Improving neighborhood safety in ways that encourage outdoor activity could also benefit women. Finally, reducing the cost of participating in leisure-time physical activity at venues where fees are charged, possibly through subsidies, could be particularly beneficial for women, as would women-only days and activities.

References

1. US Department of Health and Human Services. *Physical Activity and Health: A Report of the Surgeon General.* Hyattsville, MD: US DHHS, Centers for Disease Control and Prevention, National Center for Chronic Disease Prevention and Health Promotion; 1996.

2. Richardson CR, Kriska AM, Lantz PM, Hayward RA. Physical activity and mortality across cardiovascular disease risk groups. *Med Sci Sports Exerc.* 2004;36(11):1923–1929.

3. Carroll S, Dudfield M. What is the relationship between exercise and metabolic abnormalities? A review of the metabolic syndrome. *Sports Med.* 2004;34(6):371–418.

4. Schnohr P, Scharling H, Jensen JS. Changes in leisure-time physical activity and risk of death: an observational study of 7,000 men and women. *Am J Epidemiol.* 2003;158(7):639–644.

5. Brown DW, Balluz LS, Heath GW, et al. Associations between recommended levels of physical activity and health-related quality of life. Findings from the 2001 Behavioral Risk Factor Surveillance System (BRFSS) survey. *Prev Med.* 2003;37(5):520–528.

6. Erlichman J, Kerbey AL, James WP. Physical activity and its impact on health outcomes. Paper 1: the impact of physical activity on cardiovascular disease and all-cause mortality: an historical perspective. *Obes Rev.* 2002;3(4):257–271.

7. Haapanen-Niemi N, Miilunpalo S, Pasanen M, Vuori I, Oja P, Malmberg J. Body mass index, physical inactivity and low level of physical fitness as determinants of all-cause and cardiovascular disease mortality—16 y follow-up of middle-aged and elderly men and women. *Int J Obes Relat Metab Disord.* 2000;24(11):1465–1474.

8. Ellekjaer H, Holmen J, Ellekjaer E, Vatten L. Physical activity and stroke mortality in women. Ten-year follow-up of the Nord-Trondelag health survey, 1984–1986. *Stroke.* 2000;31(1):14–18.

9. US Department of Health and Human Services. 2008 physical activity guidelines for Americans. 2008. https://health.gov/paguidelines/guidelines/

10. Centers for Disease Control and Prevention. Physical Activity and Health. 2015. http://www.cdc.gov/physicalactivity/everyone/health/index.html?s_cid=cs_284. Accessed July 11, 2015.

11. Institute of Medicine. *Accelerating Progress in Obesity Prevention. Solving the Weight of the Nation.* Washington, DC: National Academies Press; 2012.

12. National Center for Health Statistics. *Health, United States, 2014: With Special Feature on Adults Aged 55–64.* Washington, DC: US Government Printing Office; 2015.

13. Troiano RP, Berrigan D, Dodd KW, Masse LC, Tilert T, McDowell M. Physical activity in the United States measured by accelerometer. *Med Sci Sports Exerc.* 2008;40(1):181–188.

14. 2013 National Health Interview Survey Questionnaire. Adult Health Behaviors. ftp://ftp.cdc.gov/pub/Health_Statistics/NCHS/Survey_Questionnaires/NHIS/2013/English/. Centers for Disease Control and Prevention. Accessed May 29, 2014.

15. Matthews CE, Cohen SS, Fowke JH, et al. Physical activity, sedentary behavior, and cause-specific mortality in black and white adults in the Southern Community Cohort Study. *Am J Epidemiol.* 2014;180(4):394–405.

16. Arem H, Moore SC, Patel A, et al. Leisure time physical activity and mortality: a detailed pooled analysis of the dose-response relationship. *JAMA Intern Med.* 2015;175(6):959–967.

17. Whitt-Glover MC, Taylor WC, Heath GW, Macera CA. Self-reported physical activity among blacks: estimates from national surveys. *Am J Prev Med.* 2007;33(5):412–417.

18. Belza B, Walwick J, Shiu-Thornton S, Schwartz S, Taylor M, LoGerfo J. Older adult perspectives on physical activity and exercise: voices from multiple cultures. *Prev Chronic Dis.* 2004;1(4):A09.

19. Eyler AA, Brownson RC, Donatelle RJ, King AC, Brown D, Sallis JF. Physical activity, social support, and middle- and older-aged minority women: results from a US survey. *Soc Sci Med.* 1999;49(6):781–789.

20. McNeill LH, Kreuter MW, Subramanian SV. Social environment and physical activity: a review of concepts and evidence. *Soc Sci Med.* 2006;63(4):1011–1022.

21. Kahn EB, Ramsey LT, Brownson RC, et al. The effectiveness of interventions to increase physical activity. A systematic review. *Am J Prev Med.* 2002;22(4 Suppl):73–107.

22. Centola D. An experimental study of homophily in the adoption of health behavior. *Science.* 2011;334(6060):1269–1272.

23. Hooker SP, Wilcox S, Rheaume CE, Burroughs EL, Friedman DB. Factors related to physical activity and recommended intervention strategies as told by midlife and older African American men. *Ethn Dis.* 2011;21(3):261–267.

24. Brownson RC, Eyler AA, King AC, Brown DR, Shyu YL, Sallis JF. Patterns and correlates of physical activity among US women 40 years and older. *Am J Public Health.* 2000;90(2):264–270.

25. Fleury J, Lee SM. The social ecological model and physical activity in African American women. *Am J Community Psychol.* 2006;37(1-2):129–140.

26. Shuval K, Hébert ET, Siddiqi Z, et al. Impediments and facilitators to physical activity and perceptions of sedentary behavior among urban community residents: the Fair Park Study. *Prev Chronic Dis.* 2013;10:E177.

27. Siddiqi Z, Tiro JA, Shuval K. Understanding impediments and enablers to physical activity among African American adults: a systematic review of qualitative studies. *Health Educ Res.* 2011;26(6):1010–1024.

28. Griffith DM, King A, Ober Allen J. Male peer influence on African American men's motivation for physical activity: men's and women's perspectives. *Am J Mens Health.* 2013;7(2):169–178.

29. Cogbill SA, Thompson VL, Deshpande AD. Selected sociocultural correlates of physical activity among African-American adults. *Ethn Health.* 2011;16(6):625–641.

30. Epstein JM. *Generative Social Science. Studies in Agent-based Computational Modeling.* Princeton, NJ: Princeton University Press; 2006.

31. Mattingly MJ, Blanchi SM. Gender differences in the quantity and quality of free time: the US experience. *Soc Forces.* 2003;81(3):999–1030.

32. Ainsworth BE, Wilcox S, Thompson WW, Richter DL, Henderson KA. Personal, social, and physical environmental correlates of physical activity in African-American women in South Carolina. *Am J Prev Med.* 2003;25(3 Suppl 1):23–29.

33. Baruth M, Sharpe PA, Parra-Medina D, Wilcox S. Perceived barriers to exercise and healthy eating among women from disadvantaged neighborhoods: results from a focus groups assessment. *Womens Health.* 2014;54(4):336–353.

34. Eyler AA, Baker E, Cromer L, King AC, Brownson RC, Donatelle RJ. Physical activity and minority women: a qualitative study. *Health Educ Behav.* 1998;25(5):640–652.

35. King AC, Castro C, Wilcox S, Eyler AA, Sallis JF, Brownson RC. Personal and environmental factors associated with physical inactivity among different racial-ethnic groups of US middle-aged and older-aged women. *Health Psychol.* 2000;19(4):354–364.

36. Shelton RC, McNeill LH, Puleo E, Wolin KY, Emmons KM, Bennett GG. The association between social factors and physical activity among low-income adults living in public housing. *Am J Public Health.* 2011;101(11):2102–2110.

37. US Department of Labor. Office of the Secretary. The African-American Labor Force in the Recovery. Washington, DC: DOL Office of the Secretary. http://www.dol.gov/_sec/media/reports/blacklaborforce/. Accessed February 29, 2012.

38. US Department of Health and Human Services. *Women's Health USA 2012.* Rockville, MD: US DHHS Health Resources and Services Administration, Maternal and Child Health Bureau; 2013.

39. Gaston A, Cramp A. Exercise during pregnancy: a review of patterns and determinants. *J Sci Med Sport.* 2011;14(4):299–305.

40. Taylor WC, Yancey AK, Leslie J, et al. Physical activity among African American and Latino middle school girls: consistent beliefs, expectations, and experiences across two sites. *Women Health.* 1999;30(2):67–82.

41. Vu MB, Murrie D, Gonzalez V, Jobe JB. Listening to girls and boys talk about girls' physical activity behaviors. *Health Educ Behav.* 2006;33(1):81–96.

42. Ray R. An intersectional analysis to explaining a lack of physical activity among middle class black women. *Sociol Compass.* 2014;8(6):780–791.

43. Kumanyika S. Obesity, health disparities, and prevention paradigms: hard questions and hard choices. *Prev Chronic Dis.* 2005;2(4):A02.

44. Craig P. Obesity and culture. In: Kopelman PK, Caterson ID, Dietz WH, eds. *Clinical Obesity in Adults and Children.* 3rd ed. West Sussex, UK: Wiley-Blackwell. 2010:41–57.

45. Versey HS. Centering perspectives on black women, hair politics, and physical activity. *Am J Public Health.* 2014;104(5):810–815.

46. Hall RR, Francis S, Whitt-Glover M, Loftin-Bell K, Swett K, McMichael AJ. Hair care practices as a barrier to physical activity in African American women. *JAMA Dermatol.* 2013;149(3):310–314.

47. Boyington JE, Carter-Edwards L, Piehl M, Hutson J, Langdon D, McManus S. Cultural attitudes toward weight, diet, and physical activity among overweight African American girls. *Prev Chronic Dis.* 2008;5(2):A36.

48. Evenson KR, Aytur SA, Borodulin K. Physical activity beliefs, barriers, and enablers among postpartum women. *J Womens Health.* 2009;18(12):1925–1934.

49. Evenson KR, Sarmiento OL, Macon ML, Tawney KW, Ammerman AS. Environmental, policy, and cultural factors related to physical activity among Latina immigrants. *Women Health.* 2002;36(2):43–57.

50. Miller ST, Marolen K. Physical activity-related experiences, counseling expectations, personal responsibility, and altruism among urban African American women with type 2 diabetes. *Diabetes Educ.* 2012;38(2):229–235.

51. Franzini L, Taylor W, Elliott MN, et al. Neighborhood characteristics favorable to outdoor physical activity: disparities by socioeconomic and racial/ethnic composition. *Health Place.* 2010;16(2):267–274.

52. Taylor WC, Sallis JF, Lees E, et al. Changing social and built environments to promote physical activity: recommendations from low income, urban women. *J Phys Act Health.* 2007;4(1):54–65.

53. Lovasi GS, Hutson MA, Guerra M, Neckerman KM. Built environments and obesity in disadvantaged populations. *Epidemiol Rev.* 2009;31:7–20.

54. Boone-Heinonen J, Diez Roux AV, Goff DC, et al. The neighborhood energy balance equation: does neighborhood food retail environment + physical activity environment = obesity? The CARDIA study. *PLoS One.* 2013;8(12):e85141.

55. House JS, Kaplan, GA, Morenoff J, Raudenbush SW, Williams DR, Young EA. *Chicago Community Adult Health Study, 2001–2003.* Ann Arbor, MI: Inter-university Consortium for Political and Social Research; 2012. ICPSR31142-v1.

56. Banks-Wallace J, Conn V. Interventions to promote physical activity among African American women. *Public Health Nurs.* 2002;19(5):321–335.

57. Taylor WC, Baranowski T, Young DR. Physical activity interventions in low-income, ethnic minority, and populations with disability. *Am J Prev Med.* 1998;15(4):334–343.

58. Whitt-Glover MC, Brand DJ, Turner ME, Ward SA, Jackson EM. Increasing physical activity among African-American women and girls. *Curr Sports Med Rep.* 2009;8(6):318–324.

59. Whitt-Glover MC, Crespo CJ, Joe J. Recommendations for advancing opportunities to increase physical activity in racial/ethnic minority communities. *Prev Med.* 2009;49(4):292–293.

60. Whitt-Glover MC, Kumanyika SK. Systematic review of interventions to increase physical activity and physical fitness in African-Americans. *Am J Health Promot.* 2009;23(6):S33–S56.

61. Whitt-Glover MC, Keith NR, Ceaser TG, Virgil K, Ledford L, Hasson RE. A systematic review of physical activity interventions among African American adults: evidence from 2009 to 2013. *Obes Rev.* 2014;15(Suppl 4):125–145.

62. Girl Trek Website. http://www.girltrek.org. Accessed August 23, 2015.

63. Black Girls Run! Website. http://blackgirlsrun.com. Accessed August 23, 2015.

CHAPTER 8

INDIVIDUAL, SOCIAL, AND INSTITUTIONAL PRACTICES DETERMINING SCHOOL AND COLLEGE CHOICE

Matt Kasman, PhD
Research Associate
Center on Social Dynamics and Policy
Brookings Institution

Daniel Klasik, PhD
Assistant Professor
Graduate School of Education and Human Development
The George Washington University

Acknowledgments: This chapter was supported in part by the Educational Testing Service (ETS). The views expressed here are our own and do not reflect the views of ETS. We appreciate the help and advice of Elizabeth Bruch, Rucker Johnson, Gary Orfield, Mark Long, Ross Hammond, Rachel Baker, Joe Townsend, Sean Reardon, Susanna Loeb, Terry Moe, Mark Granovetter, and Prudence Carter.

A large and consistent body of research explores the connections between high levels of education and positive health outcomes, including greater life expectancy[1]; lower levels of diabetes, heart disease, and obesity[1]; lower rates of infant mortality for more educated mothers[1]; and reduced stress.[2] These relationships have been linked to a number of potential causes. People with higher levels of education are able to live in neighborhoods with the types of resources that tend to make residents healthier—access to supermarkets with healthy food, more green space, more health care providers, and lower pollution and crime rates.[3] Furthermore, people with higher levels of education have access to large social networks that can provide information and resources to reduce hardship. Individuals with more education also have access to better jobs, which are more likely to provide comprehensive health insurance benefits.

Like many of its related health outcomes, educational quality has strong links to race and socioeconomic status. From preschool to college, students from lower socioeconomic backgrounds, as well as racial and ethnic minority groups, face obstacles that limit their access to educational opportunities. As a result, there are wide educational disparities between these groups and those who are white and of higher socioeconomic status, starting when children enter school and amplifying as students move through high school and postsecondary education. These disparities lead to dramatic income—and thus health—inequality.

Educational quality is difficult to quantify, but there is wide agreement that it broadly consists of attainment (e.g., finishing high school) and high-quality educational experiences. It is important not just whether people attend school or attain a particular educational level, but where they do so. The school that a student attends determines who their fellow students are, the teachers who instruct them, the policies and curricula that they encounter, and the resources allocated to their education; all are strongly related to educational quality and future outcomes.

There are two entry points where access to educational opportunities may be available or constrained in ways that have substantial impacts. The first is entry into grade school, usually in kindergarten. An increasing proportion of families are able to choose their children's grade schools via mechanisms that include charter schools, vouchers, and intra- and interdistrict selection.[4-6] These choices are important because they set students on a path that can have them rising above, or falling behind, their peers. Early gains and losses can determine later school and course placement and have dramatic implications for whether and where a student attends college.

The second important entry point is higher education, such as a college or university. A developing body of research connects higher levels of income not just with whether someone attends or completes any college, but with the selectivity of the college a student attends.[7-10] While attending college leads to notable economic returns, attending an more-selective college is associated with even greater returns; a degree from a top-tier university provides benefits that tend to be much larger than those from a nonselective community college. However, because of differences in educational opportunities afforded to students from differing backgrounds, not all levels of education, and certainly not all levels of college selectivity are realistic options for all students. For example, there are dramatic differences in postsecondary destinations by both race and socioeconomic status. White students are over five times more likely to enroll in a highly selective college than black students, and students from the highest income quintile are seven to eight times more likely to enroll in a highly selective college.[11]

Understanding the mechanisms that generate socioeconomic and racial disparities in educational quality at these two key points in time is not an easy task. Education lies at the intersection of a number of interests, institutions, and cultural influences. Families have a vested interest in the educational success of their offspring and the myriad benefits that this success tends to foster, including health outcomes. Similarly, society as a whole, as well as specific subentities within it, such as communities and businesses, have an interest in the amount and form of education that individuals receive. A number of institutions have been built to meet these interests: public and private schools serving kindergarten through 12th grade; pre-kindergarten centers and programs; colleges and universities that offer an astonishing variety of programs, specializations, preparatory programs, and degrees; and an array of ancillary services and organizations that includes government agencies, accrediting bodies, textbook publishers, testing companies, and a burgeoning tutoring industry.

Two cultural values have had an especially large impact on the development of the educational landscape: equality and freedom. These values often come into conflict with one another; imposing equality by necessity restricts freedom, and allowing unfettered freedom inevitably sets the stage for inequality. Equality and freedom have been uneasily reconciled at key points in time to shape educational institutions, which in turn play a role in racial and socioeconomic disparities in education. Our deep-seated belief in equality has led to the system of universal public education that Americans enjoy, where all children are guaranteed access to free kindergarten through 12th-grade education. However, there is ample room for freedom: families can select their children's schools in a variety of ways. Similarly, there is growing sentiment that some form of postsecondary education should be available to all students. Freedom plays a much larger role at this level, with students free to apply to and potentially enroll in a staggering number of colleges, and for colleges to decide whom to admit. On its surface, the question of where a particular person attends school seems simple: one of a finite, discrete number of available options. However, closer examination reveals that enrollment is the result of complex, dynamic processes. The choices that students—or families, on behalf of their children—make—are based on an evaluation of their observable options, which are determined in part by the selection and enrollment decisions made by others in the past (e.g., perception of a school's student body). Institutional rules determine whether and how schools decide between prospective students, when there are more applicants than spaces. And students then must use some set of criteria to determine how to respond to admission decisions.

To explore patterns of enrollment, we use a complex systems approach. Specifically, we use agent-based models to investigate some of the mechanisms that lead to observable racial and socioeconomic disparities in enrollment in two different settings. In this chapter, we first explore intra-district elementary school choice and then investigate some of the ways race and socioeconomic status shape patterns of college attendance.

Why Use Complex Systems Approaches?

Intra-District School Choice

Intra-district school choice, also known as open enrollment, is an increasingly common feature of large, urban school districts. These policies give families the option of selecting public schools for their children that differ from their default neighborhood schools; in some cases, open enrollment policies do away with default schools entirely and ask that every family list a set of preferred schools. Because open enrollment policies explicitly decouple school attendance from residence, many have argued that they have the potential to increase diversity within district schools by creating opportunities for families in overwhelmingly impoverished, minority neighborhoods to access schools other than highly segregated (and often low-achieving) traditional neighborhood schools. Unfortunately, in practice the impact of open enrollment policies on diversity has been underwhelming. In large urban school districts that have implemented these policies, many schools still serve a substantial majority of students from a single racial background. For example, New York City is the largest school district in the nation and strongly embraced school choice after Michael Bloomberg became mayor in 2002.[12] In the 2010–2011 school year, however, 85 percent of black students in New York City schools and 75 percent of Latino students attended schools that were composed of between 90 percent and 100 percent minority students, an increase from 81 percent and 73 percent, respectively, in the 1999–2000 school year.[13] In order for open enrollment policies to have the desired effect upon diversity, it is necessary to understand what might be limiting their impact and under what (if any) conditions they can succeed.

The student composition of schools in open enrollment districts is the result of a process that consists of three distinct stages. First, families select a set of schools in a descending order of desirability. Then, assignments are made based on these selections as well as rules that determine student priorities for seats at schools. Finally, parents can choose to enroll in their assigned school, request reassignment, or not enroll in the school district (for example, they may choose to enroll in a private school or relocate to a suburban school district). This multistage process is both complicated and dynamic. A family's school selections in a given year affect not only their own child's assignment, but also assignments for other students; space in a school that is in high demand (i.e., where there are more requests for seats than available spots) is allocated according to priority rules set by the district, and in such situations when student with higher priority selects a school, another does student to not receive a seat in that school. Similarly, enrollment decisions can affect those of other families; for example, when a family chooses not to register following assignment, that seat may go to another family that strongly desires it. Finally, the enrollment process in one year directly affects the observable composition of schools, which in turn can influence the school selection and enrollment decisions made by families the following year.

Because the open enrollment process is complex and dynamic, discerning trends in school and district composition under existing or putative conditions is not straightforward. Therefore, agent-based model simulations of the open enrollment process are an appropriate approach that can help determine diversity trends in large, urban school districts under current policy conditions as well as under experimental conditions representing policies that the district might consider implementing.

College Enrollment

Students are stratified into postsecondary education by race and family income (figures 1 and 2). Figure 1 shows the postsecondary destinations of the high school class of 2004 by college selectivity and race/ethnicity.[11] Very selective colleges (those colleges with Barron's Selectivity ratings of 1, 2, or 3 out of 6) have many more white students and many fewer black and Hispanic students than the population of 18-year-olds overall. However, despite the pattern of decreasing racial diversity with increasing selectivity, the most selective colleges (Barron's 1s) are slightly more diverse than the colleges just below them in the selectivity ratings.

In 2004, students with family incomes in the 80th percentile nationally were four times more likely to enroll in a highly selective school—one in the top two Barron's selectivity groups—than a student in the 20th income percentile (figure 2). This disparity is even more extreme for families in higher and lower income percentiles. Reardon et al.[11] showed that students from families earning more than $75,000 (in 2001 dollars) were dramatically overrepresented in the most selective categories of colleges, while students from families earning less than $25,000 were notably underrepresented at these same schools.[11] Such disparities are not new, but the underrepresentation of low-income students at highly selective schools has increased over time.[14-17]

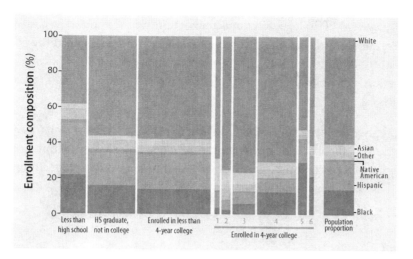

Figure 1. Racial composition of postsecondary destinations, class of 2004. Width of each bar represents percentage of college-age population enrolled the given level of school. Barron's ratings are based on measures of 4-year college selectivity; a rating range from 1, indicating the most selective colleges, to 6, indicating the least selective

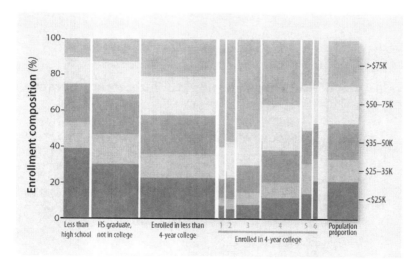

Figure 2. Income composition of postsecondary destinations, class of 2004. Barron's ratings are based on measures of 4-year college selectivity; a rating range from 1, indicating the most selective colleges, to 6, indicating the least selective

An agent-based model is ideal for answering our questions because it allows for the multistep interaction of students with colleges (application, admission, enrollment) and for both students and colleges to learn from the past. Although students in our model do not interact explicitly, their decisions do affect each other; because college seats are finite, the application decisions of each student affect the admission likelihoods of other students. By using an agent-based simulation model we were able to compare the effects of a range of practices and policies on enrollment patterns in a way that took into account how these actions would affect the entire system of colleges. By repeatedly running the model over many cohorts, we were able to study the emergent patterns of college sorting that arise from changes in the college sorting mechanisms we set out to study. Although this model is not completely realistic, it captures important dynamic features of the application, admissions, and enrollment processes, enabling us to investigate the ways that students sort into colleges.

In our work, we first set out to develop insights into which resource-based mechanisms could explain the stark racial and income-based sorting of students into colleges according to admissions selectivity. Then, we investigated alternatives to race-conscious affirmative action based on socioeconomic status.[18,19]

Methods

Intra-District School Choice

Family behavior in these simulations is based on analyses of a rich set of administrative data from a large, urban school district, which includes information on students, schools, school programs, school applications, school assignments, and enrollment. These analyses focus on students choosing kindergarten programs for the 2011–2012 and 2012–2013 school years (tables 1 and 2).

Table 1

Racial Composition of Students Choosing Kindergarten Programs (n = 8,437)

Prospective Students	(%)
Black	9.77
Hispanic	27.30
White	20.34
Asian	37.47
Other	2.52

Baseline Simulation

The baseline simulation model of the school enrollment process followed through these steps (figure 3):

Initialization: An initial set of school programs that families will be given as options is generated based on prior-year school data. A single cohort's worth of prospective students is sampled from the full set of student data. These students have three properties: race, residential location, and a latent "achievement" value assigned based on race-specific achievement distributions in the district. The attributes of school programs

Table 2

School Year Options in a Large, Urban School District

	2011–2012 (n = 69)	2012–2013 (n = 68)
Black (%)	13.2 (16.2)	13.2 (16.4)
White (%)	14.4 (13.5)	15.8 (15.3)
Hispanic (%)	26.2 (24.2)	25.6 (24.0)
Asian (%)	39.1 (25.9)	39.0 (26.0)
Eligible for free or reduced price lunch (FRPL) (%)	60.0 (21.1)	60.6 (23.4)
Enrollment	387.2 (140.1)	393.0 (138.3)
Mean English Language Arts (ELA) score	362.8 (27.8)	366.5 (29.9)
Mean math test score	394.6 (39.2)	398.7 (38.4)
Dual immersion language programs (%)	21.7	20.6
Bilingual language programs (%)	36.2	36.8
General education programs (%)	92.8	94.1

Values represent means from prior school year (except for FRPL, which is taken from 2 years prior). Standard deviations are reported in parentheses.

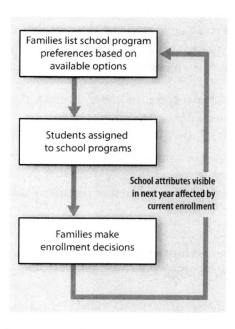

Figure 3. Stages of student enrollment process included in agent-based model

available for these simulated students include location, school achievement, school demographics, and program type (i.e., general education or language specialization).

School choice: Using race-specific estimates of participation probability (i.e., who "chooses to choose"), the set of students who will make school program selections is identified. Analyses of school selection behavior in this school district is used to inform the selections made by families in these simulations; each student who participates in the choice process makes a ranked set of school program selections.

Student assignment: Based on students' school selections and priorities (i.e., residence within an attendance zone or a low test-score area), students are assigned using a deferred-acceptance student assignment algorithm. Deferred-acceptance algorithms, which are also used to match medical school students to residencies, are computationally more complex than their predecessors, but have the advantage of not presenting any opportunities for families to try to game the school selection process. Because these algorithms incorporate temporary placement into spots in schools that can be revoked during subsequent steps, a student does not gain any advantages based on how their family ranks schools. Therefore, the dominant strategy for families is simply to list their true preferences for schools, and the assignment process is described as "strategy-proof." In addition, these algorithms are highly effective at placing students in schools, with far fewer prospective students left unassigned at the end of the process than alternative algorithms.[20,21] Students who remain unassigned as well as those who did not submit selections are randomly sorted and assigned to the closest school with an available kindergarten seat.

Student enrollment: After receiving their assignments, students' probabilities of enrolling in their assigned school are calculated based on analyses of enrollment behavior in the district.

Iteration: After students have enrolled or chosen not to enroll in district schools, schools are updated to reflect incoming kindergarten students; based on enrolling students, schools update their achievement levels, racial demographics, and percentage of students who are eligible for free or reduced-price lunch. Then the next year begins with the creation of a new cohort of students sampled from the full set of student data, who view the updated schools when making their program selections.

Output: After the model has run for a specified number of years, data from the simulation on choice, assignment, and enrollment are saved and used to calculate output metrics by year, including school segregation within the district (Theil's H), attrition rates from the district (both total and disaggregated by race), and school enrollment statistics such as distance to school and school achievement levels (both total and disaggregated by race).[1] These metrics will allow for observing trends during the course of the baseline model simulation as well as comparing simulated runs of the school selection and enrollment process.

Experimental Simulations

The simulation can be repeated, but with conditions under which the model operates that are different from the baseline. Intuition about the effect that specific interventions might have on diversity within

---

1   Theil's H is a measure that effectively represents overall school segregation,[24,25] If the composition of kindergarteners in district schools matches the overall composition of kindergarteners in the district, then this value will be 0; under conditions of complete segregation, the value will be 1.

the district is gained by comparing these scenarios to the baseline scenario, which represents the school enrollment trend under current policy conditions. Two considerations guided the alternative conditions under which the model was run. The first was relevance: these scenarios were feasible and, based on discussions with district representatives, could inform decisions about policies that might be considered in the foreseeable future. The second was parameter validity. In order to provide useful information about the outcome of the open enrollment process under specified conditions, simulations must include accurate representations of the selection and enrollment decisions that families make. For example, although it would be interesting to examine a scenario in which assignment priority based on residence in school attendance zones is eliminated, the presence of this policy would likely have a meaningful but unknown influence on observed school selection—through families choosing their residences based on school attendance zones—and outcomes from simulations that remove the policy without adjusting the school selection parameters would be unreliable.

The experimental simulations that were conducted are as follows:

1) *All families participate in the school selection process.* Because not all families participate in the school selection process, this simulation provides a plausible upper bound for the effects of interventions that are intended to increase engagement.

2) *Full participation for black and Hispanic students.* Nonparticipation is particularly prevalent among black and Hispanic families, so this represents the effects of efforts to increase engagement among traditionally disadvantaged students in the district.

3) *Changes in the information provided to families about school quality.* In these two scenarios, the achievement values of schools, which are solely based on mean scores on standardized mathematics and language-arts examinations in the baseline model, are replaced with two simple value-added measures; rather than simply reflecting levels of student achievement, which may conflate multiple sources of input, these measures are intended to specifically represent the effect of schools on students. The first measure uses only between-year gains in mathematics and English Language Arts (ELA) examination scores of students, while the second considers student race, grade level, and school year in which examinations were taken. This represents a shift in the information that is provided by the district. At present, the district publishes school reports that include mean test scores. However, it is possible for the district to follow the example of other large, urban school districts and publish more sophisticated measures of school quality. This scenario can provide insight into possible impacts on school choice and enrollment.

4) *Capacity increases in high-demand kindergarten programs.* Some schools consistently receive more selections than they can meet with assignments. This scenario explores the effects of the district taking actions that expand the number of available seats in these school programs.

5) *Changes in the priority rules used by the student assignment algorithm.* At present, the district has four levels of priority for students selecting kindergarten programs. The first tier includes children who have one or more siblings already attending a selected school. The second includes children who reside in areas designated as low test-score zones by the district. The third includes children

who reside in a school's attendance zone, and the fourth includes all other children. This priority structure is not the district's first, and it is certainly possible that it could change to meet changing political pressures or practical considerations. For example, when presented with evidence from simulations of school choice, the Boston school district recently eliminated priority for "walk zone" students in its student assignment algorithm.[22] Similarly, our scenario explores whether eliminating priority for low-test-score zone residence might have an impact on the school choice and enrollment process in the district.

College Enrollment

Baseline simulation. The same basic agent-based model, designed to provide a simple representation of the college admissions process, drove our investigation of how resource-based patterns of behavior and different affirmative-action admissions policies might affect college sorting. In this model, simulated students and schools engaged in a three-phase college admissions process: students apply to colleges, colleges admit students, and students decide where to enroll.

The students in the model had three defining characteristics: race, resources, and caliber. For simplicity we limited our model to the four largest racial groups in the United States: white, Hispanic, black, and Asian. Five percent of our students were Asian, 15 percent are black, 20 percent are Hispanic, and 60 percent were white. Our resources measure was meant to represent the economic and social capital that a student can tap when engaging in the college application process. These sources of capital, including income, parental education, and knowledge of the college application process, were grouped together because they are highly correlated, and are often conceptually linked together in higher education literature. This resource measure is based on measures of socioeconomic status from the Education Longitudinal Study of 2002 (ELS). Caliber represents the academic qualities that make a student attractive to a college, such as test scores, GPA, and high school transcripts. We constructed our sample of simulated students to match the joint distribution of race, socioeconomic status, and composite math and reading scores in the ELS sample. We converted the scores from the original ELS test-score scale to a scale that approximates the 1,600-point SAT because of the ubiquity of this scale.

In our model, colleges had just one characteristic, which we call "quality." This is simply the average caliber of the students who enrolled in that school in the prior year. In the real world, this mean student caliber is probably correlated with, but not the same as, the quality of educational experience for students at a given college.

As the model iterated through the three admissions stages, many features helped it behave in a way that supported comparisons to real-world college choice behavior. In the first stage, students decide where to submit their applications. They do not apply to every college, so they have to decide which ones to apply to. Our students were relatively sophisticated; they decide where to apply based on a procedure that weighs the estimated likelihood a student will get into a particular school—determined by the results of applications of students with similar caliber to that school in previous iterations of the model—and the quality of a given school. However, as with students in the real world, our students did not have a consensus about what the "best" college is. Rather, they viewed the quality of a college with a certain amount of distortion, with widely varying preferences for different colleges.

Just as students have their own preferences for colleges, colleges have their own preferences for students. In other words, in the second phase of our model, when colleges decide which students to admit, they view a student's caliber with a certain level of idiosyncrasy. This idiosyncrasy reflects the different priorities and needs of college campuses—some students might, for example, get an admissions boost for being an excellent athlete at some colleges, but not others. Colleges also must focus on filling their incoming classes. Each college has a fixed number of seats that they do not want to over- or underfill. Colleges do not know how many of the students that they admit will enroll, so they estimate based on their yield from prior iterations of the model.

In the final stage of our model, students simply looked at the colleges to which they were admitted and enrolled in the one that had the highest perceived quality, according to the individual student's perception of college quality.

Our models did not address issues of cost or financial aid. It is unclear how cost and financial aid decisions should affect the stratification that we observed in our models. On the one hand, more selective colleges cost more to attend than less selective ones, perhaps exaggerating resource-based stratification. On the other hand, financial aid can temper some of these cost differences, perhaps reducing resource-based stratification. Because financial aid considerations are well studied elsewhere, our goal at least in these versions of our model was to focus on the enrollment effects of mechanisms other than cost and aid.

Because there is a certain amount of learning that happens in the model—colleges learn to anticipate yield rates, students learn how likely they are to be admitted to particular colleges—we ran the model for up to 30 years in order for this learning to occur and the model to stabilize. Note that these learning processes were identical for all colleges and students. In each of these iterations, the 40 colleges in our simulated world stayed the same and tried to fill a class of 150 students out of a new set of 10,000 students each.

Starting from this basic model, we added and subtracted certain student and college behaviors to help us answer our two main research questions:

College sorting and family resources. Although many researchers have studied the connection between family resources and whether students attend *any* college, we do not know specifically why resources appear so instrumental in determining *which* college students attend. Resources may affect college sorting in a number of ways. Perhaps most significantly, academic achievement is strongly associated with resources, particularly family income and socioeconomic status; high-income students have much higher scores on standardized tests (including the SAT and ACT) than middle- and low-income students, and this gap has been growing over time.[23] Because academic achievement is a key criterion for admission to selective schools, it is not surprising that high-resource students are more likely to be admitted to such schools.

The college admissions process, however, is complex and—as with educational attainment in general—the relationship between resources and achievement may only partly explain the apparent resource advantage in college enrollment. Many other mechanisms may play important roles. High-resource students may engage in activities that make them more attractive to colleges, such as using admissions consultants or spending more time pursuing extracurricular interests. These students may be more knowledgeable about choices in the market for postsecondary education; may tend to submit more applications; or may evaluate the benefits of college attendance differently. Colleges themselves may also play a role by using recruitment or admissions strategies based on nonacademic factors related to resources, for example by giving preference to legacy admissions, or, conversely, to qualified low-income students. How the many factors related to socioeconomic status may affect college attendance is unclear.

By altering the distribution of student characteristics and the factors that govern their application behaviors, we use the model to explore the relative effects of these five mechanisms on college enrollment patterns:

1) *Differential high school achievement.* We examined the difference on model outcomes between when we set the correlation between resources and caliber to roughly reflect the real world (about r = 0.3) and when set to 0.

2) *Application enhancement.* We tested our application enhancement hypothesis by altering the caliber of students that colleges use to evaluate applications. We started with the distorted caliber perception we used to simulate idiosyncratic preferences for students and then added or subtracted up to 0.1 standard deviations of caliber as a function of family resources. Students with the lowest resources had their perceived caliber lowered by 0.1 standard deviations, while those with the highest caliber have their perceived caliber enhanced by 0.1 standard deviations. Students with average resources do not have their caliber changed at all.

3) *Unequal information.* We model unequal information by adjusting how reliably students perceive college quality. We have built into our model a parameter that causes students to view college quality with a certain amount of noise. When we test the effects of unequal information by resources, we decrease the reliability with which low-resource students perceive college quality, while higher resource students are more likely to have an accurate assessment of a college's quality.

4) *Perceived utility of college enrollment.* Part of how students decide where to submit their application depends on how they weigh the value of attending a more selective institution against the risk of not being admitted. If high resource students value high-quality schools more, they will be more likely to apply to these colleges. We model this phenomenon by making the parameter that determines quality valuation a function of students' resources.

5) *Number of applications.* On average, both in our model and in the real world, college applicants submit about four applications. We model the tendency of higher resource students to submit more applications by adding half the standardized value of students' resources (rounded to the nearest integer) to this base value of 4. Thus, a student with resources 2 standard deviations above the mean would submit five applications.

College sorting and affirmative action. With increased legal pressure against the use of race-conscious affirmative action policies in college admissions, there is growing concern that these practices will not be available for colleges to use as a tool to increase racial diversity on their campuses. The elimination of race-conscious admissions practices could mean even lower representation of racial and ethnic minority students at the nation's most selective colleges. In response, scholars and policymakers have started to look for race-neutral alternatives to race-conscious affirmative action. One of these is to give admissions preferences based on family income rather than race, based on the theory that due to the strong relationship between race and family income, selecting students based on family income could help to increase racial diversity.

The challenge with such proposals is that it is difficult to assess their effectiveness through real-world experimentation—tinkering with established admissions policies has real consequences for students seeking college enrollment. Thus, an agent-based model presents a valuable tool in assessing the promise of race-neutral admissions alternatives.

We started with our base college-sorting model, including all of the resource mechanisms described above. We then created rules in which certain sets of colleges (e.g., just the top four colleges, half of all colleges, etc.) give admissions preferences to students based either on their race, resources, or both. Recall that the students in our model had race and resource characteristics that mirror the U.S. college-age population, so the same associations between race and resources that exist in the real world were present in our model. We systematically had colleges give students no, moderate, or strong race and/or resource preferences. The magnitude of the moderate preferences was aligned with the implicit weight selective colleges give to racial minority students during the admissions process and was operationalized as an explicit value added to the caliber of students that colleges see when they are making their admissions decisions. For race, students would have a fixed weight added to their apparent caliber according to their race, while the weight for resources was a linear function of student resource levels.

Results

Intra-district School Choice

Trends in baseline simulation. We observed enrollment trends during a 10-year run of the baseline simulation, disaggregated by race. Figure 4A shows trends in school achievement levels enrolled in by students of different races. Overall, there was not much change during the course of the simulation. The largest change was for black students, who tended to enroll in slightly lower-achieving schools at the end of the simulation than at the start. Figure 4B shows trends in the percentage of students of the same race attending the schools in which students enroll; there is a moderate increase for white students that levels out at around year 7, and slight decreases for black and Asian students. The stability in these trends seems plausible given the long history of school choice in this district; any sorting by race that is likely to occur had plenty of time to happen.

Comparing the baseline simulation to experimental simulations. The experimental runs provided insights into the effects that different policy conditions could have on racial diversity in district schools, specifically, (1) the number of predominantly single-race schools (either over 60 percent single-race or over 80 percent single-race, cut points that are used by the district) and (2) Theil's H, an index that effectively portrays

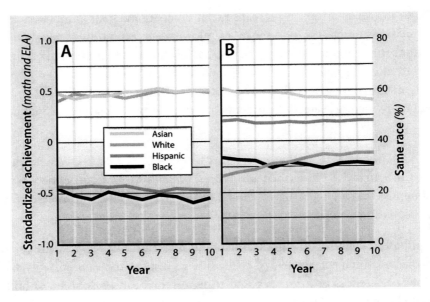

Figure 4. Trends in (A) standardized school achievement levels and (B) racial composition of enrolled schools in baseline simulation

racial segregation in the district and will equal 0 when the racial composition of all schools matches that of the district as a whole and 1 under conditions of total racial segregation.[24,25] Figure 5 shows these values at the end of each simulation. Full school-choice participation yielded the greatest increase in racial diversity in district schools relative to the baseline simulation; this intervention reduced the number of schools that would be over 60 percent single-race from 32 to 27, the number of schools that would be over 80 percent from 10 to 8, and the segregation index from 0.241 to 0.226. By definition, in this scenario more families participated in the choice process and provided the district with ranked preferences than in the baseline scenario, and fewer families (although still some) are "manually" placed in their neighborhood or closest school. As a result, fewer students were assigned to and enrolled in schools with high concentrations of students of the same race; the average racial compositions of the schools that students of different races enrolled in were similar in this and the baseline scenario, but the full participation scenario experienced a reduction in the number of schools that were predominately attended by Hispanic and Asian students. Conversely, removing assignment priority for residents in a low test-score zone resulted in the largest decrease in racial diversity in district schools; at the end of this simulation, we observed 34 schools that were over 60 percent single-race, 11 over 80 percent, and a segregation index value of 0.255. As with the achievement gap, this reflects a change in the ability of the disproportionately black and Hispanic residents of low test-score zones to obtain assignment in schools that are higher-achieving and serving greater proportions of white and Asian students.

College Enrollment

College sorting and family resources. Figure 6 shows the average quality of a college in which students from different resource levels enroll when certain resource-based mechanisms are eliminated. All of our

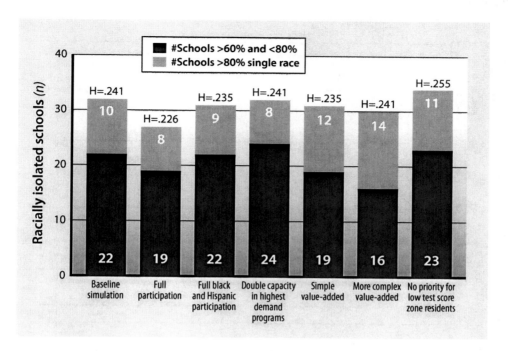

Figure 5. Comparison of racial isolation (measured using predominantly single-race school counts and Theil's H) across simulations in year 10

hypothesized connections between resources and college sorting contributed to the stratification of high- and low-resource students into high- and low-quality colleges, with the exception of the differential valuation of the value of college quality. The relationship between resources and caliber had the largest impact on the likelihood that low-income students would enroll in highly selective colleges: the elimination of this correlation had a similar impact to eliminating all of the other four mechanisms. While it is difficult to directly address the correlation between resources and caliber in real life, it does seem possible to use policy to address the other mechanisms we test. For example, efforts to encourage low-income students to submit more college applications or to provide them with more information about college could help to reduce enrollment gaps between high- and low-resource students.

Affirmative action. Figure 7A and B showed, perhaps not surprisingly, that each type of admission preference was good at creating diversity along the measure that is given the preference. In other words, race preferences did well at creating racial diversity (figure 7A), while resource preferences create resource diversity (figure 7B). However, the relationship between race and resources was not strong enough for resource preferences to create a notable amount of racial diversity, and vice versa.

We also looked at whether there was evidence that colleges that used affirmative action did a disservice to the students that benefit from such policies by putting them in an environment where their peers academically outmatch them. We found no evidence of any notable change in academic mismatch as a result of any affirmative action policy (figure 8).

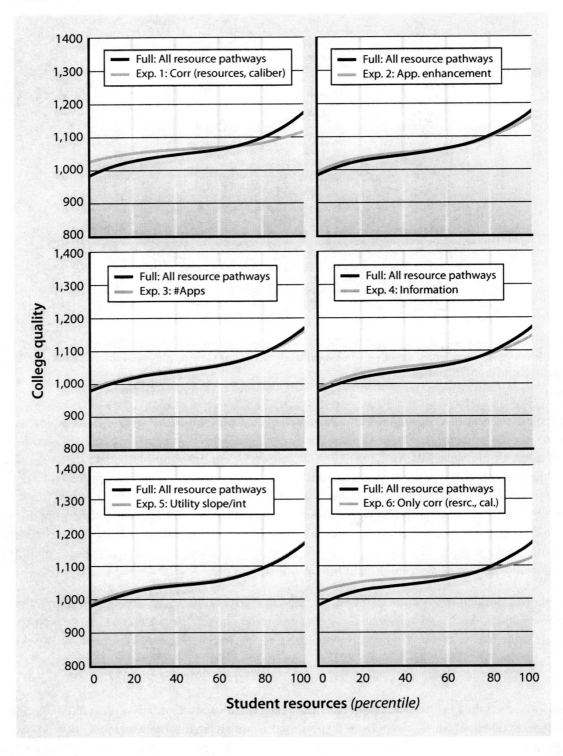

Figure 6. Quality of college in which student enrolls, by student resource percentile. Quality is determined by the average caliber of students enrolled in previous years

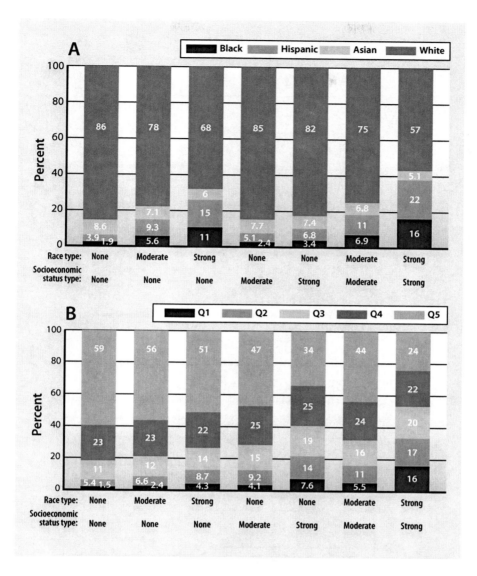

Figure 7. (A) Racial composition and (B) socioeconomic composition of colleges using affirmative action. Race- and SES-type indicate whether colleges in the model used race or socioeconomic status forms of admissions preferences and, if so, whether the moderate or strong versions were used

Conclusion

Agent-based modeling provided us with a strong tool for understanding school choice and college sorting. In each context that we explored, our models were able to account for the complex interactions of individual and institutional actors that determine where students go to school. In doing so, we believe we have built tools that can provide powerful insights into the potential long-term and large-scale effects of policies that are the focus of enormous interest and scrutiny at present, such as intra-district choice at kindergarten through high school levels and affirmative action at the college level.

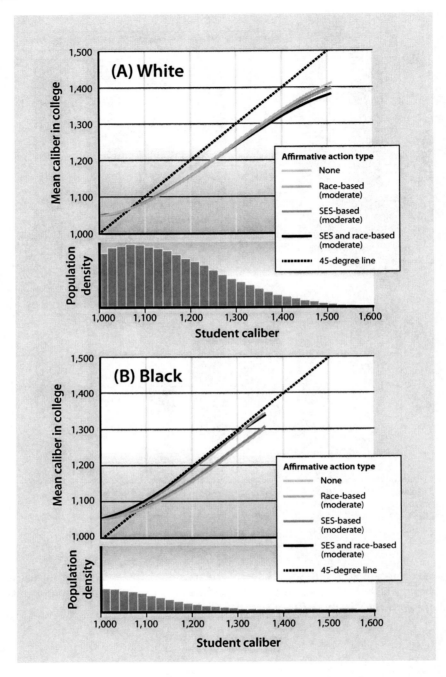

Figure 8. Mean caliber of students in own college, by race and affirmative action type for (A) white and (B) black students; top four schools use affirmative action

Agent-based models provide an opportunity to build upon and supplement existing evidence from observational approaches. These models allow for the development of intuition about school choice processes in ways that would not be possible in an observational study. It is difficult to manipulate, for example, the admissions conditions that college applicants face. It would be difficult to convince colleges to cooperate and a challenge to assure that students would not face worse college enrollment options than under *status quo* conditions.

By building on existing empirical models to explore mechanisms and policy effects, we can make statements about why persistent disparities in educational enrollment at different levels occur and how policymakers and other interested parties can address them. Often these results are somewhat surprising or counterintuitive. In the school choice model, we saw that the largest increase in racial diversity within public schools was obtained by increasing participation in the choice process, rather than by making changes to assignment or school capacities. In the college sorting model, we learned that eliminating the correlation between resources and student caliber would have an equivalent effect on equity in college enrollment as policy measures that address all of the other resource-based mechanisms included in the model. We also learned that even extreme versions of affirmative action based on socioeconomic status would not be able to replicate the racial diversity in colleges that use race-based affirmative action. These are important policy lessons that could not be practically studied in an observational setting.

These findings have important implications for policymakers who wish to undertake the extremely challenging work of promoting equitable access to educational opportunity. A greater understanding of the complex mechanisms that drive elementary school and college choices and enrollment can help them to avoid making decisions that are costly but not effective, squandering resources and blunting zeal for further action, and to instead focus their energies on efforts that have to potential to actually decrease educational stratification.

References

1. Robert Wood Johnson Foundation. *Education and Health*. Princeton, NJ: Robert Wood Johnson Foundation; 2011.

2. Pampel FC, Krueger PM, Denney JT. Socioeconomic disparities in health behaviors. *Annu Rev Sociol.* 2010;36:349–370.

3. Why education matters to health: exploring the causes. Center on Society and Health Website. http://society-health.vcu.edu/work/the-projects/why-education-matters-to-health-exploring-the-causes.html. Accessed June 30, 2015.

4. Buckley J, Schneider M. *Charter Schools: Hope or Hype?* Princeton, NJ: Princeton University Press; 2007.

5. Henig J. *Rethinking School Choice: Limits of the Market Metaphor*. Princeton, NJ: Princeton University Press; 1994.

6. Schneider M, Teske P, Marschall M. *Choosing Schools: Consumer Choice and the Quality of American Schools*. Princeton, NJ: Princeton University Press; 2000.

7. Black D, Smith J. How robust is the evidence on the effects of college quality? Evidence from matching. *J Econom.* 2004;121:99–124.

8. Dale S, Krueger AB. *Estimating the Return to College Selectivity over the Career Using Administrative Earnings Data*. National Bureau of Economic Research Working Paper No. 17159; 2011.

9. Hoekstra M. The effect of attending the flagship state university on earnings: a discontinuity-based approach. *Rev Econ Stat.* 2009;91(4):717–724.

10. Long MC. College quality and early adult outcomes. *Econ Educ Rev.* 2008;27:588–602.

11. Reardon SF, Baker RB, Klasik D. *Race, Income, and Enrollment Patterns in Highly Selective Colleges, 1982–2004*. Stanford, CA: Center for Education Policy Analysis; 2012.

12. O'Day JA, Bitter CS, Gomez LM. *Education Reform in New York City: Ambitious Change in the Nation's Most Complex School System*. Cambridge, MA: Harvard Education Press; 2011.

13. Kucsera J, Orfield G. *New York State's Extreme School Segregation: Inequality, Inaction and a Damaged Future*. Los Angeles, CA: The Civil Rights Project; 2014.

14. Alon S. The evolution of class inequality in higher education: competition, exclusion, and adaptation. *Am Sociol Rev.* 2009;74:731–755.

15. Astin A, Oseguera L. The declining "equity" of American higher education. *Rev High Educ.* 2004;27(3):321–341.

16. Belley P, Lochner L. The changing role of family income and ability in determining educational achievement. *J Hum Cap.* 2007;1(1):37–89.

17. Karen D. Changes in access to higher education in the United States: 1980–1992. *Sociol Educ.* 2002;75(3):191–210.

18. Reardon SF, Kasman M, Klasik D, Baker R. Agent-based simulation models of the college sorting process. *J Artif Soc Soc Simul.* 2016;19(1):8.

19. Reardon SF, Baker RB, Kasman M, Klasik D, Townsend JB. *Simulation Models of the Effects of Race- and Socioeconomic-based Affirmative Action Policies.* Stanford, CA: Center for Education Policy Analysis; 2015.

20. Abdulkadiroğlu A, Pathak PA, Roth AE. The New York City high school match. *Am Econ Rev.* 2005;95(2):364–367.

21. Toch T, Aldeman C. *Matchmaking: Enabling Mandatory Public School Choice in New York and Boston.* Washington, DC: Education Sector; 2009.

22. Dur UM, Kominers SD, Pathak PA, Sönmez T. *The Demise of Walk Zones in Boston: Priorities vs. Precedence in School Choice.* Cambridge, MA: National Bureau of Economic Research; 2013. No. W18981.

23. Reardon SF. The widening academic achievement gap between the rich and the poor: new evidence and possible explanations. In: Duncan GC, Murnane R, eds. *Whither Opportunity?* New York: Russell Sage Foundation; 2011:91–116.

24. Iceland J. *The Multigroup Entropy Index (also known as Theil's H or the Information Theory Index).* US Census Bureau; 2004.

25. Reardon SF, Firebaugh G. Measures of multigroup segregation. *Sociol Methodol.* 2002;32(1):33–67.

CHAPTER 9

CONTINGENT INEQUALITIES: AN EXPLORATION OF HEALTH INEQUALITIES IN THE UNITED STATES AND CANADA

Michael Wolfson, PhD
Canada Research Chair in Population Health Modeling/Populomics
School of Epidemiology, Public Health and Preventive Medicine, Faculty of Medicine
University of Ottawa

Reed F. Beall
Vanier Scholar and PhD Candidate in Population Health
Faculty of Health Sciences,
University of Ottawa

Acknowledgments: This research was funded and developed as part of the NIH-funded Network on Inequality, Complexity and Health (NICH) led by George A. Kaplan. We are deeply indebted to NICH colleagues for many valuable discussions and to Steve Gribble for his usually remarkable software and modeling work.

"An aggregate relation between income inequality and health is not necessary—associations are contingent."[1]

Income inequality is pervasive and has generally increased over recent decades in most countries of the world.[2] At the same time, and clearly in modern high-income societies, there is a pervasive individual-level income gradient in health: not only are there large variations in health status and longevity across members of a population, but these basic health measures are also inversely correlated with income and other measures of socioeconomic status. At another level, there is provocative evidence that for population groups, whether countries, states, or cities, there are correlations between income inequality and average measures of health for these populations.

In much of the recent debate about the relationship between income inequality and population health, the methodological analysis has moved toward sophisticated econometric analysis, using time series of cross-sectional data, for example on sets of countries.[3] These analyses attempt to determine whether in a regression there is a significant coefficient on the income inequality variable (e.g., a Gini coefficient), with various measures of mortality or life expectancy as the dependent variable. Some studies find a statistically significant relationship, while others, when further covariates are added, do not. This literature on whether or not there is even a correlation between income inequality and health, let alone a causal relationship, raises fundamental empirical and conceptual questions:

> As long as there are some potential confounders that have not been or cannot be measured and included in analyses, this research endeavor will be hung over with question marks ... The literature has accordingly reached an empirical impasse. It will never be possible to adequately control for all the time-varying confounders that will be viewed as plausible, and it will never be possible to show that all potential confounders are true confounders and, therefore, to rule out the possibility that income inequality truly does affect population health.

> One way to resolve this problem would be to articulate a sufficiently cogent and thorough theoretical framework so that the number of potential confounders is theoretically constrained. Not only has no such framework yet been advanced, but also its absence points up an important conceptual impasse in the literature. ... The literature on income inequality and health has accordingly reached a conceptual impasse to match its empirical one.[4]

One major confounder in ecological (i.e., population group level) studies of the relationship between income inequality and health is the gradient in health at the individual level: higher incomes are associated with better health (figure 1). The reasons for this income–mortality association are contested; some suggest "reverse causality," with the main causal pathway running from poor health to lower income. However, Wolfson et al.[5] provide strong evidence that, at least for Canadian males, the majority of this association is likely causal, from income to health rather than the reverse.

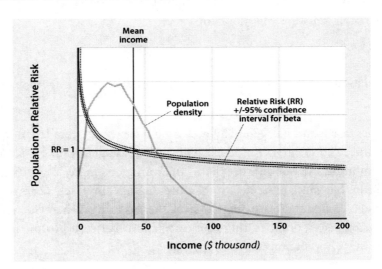

Figure 1. Income distribution and mortality relative risk in the United States, 1990. N.B. indicates proportion of population for density curve and relative risk for risk curve. Adopted from Wolfson (2016), and used with permission[6]

At the same time, figure 1 provides one basis for observing not only an individual-level association between income and health (whether measured by mortality rates or some other indicator of individuals' health), but also an association between two population-level attributes: income inequality and average health. Because the individual-level income gradient is nonlinear, as individuals become more spread out along the horizontal axis (i.e., as income inequality increases) average health (however measured) necessarily must decline, which is represented by increasing mortality rates in the context of figure 1. Based on this well-known mathematical property, Gravelle argued that the fact higher income inequality is associated with higher mortality is nothing more than a statistical artefact.[7] While this is logically correct, Wolfson et al.[8] showed that something further must be at work; the curvilinear relationship shown in figure 1 by itself was not close to being sufficient to account for the observed correlation between income inequality and mortality among the 50 U.S. states.

Deaton and Lubotsky[9] claimed that the associations observed in the United States failed to account for race. But in a multilevel analysis, Backlund et al.[10] showed a statistically significant relationship between income inequality and mortality rates at the state level in the United States, even after controlling for race at both the individual and state levels. Wilkinson and Pickett[11], in their popular book, strongly argued (albeit controversially) that income inequality is bad not only for health, but also for a wide range of social ills.

Importantly, the data shown in figure 2[12] for Canada and the United States clearly suggest that the correlation between inequality and average working-age mortality is "contingent." We observe a strong correlation between a measure of city-level[3] income inequality (measured by median share of income accruing to the bottom half) and working-age mortality rates in the United States. However, in Canada, there is no correlation. More extensive results for five countries are given in Ross et al..[13] In that case, both the United States and United Kingdom showed a strong correlation between income inequality and mortality at the city level, while Canada, Sweden, and Australia did not. These clear differences suggest that there are other major country-specific factors on which the relationship is contingent.

This contingent correlation of income inequality and mortality at the metropolitan or city level—yes in the United States and not in Canada—is suggestive, considering the controversies surrounding the U.S. state and international country-level regression analyses noted by Zimmerman above.[4] It should not be surprising that there are conflicting empirical results in the literature, when figure 2 clearly shows that other major factors must be affecting the empirical associations between income inequality and health. In econometric or regression terms, there must be major confounding variables in this relationship, and these confounders must vary between countries.

Why Complex Systems Methods

As noted, the literature on income inequality and its relationship to population health is at both an empirical and conceptual impasse.[4] Furthermore, conventional econometric methods are unlikely to resolve matters. Instead, a new kind of approach is required, one that starts with an explicit theoretical and conceptual

---

3   U.S. data refer to Standardized Metropolitan Statistical Areas (SMSAs).[13] The Canadian data were specifically constructed to be as similar to the U.S. data as possible.

framework, draws on empirical observations to the extent feasible, abandons "one equation for everything" econometrics, and draws on modern computer simulation techniques to examine the multiple co-evolving and mutually interacting factors embodied in the theory.

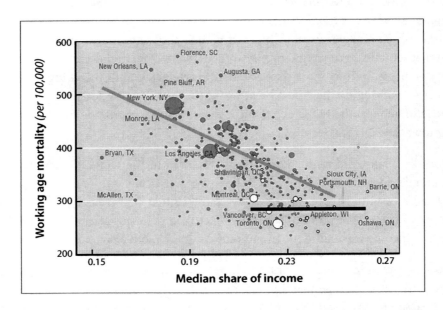

Figure 2. Working-age mortality (per 100,000) and median shares of income for U.S. and Canadian metropolitan areas. (Colors are visible at http://bit.ly/2hzGBaG, Wolfson (2016), used with permission

There are a number of candidate factors that might account for the different patterns of association. However, a great deal of the relevant data is missing. Moreover, a convincing account of these provocative contingent correlations requires a theory operating at multiple levels—from individuals to families to neighborhoods to cities—reflecting the reality that factors at these different levels of aggregation mutually interact and dynamically coevolve. In order to incorporate these realities, this analysis explores the observed contingent correlations in a quasi-theoretical manner, using complex system methods. Specifically, we construct an agent-based model, the Theoretical Health Inequality Model (THIM) to explore these relationships, with a focus on Canada and the United States.

In order to articulate a theory that can account for the observations in figure 2, several hypotheses can be considered. One is that the main factor accounting for the existence of a correlation between income inequality and mortality at the city level, or more precisely metropolitan area, in the United States but not in Canada is the nature of economic segregation within metropolitan areas. For example, anecdotally, large U.S. cities have far more gated communities than Canadian cities, where the very rich live, as well as more ghetto areas of mainly poor people. Likewise, disparities in average incomes between these different neighborhoods are greater in the United States than in Canada, while income heterogeneity within U.S. neighborhoods is less than in Canada. However, comparable data to substantiate directly this impression of significantly different spatial income segregation in the two countries are not available.

Neighborhood segregation is most visibly associated with race in the United States, less so in Canada. But racial segregation in U.S. cities is also strongly associated with income segregation.[14] As a result, in this abstract model, we focus only on income segregation, without reference to racial segregation, to maintain simplicity and facilitate comparability between the cities in the two countries.

In addition to neighborhood income segregation, another important consideration is the likely effect that the average income of a neighborhood has on the quality of education, where levels and variations in local school quality represent one of the factors differentiating Canadian and U.S. cities.[15,16] Another major factor differentiating Canada and the United States may be the roles played by parental socioeconomic position in transmitting social advantage and disadvantage from one generation to the next; for example, whether intergenerational income mobility is higher in one country or relatively lower.[17]

Even if high-quality comparable data for the two countries existed, there is no straightforward statistical method of testing or assessing their significance. The reason is the multilevel, interacting, and dynamic character of these various hypothesized factors. They form, in combination, a complex system or "web of causality."[18] As a result, effective theorizing, and in turn a plausible account, requires some sort of simulation modeling, our raison d'être for creating THIM. At the same time, in order for the analytical results to be plausible, it is preferable, to the extent possible, for the simulation modeling to align well with known statistical observations, i.e., the various "stylized facts."

The first challenge is whether, with our relatively simple theoretical model, it is even possible to generate the different patterns shown in figure 2. The main focus of our THIM simulations was to represent stylized versions of cities in the United States (U) and Canada (C). If THIM can successfully reproduce the contingent correlation observed (and it can), the second challenge is to determine which factors included in the model are key to the contingency of the correlation.

THIM Structure

To assess a set of hypothesized factors that could account for the differences between Canadian and U.S. cities (figure 2), we constructed an agent-based model. THIM incorporates simplified, stylized (yet plausible), empirically based individual-level relationships among health status, education, income, mortality rates, and neighborhood mobility. In turn, the latter affects the extent of neighborhood income segregation.

THIM has a population of individual unisex agents. They are born to a parent; live in neighborhoods; go to school; start working and earning income; have their health status affected by a combination of their education, own income, and average neighborhood income; and then face mortality rates that depend on their age, health, and income.

In diagrammatic form, each agent has a number of characteristics (figure 3). The arrows indicate that each agent starts life with a predestined level of education (E). E is a measure (in years) not only of formal education, but also social skills and the cumulative results of informal "home curriculum," cultural upbringing, and neighborhood barriers and facilitators, all factors that can make a difference in one's eventual earning potential as an adult. As shown by the arrow in figure 3 from E to Y, education (as just broadly defined) is assumed to influence income (Y, in dollars, the commonly used variable name for income by economists) directly, and health status (H, a number ranging between zero for dead and one for full health), and mortality (D = death) indirectly via income. Income also influences residential location (L) among neighborhoods.

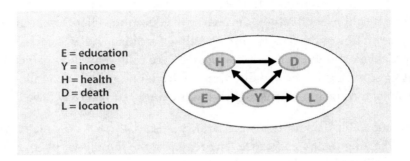

Figure 3. Sims attributes and their relationships. E = education, Y = income, H = health, D = death, L = location

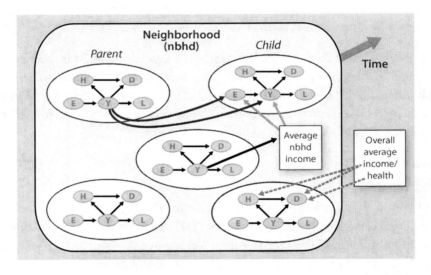

Figure 4. Sims in a neighborhood. E = education, Y = income, H = health, D = death, L = location

Furthermore, the individual agents in THIM have multilevel relationships: every agent is a member of a parent-child dyad (at least when one is a child), and agents interact with other agents in their neighborhoods and within their city (or metropolitan area), giving rise to additional posited causal influences. In particular, there are parent-to-child effects via parental income (Y) affecting child agents' education (E) and income (Y) (figure 4). THIM also posits neighborhood effects where average neighborhood income affects both agents' education and their income, and hence indirectly their health, mortality, and neighborhood location.

Finally, a third level, the city, is comprised of multiple neighborhoods (figure 5). One key factor at this broader level is geographic mobility. Adult agents are posited to have a general propensity (of variable strength) to move to neighborhoods where their own income is closer to the neighborhood average (i.e., income homophily). Depending on the strength of this propensity, neighborhoods can either be quite heterogeneous in terms of residents' incomes and levels of education, or more segregated with neighborhoods more internally homogenous, but more polarized compared one to another (e.g., more "gates" and "ghettos" as in the United States compared to Canada).

Finally, there is widespread evidence that the individual-level socioeconomic gradient in health shown in figure 1 is pervasive both across jurisdictions and over time. Furthermore, there is strongly suggestive evidence that what matters is not absolute levels of income or health, but rather income and health relative to the averages of the society in that time and place. For example, even going back centuries, there is evidence of individual-level gradients in health.[19]

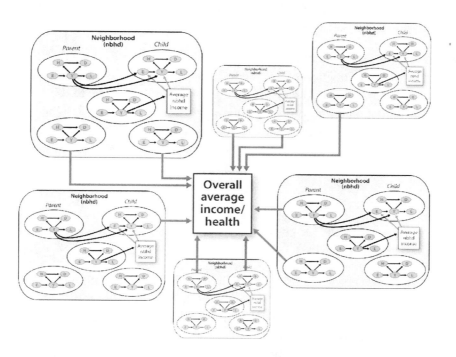

Figure 5. A THIM city with multiple neighborhoods, and multiple sims within each neighborhood. E = education, Y = income, H = health, D = death, L = location

In a more mathematical (or pseudo code) form, the model can be summarized by a set of equations. These equations may look simple, but in fact they describe a quite complex system. At its foundation, THIM is an agent-based model working at the individual level. However, the model has parent-child dyad-level, neighborhood-level, and city-level calculations built into its equations (figures 4 and 5). This is indicated by the fonts in the text below, where bolded variables represent characteristics of the agent's parent, and bolded and italicized variables are characteristics of the neighborhood where the agent currently lives, or attributes of the society (city) overall. The equations are also enriched by the fact that the first four also include as inputs random variables drawn from specified distributions. As a result, even though THIM is based on only a handful of equations, it is potentially capable of complex behavior.[20]

1. Fixed at birth for each agent

- Education (E) = fcn (**parent's income,** *average neighborhood income*, random variation) [measured in years]

    o Interpretation: When an agent is born, its education level (e.g. an integer between 0 and 20) is determined as a function of its parent's income, the average income in its neighborhood, and random variation (e.g., drawn from a uniform distribution centered at 10 years).

- Potential income (Y*) = fcn (education, **parent's income,** *average neighborhood income*, random variation reflecting various degrees of "innate" inequality) [measured as a strictly positive index with mean = 1, and positively skewed as widely observed empirically]

    o Interpretation: When an agent is born, its potential income (n.b. not actual income; see below) is determined next as a function of its (predestined) education, its parent's income (relative to the neighborhood average), its average neighborhood income (relative to the overall average across all neighborhoods), and random variation drawn from a specially designed distribution representing innate or exogenous inequality factors (described further below in connection with table 2, figure 9).

2. Evolving over time/age

- Income (Y) = average income for given age × individual's potential income (Y*) × annual random variation [measured in dollars]

    o Interpretation: Each year, an agent's actual dollar income is determined by multiplying its innate income earning potential (Y*), by a stereotypical (average) age-income profile and by a random variable drawn from an independent lognormal distribution, such that the agent's income over time will have high autocorrelation but will show skewed variability each year around the age-income profile value at that age, resulting in empirically realistic though completely synthetic individual-level income trajectories.

- Change in health (H) = random drift (mostly down, piecewise linear density) + fcn (own income/ *average incomes of those at similar ages across all neighborhoods*) [measured by an index in the [0,1] interval where 1 is full health, and 0 is dead]

    o Interpretation: Each agent's health status (a number between 0 and 1) in a given year is calculated by incorporating a random drift (usually downward, though occasional improvements in health can also occur); the pace of this mostly downward drift is modulated as a function of the agent's income in the current year relative to the average incomes of all other similarly aged agents, with slower declines associated with higher relative incomes.

- Mortality risk (D) = average mortality rate for given age × fcn (own income/*average incomes of those at similar ages across all neighborhoods*, own health/*average health across all neighborhoods*) [measured as a relative risk]

  o Interpretation: Each agent's risk of dying in a given year is calculated by first referencing a standard mortality rate schedule for the agent's current age, then multiplying by a relative risk determined by a combination of the agent's own income relative to all other similarly aged agents and its health status relative to all other similarly aged agents.

- Neighborhood mobility (ΔL) = fcn (own income, *own neighborhood average income, other neighborhoods' average incomes*) [where L indexes the neighborhood, and the total number of neighborhoods is a parameter]

  o Interpretation: Coinciding with its birthday, an agent will try to change neighborhood if its own income is sufficiently discrepant (either above or below) the average income of its current neighborhood. If the agent is trying to move, the agent will move into the neighborhood with an average income that is the most similar to its own and that has space available. The simulation user can set parameters, including the number of neighborhoods, the limit on the occupancy of each neighborhood, and the threshold that determines when an agent tries to move.

The model source code is available at the moment from the author and will eventually be posted online. An executable version of the model is available at:

http://microsim.beyond2020.com/demomodels/Browse/Scenarios.aspx.

Method—Selecting Parameters

While THIM is an abstract theoretical model, in order for its results to be as meaningful as possible, the parameters have been based on stylized facts—observed empirical relationships for the United States and Canada.

Our development of THIM was motivated by observations regarding the correlation between income inequality and health (figure 2). Because this is a contingent correlation, it varies by country, and therefore depends on a range of other factors.

For many aspects of THIM, we lack data of sufficient quality to inform parameter choice. Still, a number of pieces of empirical evidence have been sufficient for general guidance on setting THIM parameters.

Individual income and health: Individual-level relationships between income and health (figure 1) were one of the factors with the potential to drive differences in the city-level income inequality-mortality relationship observed between Canada and the United States (figure 2). A central question, therefore, is whether this relationship is stronger in the United States than in Canada. High-quality comparable

Canada-U.S. data on health status are limited. The most comparable data are from the Joint Canada-U.S. Survey of Health,[21] which suggests that the individual-level gradient is generally steeper in the United States than in Canada.

City income inequality: U.S. cities have a wider range of within-city income inequality than those in Canada (figure 2). This observation is consistent with the general observation that the United States has higher income inequality (using a variety of measures) than Canada. In THIM, the initial driver of income inequality among individual agents is the input parameter (actually a nonparametric density function) for the distribution of potential income (Y*). We explored a range of these Y* distributions, with Gini coefficients in the range 0.1–0.5 (see below).

Age and income: THIM posits a number of other factors that determine actual incomes. One is a stylized average age-income profile (figure 6). (Like many THIM parameters, this is described in general, nonparametric terms by an arbitrary piecewise linear function.) While evidence suggests that such profiles may be steeper in the United States than in Canada at younger ages, and relatively lower among the elderly, this profile is assumed to be identical for our representative cities in the United States and Canada.

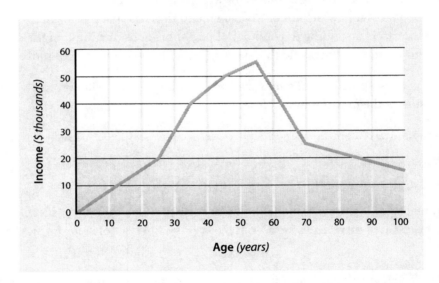

Figure 6. Simplified baseline average age-income profile. Wolfson (2016), used with permission[6]

Other factors determining an agent's actual income at any given age are the parental, neighborhood and educational influences acting at birth, as well as a stochastic term over the entire lifetime, each described shortly.

Mortality: THIM posits a standard baseline pattern of mortality rates and associated survival curves. The *shapes* of the survival curves in Canada and the United States is not notably different, so the same age-specific mortality rates, hence survival curves, are used for both countries (figure 7).

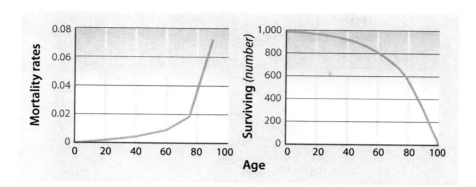

Figure 7. Baseline age-specific mortality rates and corresponding survival curve. Wolfson (2016), used with permission[6]

Of course, actual life expectancies differ, with the U.S. life expectancy more than 2 years lower than in Canada. However, we start with identical baseline mortality rates precisely in order to use THIM to see whether a differential life expectancy emerges from the simulations, as a result of the other factors included the model.

Health care system: In the literature, comparisons of health in Canada and the United States almost always mention differences in the two countries' health care sectors. The United States is a dramatically high outlier in terms of health care spending, while Canada is in the upper-middle range among countries in the Organisation for Economic Co-operation and Development (OECD). Yet, U.S. life expectancy is lower than in Canada. If anything, aggregate data show that for countries spending more than $2,000 per capita on health care, more health care spending appears to be associated with reduced life expectancy.[22]

Health care in the United States may be a significant disequalizing factor compared to Canada. For about the upper half of the income spectrum in the two countries, health care has roughly the same impacts on health; in other words, for all the extra spending, the rich in the United States are not significantly healthier than their Canadian counterparts.[21] However, the poor in the bottom income quintile in United States are significantly worse off. Empirically, it is difficult to determine whether this difference is due to poorer access to health care, or to differences in the fundamental determinants of health. Health care per se is not explicitly included in THIM. But we explore its role implicitly in several aspects of the parameterization of the THIM simulations presented below.

Education: THIM explicitly allows for a causal pathway whereby parental income can influence children's education. One source of information on this relationship is the OECD (2012) PISA (Program for International Student Achievement) study, which includes data on math scores by the SES of children's parents (figure 8).[23] Canadian children performed better overall, with higher scores at all levels of parental SES. Furthermore, the correlation between PISA scores and parental SES in Canada was about half that for the U.S. children who had a wider dispersion in their math scores. These results for math scores at age 15 are corroborated by similar results for adult literacy, where the United States has lower average adult literacy scores and a substantially higher correlation of these literacy scores with an indicator of socioeconomic factors.

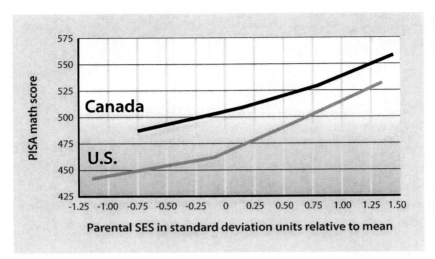

Figure 8. PISA math scores by parental SES, in standard deviation units relative to the mean. Wolfson (2016), used with permission[6]

The OECD (2012) PISA study also provides a comparable Canada-U.S. indication of neighborhood influences on educational outcomes, showing math scores by the average SES of all the children's parents in a given child's school. Using the school as a marker for neighborhood influences, there is a wider gap in math scores between Canada and the United States for the disadvantaged schools than for schools whose parents have average socioeconomic backgrounds. This suggests a substantially larger adverse impact on children's educational outcome in the United States compared to Canada from living in a poorer neighborhood.

Parental income: Another factor affecting children's incomes is their parents' incomes. The parent to child elasticity of income in the United States (i.e., the amount statistically that a son's income increases per one-unit increase in the father's income) is about twice that of Canada, indicating much lower intergenerational income mobility in the United States, and correspondingly a much stronger influence of parental incomes on child incomes.[17]

Modeling Scenarios

Based on these kinds of stylized results, the THIM parameters have been divided into three groups:

- Those that are the same in all simulations;

- Those taking either a C or a U value; and

- Inequality in potential income, Y*.

Table 1 shows values for the second group of parameters for each of five scenarios:

- Baseline scenarios for the hypothetical Canadian (C) and U.S. (U) cities (columns 1 and 2);

- Scenarios in which differences between the Canadian (C*) and U.S. cities (U*), other than for the last three parameters affecting neighborhood income segregation, are reduced or eliminated (columns 3 and 4); and

- Scenario in which the last three parameters affecting neighborhood income segregation in the U cities are made identical to those for scenario C (U**).

The first two sets of U/C parameters were designed to assess our first hypothesis, that the (highly simplified) theory and stylized facts embodied in THIM are sufficient to account for the observed difference in correlation between measures of income inequality and average health (figure 2).

This pair of scenarios seeks to establish our first hypothesis, that the factors and causal pathways included in THIM and their stylized quantification are indeed capable of reproducing the observed contingent correlation. (Note that sufficiency does not entail necessity; there may be other sufficient theories.) The three other parameter scenarios (assuming the first hypothesis is correct) are then designed to assess the second hypothesis: that these observed differences are primarily the result of the greater income segregation across neighborhoods in the United States as compared to Canadian cities.

We explore this second hypothesis by partitioning the parameters in into four sub-sets (table 1):

- Education, including parental and neighborhood influences,

- Income, including parental and neighborhood influences,

- Mortality, including health and income influences, and

- Parameters that drive patterns of neighborhood income segregation in THIM.

The plausible view that the U.S. correlation is mainly driven by differences in neighborhood income segregation is tested by comparing the results of THIM simulations for the U and U** parameter sets.

However, a second possibility is that the contingent correlation observed in figure 2 is not primarily the result of neighborhood income segregation per se, but rather is due to other key societal differences between Canada and the United States; for example, local school quality and the tendency of parents to pass social advantage and disadvantage to their children. This alternative hypothesis is tested by comparing the C*/U* patterns with the C/U patterns.

It is important to emphasize that there is no necessary correlation between neighborhood income segregation and local school quality. Most large Canadian cities, for example, have one school board for the entire city, spanning both poor and rich neighborhoods, and school board policy typically ensures substantial equity in school quality, regardless of parents' income levels. In contrast, wealthier city neighborhoods in many U.S. cities (typically suburbs or exurbs) often have their own local school board separate from the larger central city's school district, and therefore are under no obligation to redistribute resources to poorer, often inner city, schools. Similarly, neighborhood income segregation and the passing of social advantages and disadvantages from parents to children are not necessarily correlated, for example if the public school system really operates to level opportunities across an entire city.

Table 1

THIM Parameters for Scenarios

Parameter	Interpretation	C	U	C*	U*	U**
# neighborhoods	Number of neighborhoods	3	12	3	12	**3**
StayPropIncDiff	Threshold at which an agent's income as a proportion of neighborhood average below which agent stays in its neighborhood	0.75	0.15	0.75	0.15	**0.75**
MovePropIncDiff	Threshold at which an agent's income as a proportion of neighborhood average income above which agent moves	0.95	0.25	0.95	0.25	**0.95**
Esigma	Level of random variation from average in education assignments	2	4	**3**	**3**	4
EBetaIncPar	Level of influence of parental income on its child's education determinant at birth	1	2	**1.2**	**1.8**	2
EBetaIncNbhd	Level of influence of neighborhood's average income on child's level of education	0.5	1	**0.6**	**0.9**	1
YBetaEduc	Level of influence of education on an agent's potential income earning determination at birth	0.2	0.6	**0.2**	**0.5**	0.6
YBetaIncPar	Level of influence of the parent's income on its child's potential income earning determination at birth	0.2	0.6	**0.2**	**0.5**	0.6
YBetaIncNbhd	Level of influence of an agent's neighborhood's average income on that agent's potential income earning power determination	0.2	1	**0.4**	1	1
Ysigma	Level of random variation of income earnings in a given year from the standard life course	0.05	0.15	**0.1**	**0.1**	0.15
HIncParm	Level at which an agent's income influences its health	0.001	0.006	**0.008**	**0.008**	0.006
MBetaH	Level at which an agent's death is determined by its health status	0.25	0.75	**0.3**	**0.3**	0.75
MBetaIncNear	Level at which income is a determinant of when an agent dies	0.08	0.24	**0.1**	**0.1**	0.24

Bolded values highlight parameters that have changed from corresponding U and C values in the first two columns.

C = baseline Canadian parameters.
U = baseline U.S. parameters.
C* = baseline Canadian parameters, except weaker differences between Canada and the United States in factors other than neighborhood mobility.
U* = baseline U.S. parameter, except weaker differences between Canada and the United States in factors other than neighborhood mobility.
U** = baseline U.S. parameters, except Canadian neighborhood mobility.

Other policies that need not be correlated with neighborhood income segregation include the generosity of basic income guarantees via programs such as welfare, unemployment insurance, and public pensions, as well as labor market regulations regarding parental leave. In general, Canadian policies are more generous than those in the United States. Some combination of these differences between the United States and Canada likely accounts for the much higher intergenerational income mobility found by Corak (2013).[17] These factors can in principle all operate independently of neighborhood income segregation.

These possibilities are reflected concretely in the parameters in table 1. The first set of three parameters characterizes the neighborhood structures for the C and U cities. In line with the greater fragmentation of governance structures in U.S. cities—which often reflects the ability of wealthier neighborhoods to "opt out" of collective local public goods, including education, that would otherwise flow to poorer neighborhoods—we posit a larger number of neighborhoods for the U.S. cities (12) than the Canadian cities (3).

Mobility: THIM posits a general desire to live in a neighborhood whose average income is as close as possible to the agent's own income. However, such mobility is only allowed if the absolute difference between the agent's income and that of the neighborhood where it resides is above some threshold. If this threshold is high, there is less movement between neighborhoods. In turn, high parameters reflect the willingness of higher income agents to live in a neighborhood with more income variation and a greater tolerance for income diversity. At the same time, lower income agents do not have as strong a need to move to a neighborhood with lower average income when their own income is well below the neighborhood average. Such a high mobility threshold embodies the premise that neighborhood gentrification exerts less pressure on lower income agents to move out.

In contrast, lower mobility thresholds combined with a larger number of neighborhoods will lead to more income homogeneity within neighborhoods, and larger income differences between neighborhoods. In turn, to the extent that a neighborhood's average income affects agents' educational and income prospects, there will be greater inequality in these outcomes between neighborhoods. These three "neighborhood income segregation" parameters enabled us to assess the hypothesis that the different correlations between a health measure (working age mortality in the case of figure 2) and an income inequality measure (median share in figure 2) are primarily a result of greater neighborhood (income) segregation in the United States than in Canada.

Education: Next, we posited that agents living in U.S. cities have parental and neighborhood income influences on educational attainment (EBetaIncPar and EBetaIncNbhd) that are twice those in the Canadian cities (table 1). Furthermore, there is twice the variability in outcomes (Esigma) in U versus C cities. These parameter settings are generally in line with the empirical evidence cited above. In the C*/U* scenarios, the differences between the C and U cities are reduced to half again rather than twice as large for the parental and neighborhood income influences on educational attainment, and the C/U parameter difference is eliminated for the variability in educational attainment outcomes (Esigma).

Income: The YBetaEduc/YBetaIncPar/YBetaIncNbhd parameters reflect the impacts (elasticities) of own education, parental relative income and neighborhood relative average income (respectively) on potential income throughout the agent's life (table 1). YSigma is the annual lognormal variability in actual income, drawn independently from one year to the next. The U values are all posited to be significantly higher than the C values, with the differences between C and U scenarios larger than those in the C* and U* scenarios.

Health transitions and mortality rates: The U cities' parameters embody a larger impact of income (MBetaIncNear) and health (MBetaH) on mortality than those for the C cities, and income also has a larger impact on health transitions (HIncParm). This latter difference can be seen in part as an implicit reflection of the differences in access to health care between Canada and the United States; significant segments of the lower income population in the United States, do not have effective access to care, far more so than in Canada, with its universal, publicly funded hospital and physician care.

Income inequality: There is a wide variation in median income shares across cities, with U.S. metropolitan areas spanning a wider range (figure 2). In THIM, the distribution of income is an output, not an input. An agent's actual income at any given age is the product of a series of factors. But one parameter (actually a set of parameters representing a density function) affords an important further influence on this key output, the distribution of agents' potential income (Y*). This distribution (nonparametric density function, see below) parameter reflects variations in innate ability, personality, and other characteristics that remain fixed throughout life. It is inherently unobservable, though widely posited in the economics literature.

Instead of being the same for everyone, Y* is a scalar drawn randomly from a skewed distribution. We posited eight such distributions for Y*, designed to generate a range of income inequality that is wider than that observed in Canada and the United States, both overall and in the cities (figure 2). Including simulations with a more extreme range of potential income (Y*) inequality enables a stronger set of tests of the C versus U parameter sets.

The Gini coefficient is the most widely used measure of income inequality. However, the comparable income inequality data at the city level (figure 2) was based on median shares. It is a conceptually simpler measure defined as the share of income accruing to the bottom half of the population ranked by income.[4] Still, any income-distribution density function embodies an infinity of points, so the "shape" of any given density can be summarized in an index in numerous ways. Indeed, some features of income distributions are broadly associated in the public's mind with inequality, but are mathematically inconsistent with the usual axiomatization underlying most commonly used income inequality measures like the Gini coefficient. A specific and important case is polarization.[24,25] To assess the robustness of our results, we focused on three summary measures of income inequality: the Gini coefficient, the median share, and the polarization index. Figure 9 illustrates the range of Y* inequality scenarios by showing the density function and Lorenz curves for the first and eighth input distributions.

Furthermore, inequality measures for a set of income distributions need not be correlated in rank order. For example, even though two income distributions may have identical Gini coefficients, they can still have quite different shapes, such as one having more inequality at lower incomes while the other has more inequality at higher incomes. In the economics literature on inequality measures, these kinds of situations

---

4   Strictly speaking, the median share should not be called an inequality measure because it need not be consistent with the partial ordering of income distributions induced by the criterion of Lorenz domination, i.e. that one Lorenz curve is everywhere closer to (or everywhere further from) the 45* line.[26]

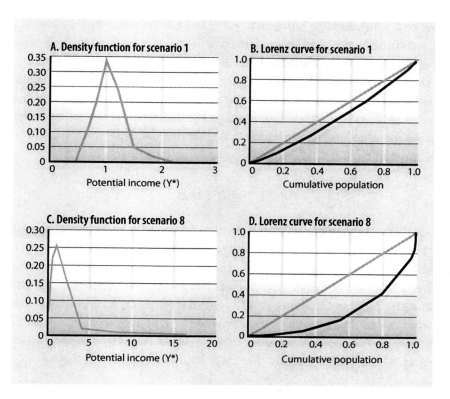

Figure 9. Density functions and Lorenz Curves for Y* distribution of (A) scenario 1, (B) Lorenz curve for scenario 1; (C) density function for scenario 8 and (D) Lorenz curve for scenario 8, per (table 2). Wolfson (2016), used with permission[6]

Table 2

Inequality Measures for Eight Y* Input Distributions

Simulation Number	1	2	3	4	5	6	7	8
Y* Gini coefficient	0.093	0.269	0.358	0.408	0.425	0.471	0.556	0.571
Y* median share	0.450	0.314	0.238	0.223	0.123	0.177	0.127	0.098
Y* polarization	0.015	0.206	0.330	0.291	0.657	0.350	0.380	0.467

From Wolfson (2016), used with permission.[6]

are typically associated with crossing Lorenz curves.[26] In order to encompass this reality, the eight Y* distributions that we constructed included situations where the three inequality measures are not rank order correlated. Accordingly, table 2 shows these three measures for each of the eight Y* distributions used as input parameters (with each distribution represented as a vector pair). By construction, the Gini coefficients increase monotonically from left to right across the eight posited Y* distributions. But this is deliberately not the case for either the median share or the polarization index. Formally, it demonstrates the theoretical points just noted, while practically it is intended to ensure the robustness of our results by including in our simulations a variety of plausibly unequal income distributions.

Findings

Given THIM as our theory of the potential determinants of the patterns observed in figure 2, we first examined whether the factors included were sufficient to reproduce the observed contingent correlations. It is certainly possible that THIM is unable to do this, implying the underlying theory is lacking key factors and/or causal pathways. But as we will discuss in more detail, we have found that THIM is indeed able to reproduce patterns similar to those in figure 2. As a second step, we explored which of the various posited causal pathways were most important, in particular whether neighborhood income segregation was the key factor. Of course, there may be other theories that can also account for the patterns observed in figure 2; all we are exploring with THIM is whether there is at least one satisfactory theory.

To start, we examined several simulation results from the perspective of face validity. While THIM is theoretical, it is based to a substantial degree on empirical evidence, albeit summarized in the form of stylized facts. THIM simulations have all been run for 500 "years." This length of simulation is admittedly arbitrary. It has proven long enough that any artifacts from choice of initial conditions have died out; it allows for at least five generations of agents (the maximum age is 100); and it enables the results for various decades over this timespan to be checked for stability. (These stochastic elements also give rise to Monte Carlo error; the THIM results presented have been assessed to ensure that this source of error is not material.)

One example is the series of univariate distributions of health status for each of several age groups. In THIM, this is not an input, but rather the outcome of many interacting factors in a simulation. Figure 10A shows count frequencies for levels of H (the summary index of health in the [0,1] interval used in THIM) by age group, as generated by a typical THIM simulation. The horizontal axis is first broken down into a series of five-year age groups, and then within each of these age groups by levels of H ranging from zero to one in 20 intervals of width 0.05. Multiple curves are shown. These curves are from various decades over the 500-year simulation period. Since they lie almost on top of one another, it shows that this simulation's outputs from THIM are stable over time.

Qualitatively, the distributions become less tall and more negatively skewed (i.e., less concentrated at high levels of H) as we move from left to right up the age spectrum, indicating both a general decline in health and a decline in the total population as a result of higher (cumulative) mortality with higher age. These distributions are similar to those observed in Statistics Canada's National Population Health Survey for the McMaster Health Utility Index (HUI),[27] the real world counterpart of the H variable in THIM.

A

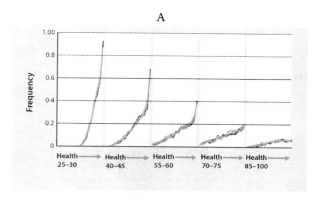

B

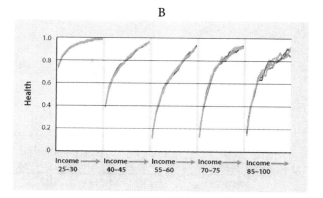

Figure 10. Cumulative health status distributions of (A) population counts and (B) income for selected age groups in a THIM simulation. In (A), the horizontal axis consists of 5-year age groups, and within each age group 20 intervals of H, each 0.05 wide. In (B), the horizontal axis consists of 5-year age groups, and then within each age group a series of income intervals of increasing width. Both simulations span 500 years. The legend indicates decades over the 500 years that are shown. Despite some variability, the time series of these distributions is quite stable. Wolfson (2016), used with permission[6]

THIM also produces plausible individual-level health-income gradients (figure 10B).[27] The horizontal axis is again first broken down by five-year age groups, but this time within age groups by income. The vertical axis is the average level of H within each age/income interval. Again, multiple curves are shown from decades over the 500-year simulation period. Since they lie close to one another, these simulation results are also stable over time.

The plausibility of these simulation outputs is evident by comparing figure 10B to figure 1: the health indicator becomes worse for those with lower income and better for those with higher income (though all age groups are combined in figure 1 while they are separated in figure 10B, and figure 1 shows mortality while figure 10B shows H, the curves sloping downward rather than upward). This same pattern can also be seen in McIntosh et al.[28]

In this case, moving from left to right to higher age groups, the gradients become steeper and somewhat more variable and noisy. This noisiness is due to the decreasing numbers of individuals at higher ages. (The absence of individuals with low health status H in the 85-to-90 age interval is due to the mortality selection, as posited, with mortality rates depending on H.)

Table 3 presents our first set of main results. The top three rows, showing inequality indices for the input Y* *potential* income distributions are identical to table 2. However, the resulting simulation output income inequality values in the following six rows are considerably different. The reason is that actual incomes depend not only on potential income Y*, but also the influences of parental and neighborhood factors working via the causal pathways embodied in our theory through education, systematic variations in income over the lifecycle based on a typical average age-income profile, an annual stochastic disturbance reflecting short-term income volatility, plus the possibility of mortality selection by income, especially for higher ages.

Table 3

Income Inequality's Path from Y* to Final Population Income Inequality for Three Inequality Measures, Five Y* Scenarios, and U Versus C Parameters

Simulation Number	1	2	3	4	5	6	7	8
Y* Gini coefficient	0.093	0.269	0.358	0.408	0.425	0.471	0.556	0.571
Y* median share	0.450	0.314	0.238	0.223	0.123	0.177	0.127	0.098
Y* polarization	0.015	0.206	0.330	0.291	0.657	0.350	0.380	0.467
C Gini coefficient	0.281	0.383	0.441	0.477	0.403	0.496	0.511	0.530
C median share	0.298	0.233	0.187	0.174	0.202	0.165	0.160	0.152
C polarization	0.140	0.190	0.266	0.270	0.247	0.280	0.276	0.287
U Gini coefficient	0.393	0.409	0.416	0.420	0.420	0.467	0.514	0.474
U median share	0.225	0.213	0.208	0.206	0.206	0.178	0.155	0.179
U polarization	0.192	0.213	0.219	0.221	0.221	0.259	0.291	0.249

From Wolfson (2016), used with permission.[6]

For example, the most equal potential income Y* scenario has a Gini coefficient of 0.093 for Y*. But when this is played out in a THIM simulation, the income distribution Gini coefficients for the C and U cities end up much more unequal at 0.264 and 0.370, respectively. At the other end of the posited Y* inequality scenarios, the highly unequal input distribution of Y* with a Gini coefficient of 0.571 ends up generating, in the context of all the other C/U parameters, somewhat less unequal Gini coefficient coefficients of 0.530 and 0.474 for C and U cities, respectively.

Interestingly, the C city parameters can actually result in a higher Gini coefficient (a smaller reduction from the Gini coefficient of the Y* input distribution in the first row) than the U city parameters (fourth and seventh rows). Still, for four of the Y* scenarios, the C Gini coefficient ends up being lower than the U Gini coefficient, while for three of these scenarios, the median share and polarization index show lower inequality for the C cities. The extent to which inequality in potential income Y* is translated by the model into inequality of the actual population distribution of income is not always the same when comparing U city scenarios to C city scenarios (figures 11–13, discussed further below).

Our key health outcome measures in THIM are life expectancy (LE) and health-adjusted life expectancy (HALE). HALE is life expectancy adjusted for years lived in less than full health. While LE is simply based on the length of life (1 when alive, 0 when dead), HALE is based on health status while alive (H when alive, 0 when dead). Since THIM simulates individuals throughout their life courses, both LE and HALE are built using individual microdata in exactly the same way that a national statistical office would do the calculation if it had the relevant data for the actual population using cross-sectional data from overlapping birth cohorts and the Sullivan method.[29] LE and HALE are both broader population health measures than the working age mortality used in figure 2, especially HALE.

These outcomes are plotted for each inequality measure in figure 11 with the (output) income inequality measures along the horizontal axis. (While the vertical axes in the three graphs are identical, the horizontal axis scales are specific to each inequality measure. But each of the three horizontal axis scales is the same as in the corresponding graphs for the two other scenarios shown in figures 12 and 13.)

Recall that the input baseline age-specific mortality schedule is associated with a conventional life expectancy of 77 years. The graphs, however, show that a range of LEs resulting from the THIM simulations, with some of these outcomes a bit higher and most somewhat lower.

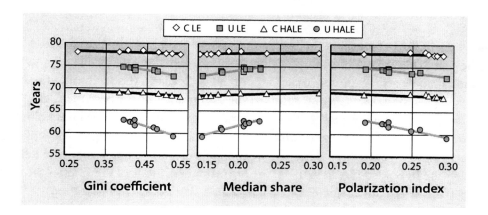

Figure 11. LE and HALE for U and C cities, by Gini, median share, and Polarization Index

The first observation is that in all cases, the LEs and HALEs (both measured in years) of the C cities are higher everywhere than those for the U cities. This result corresponds to the observation in figure 2 that Canadian cities generally have lower working-age mortality rates at similar levels of the median share inequality indicator.

The "realized" levels of income inequality are noticeably different for the U and C cities, even though each pair of scenarios (for a U and a C city) starts with the same levels of potential income (Y*) inequality (table 3). Figure 11 shows the C cities spanning a wider range of inequality levels across the horizontal axis than the U cities. Furthermore, the U cities tend to cluster at higher income inequality levels (i.e., higher Gini coefficient, lower median share, and higher polarization index) than the C cities. These tendencies reflect the complex and intertwined underlying processes in THIM.

Most importantly, from the viewpoint of our main hypothesis, the slopes of the relationships are systematically different. In all cases, there is an almost flat relationship for both LE and HALE with all three of the inequality measures for the C cities. But for the U cities, in all cases a slope is evident.

Furthermore, all slopes for the U cities are steeper for the HALE outcomes than for LE outcomes. This difference in slopes results from the socioeconomic processes posited in THIM having more extensive impacts for HALE (which is based on both mortality rates and health status) as compared to LE (which is affected only by mortality rates).

We have therefore established that THIM can indeed reproduce contingent correlations and can account for the results shown in figure 2—in effect a "proof by construction."

We next begin assessing which factors in THIM are most important. This pertains to our second hypothesis, that neighborhood income segregation is the key factor driving the observed Canada-U.S. differences, in contrast to an alternative hypothesis that the complex of direct and indirect education and income effects, irrespective of neighborhood income segregation, are most important. To assess these competing hypotheses, we divided the parameters in table 1 into sets, where the first set of three parameters is related directly to neighborhood income segregation.

Figure 12 shows the results comparing the U and U** scenarios, defined by the parameters in the corresponding columns in table 1. Recall that the key difference between these two scenarios was the propensity for neighborhood income segregation to arise. Under the U** scenario (last column, first three rows), the only change was to give the U city (second column) the same values as the baseline C city (first column). The results are clear. Changing the neighborhood income segregation parameters has no noticeable effect on the *slopes* for the U cities for all three inequality measures, as is shown in figure 12. Still, when these U city neighborhood income segregation parameters are changed to the C city values (the differences in the parameter settings are in bolded text in table 1), the horizontal positions of the U cities are shifted toward lower inequality (i.e., lower Gini coefficients, higher median shares, lower polarization).

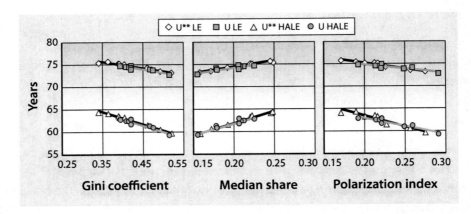

Figure 12. LE and HALE for U and U** cities by Gini, median share, and Polarization Index

Thus, based on these THIM simulations, neighborhood income segregation has a noticeable impact on overall income inequality as measured by any of our three indicators. But this change in inequality does not change the slopes of the LE or HALE health indicators in relation to income inequality; hence the U cities do not appear like C cities with regard to an absence of correlation between inequality and health.

In other words, income segregation, at least within the theory embodied in THIM, is not the key factor in accounting for the contingent correlation observed in figure 2.

But can anything else embodied in THIM's theory account for the observed contingent correlation? To address this question, we can weaken the range of posited differences in the remaining factors—specifically by moving from the C/U (first two columns of table 1) to the C*/U* pair of scenarios (third and fourth columns in table 1).

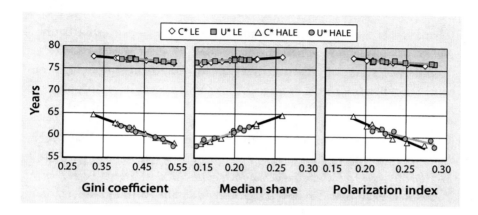

Figure 13. LE and HALE for C* and U* cities by Gini, median share, and Polarization Index

The results are shown in figure 13. Both U and C cities now have similar slopes. Compared to figure 12, the U city slopes in figure 13 are not as steep. But now, C city slopes have emerged, and are virtually identical to those for the U cities. The main difference in the comparison between the C* and the U* cities is that the differences between U and C cities in the posited impacts of all factors *other than* neighborhood income segregation have all been weakened. It is also notable that for each given Y* distribution, the C* cities generally have lower inequality than the corresponding U* cities.

Thus, differences in factors other than neighborhood income segregation, given the theory embodied THIM, can account for the difference observed in figure 2.

Implications

We have constructed a theory to account for the observation that correlations between income inequality and health appear to be contingent on country-specific factors. This theory is embodied in THIM, an agent-based microsimulation model. As with virtually all theories, major simplifications were made. At the same time, we appealed to real-world observations to infer a set of stylized facts, which have been incorporated into THIM with face validity, in that it can generate realistic patterns of outputs.

Our first major result shows that, given an appropriate set of input parameters, THIM is able to generate contingent patterns of correlation between income inequality and health similar to those observed, specifically between Canada and the United States. THIM may not provide the only plausible theory that accounts for the observations in figure 2, but we have shown that it is possible, in a relatively parsimonious manner using an agent-based model, to construct at least one adequate theory.

The second major result focuses on whether the observed contingent correlation when comparing Canada and the United States is the result of greater income segregation in the United States, which in turn is strongly related to racial segregation. Our answer is no. When we simulate a U.S.-style city but with Canadian-style neighborhood income segregation, the U.S. pattern of correlated health and income inequality indicators does not disappear.

Our third major result is that there are other Canada-U.S. differences that can account for the observed differences in correlations between income inequality and health measures across cities in the two countries. These include differences in the parent-to-child transmission of income and education advantage or disadvantage, the impact of neighborhood average income on local school quality and educational opportunities more generally, and the strength of income effects on health (among others).

Of course, there can be a relationship between these factors and neighborhood income segregation. However, there is no necessary correlation. Thus, our finding that overt neighborhood income segregation cannot account for the observed Canada-U.S. contingent correlations between income inequality and health (figure 12) does not mean that it is operating more indirectly through the factors that can account for the contingent correlation.

For example, a child's education depends jointly on both parental and neighborhood average relative incomes. As a result, high levels of income segregation will result (endogenously to the model) in larger differences of local school quality in THIM (as reflected in levels of E), so there can be some correlation between neighborhood income segregation and school quality.

However, in most large Canadian cities, school board catchment areas span the entire metropolitan area, including both poor and rich neighborhoods, and school board policies typically ensure substantial equality of school quality no matter the income levels of the students' parents.[c] For example, Canadian school boards typically ensure similar levels of library and athletic facilities, and rotate teachers and principals to ensure fairly even quality. Similarly, municipal amalgamation is more prevalent in Canada. With a broader geographic span for municipal governments, it is more likely that local public goods are more equally distributed, notwithstanding differences in neighborhood income.

In contrast, in the United States new and typically wealthy suburbs create their own local governments and school boards, thereby opting out of citywide responsibilities and avoiding obligations to redistribute resources to poorer (often inner city) schools.[30] Indeed, large U.S. metropolitan areas can have dozens, even more than a hundred in some cases, local governments.

Our THIM simulations suggest that having institutions such as citywide school boards and amalgamated municipal governments that can redistribute in-kind public goods (e.g., school quality) across neighborhoods, no matter how segregated these neighborhoods are in terms of incomes, is highly important, and indeed more important than neighborhood income segregation per se.

Similarly, our THIM simulations suggest that the tendency of parents to pass social advantage and disadvantage to their children is also more important than neighborhood income segregation. Again, while these tendencies may be correlated with neighborhood income, there are many other public policies that enhance equality of opportunity and hence intergenerational income mobility where, as observed,[17] Canada has twice the rate of intergenerational mobility as the United States. One such policy is the broader geographic span of school boards; other relevant policies include the generosity of basic income guarantees via programs such as welfare, unemployment insurance, and public pensions, as well as regulations in areas such as parental leave. In general, Canadian policies are more generous than those in the United States.

The strength of the causal effect from income to health status and mortality can also be independent of neighborhood incomes. In terms of health care, the differences between Canada and the United States are obvious; gaps in insurance coverage are far more stratified by individual incomes in the United States than in Canada, with negligible relationship to neighborhood income segregation. To the extent that causal pathways from income to health status and mortality operate via psychosocial[31] or neo-material[1] pathways, these too can be largely independent of neighborhood income segregation.

These implications, combined with our THIM results, suggest an important and possibly under-appreciated policy implication. Rather than moving people around to reduce racial and income segregation in schools and neighborhoods, policy interventions designed to weaken the correlation between city-level income inequality and health may be more effective. Such interventions would support local government structures that prevent the wealthy from opting out of the redistribution of citywide public goods (e.g., education, libraries, parks, and other recreation facilities) and increase the access of lower-income individuals to citywide amenities through more effective public transit and appropriate planning and zoning.

Notwithstanding the "American Dream" mythology of Horatio Alger (and, more recently, Bill Gates and Mark Zuckerberg), that by trying hard anyone can rise up through society's ranks, parents in the United States are more likely to pass their social and economic advantages and disadvantages on to their children than in Canada. In our THIM simulations, this pathway is more important than neighborhood income segregation. As a result, policies that truly provide a more level playing field, and in turn, greater equality of opportunity, are also potentially more important than policies focusing on neighborhood income segregation.

In all of these cases, THIM has generated empirically testable hypotheses. An important challenge has been the lack of appropriate data, especially neighborhood-level data for a sample of Canadian and U.S. cities. For example, there is nothing of the quality of the international PISA data on education.

Finally, THIM represents a step forward in modes of theorizing in social epidemiology. By using a quantified agent-based microsimulation model, we have brought together into a coherent framework many diverse elements of current social science and epidemiological research. There is an obvious and much older parallel to the field of astronomy where, historically, there has been a healthy iteration between observation and theory—new and more powerful telescopes have sparked new theories, which in turn have led to the design and funding of new kinds of astronomical observations. Recently, with the growth of all-sky surveys, astronomical theories are more commonly embodied in computer simulation models, for example of millions of stars in interacting galaxies (https://www.youtube.com/watch?v=D-0GaBQ494E) By analogy, the theoretical conclusions derived here with THIM can and should spark the development of the new observations needed for a more robust empirical assessment of our theory.

References

1. Lynch JW, Smith GD, Kaplan GA, House JS. Income inequality and mortality: importance to health of individual income, psychosocial environment, or material conditions. *BMJ.* 2000;320(7243):1200–1204.

2. Organisation for Economic Co-operation and Development (OECD). *In It Together: Why Less Inequality Benefits All.* Paris: OECD Publishing; 2015.

3. Hu Y, van Lenthe FJ, Mackenbach JP. Income inequality, life expectancy and cause-specific mortality in 43 European countries, 1987–2008: a fixed effects study. *Eur J Epidemiol.* 2015;30(8):615–625.

4. Zimmerman FJ. A commentary on "Neo-materialist theory and the temporal relationship between income inequality and longevity change". *Soc Sci Med.* 2008;66(9):1882–1894.

5. Wolfson M, Rowe G, Gentleman JF, Tomiak M. Career earnings and death: a longitudinal analysis of older Canadian men. *J Gerontol.* 1993;48(4):S167–S179.

6. Wolfson MC. Exploring Contingent Inequalities – Algorithm Description for the Theoretical Health Inequality Model (THIM). 2016. https://goo.gl/4M5iuP.

7. Gravelle H. How much of the relation between population mortality and unequal distribution of income is a statistical artefact? *BMJ.* 1998;316(7128):382–385.

8. Wolfson M, Kaplan G, Lynch J, Ross N, Backlund E. Relation between income inequality and mortality: empirical demonstration. *BMJ.* 1999;319(7215):953–955.

9. Deaton A, Lubotsky D. Mortality, inequality and race in American cities and states. *Soc Sci Med.* 2003;56(6):1139–1153.

10. Backlund E, Rowe G, Lynch J, Wolfson MC, Kaplan GA, Sorlie PD. Income inequality and mortality: a multilevel prospective study of 521,248 individuals in 50 US states. *Int J Epidemiol.* 2007;36(3):590–596.

11. Wilkinson RG, Pickett K. *The Spirit Level: Why Greater Equality Makes Societies Stronger.* New York, NY: Bloomsbury Press; 2009.

12. Ross NA, Wolfson MC, Dunn JR, Berthelot J-M, Kaplan GA, Lynch JW. Relation between income inequality and mortality in Canada and in the United States: cross sectional assessment using census data and vital statistics. *BMJ.* 2000;320(7239):898–902.

13. Ross NA, Dorling D, Dunn JR, et al. Metropolitan income inequality and working-age mortality: a cross-sectional analysis using comparable data from five countries. *J Urban Health.* 2005;82(1):101–110.

14. Walks RA, Bourne LS. Ghettos in Canada's cities? Racial segregation, ethnic enclaves and poverty concentration in Canadian urban areas. *Can Geogr.* 2006;50(3):273–297.

15. Organisation for Economic Co-operation and Development (OECD). *OECD Skills Outlook 2013: First Results from the Survey of Adult Skills. Figure 3.8c.* Paris: 2013.

16. Organisation for Economic Co-operation and Development (OECD). Table II.2.10: Parents' education and occupation, and students' home possessions, by schools' socioeconomic profile. In: OECD, ed. PISA 2012 Results: Excellence through Equity Giving Every Student the Chance to Succeed; Vol. 2. OECD Publishing; 2013:205.

17. Corak M. Income inequality, equality of opportunity, and intergenerational mobility. *J Econ Perspect.* 2013;27(3):79–102.

18. Krieger N. Epidemiology and the web of causation: has anyone seen the spider? *Soc Sci Med.* 1994;39(7):887–903.

19. Smith GD, Carroll D, Rankin S, Rowan D. Socioeconomic differentials in mortality: evidence from Glasgow graveyards. *BMJ.* 1992;305(6868):1554–1557.

20. Wolfson M, Gribble S, Beall R. Exploring contingent inequalities: building the theoretical health inequality model. In: Grow A, Van Bavel J, eds. *Agent-Based Modeling in Population Studies: Concepts, Models, and Applications.* Berlin: Springer International Publishing; 2017.

21. Sanmartin C, Ng E, Blackwell D, Gentleman J, Martinez M, Simile C. Joint Canada/US Survey of Health. 2002–3. National Center for Health Statistics and Statistics Canada; 2004. http://www.cdc.gov/nchs/data/nhis/jcush_analyticalreport.pdf.

22. Joumard I, André C, Nicq C. *Health Care Systems: Efficiency and Institutions.* Vol. 769. Paris: OECD Publishing; 2010.

23. Organisation for Economic Co-operation and Development (OECD). Table II.2.6: relationship between mathematics performance and elements of socioeconomic status. In: OECD, ed. PISA 2012 Results: Excellence through Equity Giving Every Student the Chance to Succeed. Vol. 2. Paris: OECD Publishing; 2013:193.

24. Wolfson MC. When Inequalities Diverge. *Am Econ Rev.* 1994;84(2):353–358.

25. Foster JE, Wolfson MC. Polarization and the decline of the middle class: Canada and the U.S. *J Econ Inequal.* 2010;8(2):247–273.

26. Atkinson AB. On the measurement of inequality. *J Econ Theory.* 1970;2(3):244–263.

27. Feeny D, Furlong W, Torrance GW, et al. Multiattribute and single-attribute utility functions for the health utilities index Mark 3 system. *Med Care.* 2002;40(2):113–128.

28. McIntosh C, Finès P, Wilkins R, Wolfson M. *Income Disparities in Health-Adjusted Life Expectancy for Canadian Adults, 1991–2001.* Ottawa: Statistics Canada; 2009.

29. Sullivan DF. A single index of mortality and morbidity. *HSMHA Health Rep.* 1971;86(4):347–354.

30. Orfield G, Eaton SE. *Dismantling Desegregation: The Quiet Reversal of Brown v. Board of Education.* New York, NY: New Press; 1997.

31. Marmot M, Wilkinson RG. Psychosocial and material pathways in the relation between income and health: a response to Lynch et al. *BMJ.* 2001;322(7296):1233–1236.

CHAPTER 10

MODELING THE UNDERLYING DYNAMICS OF THE SPREAD OF CRIME: AGENT-BASED MODELS

Carl P. Simon, PhD
Professor of Mathematics, Complex Systems and Public Policy
University of Michigan

David B. McMillon
Doctoral student
Center for the Study of Complex Systems
University of Michigan

Jeffrey Morenoff, PhD
Professor
Department of Sociology and Population Studies Center
University of Michigan

William M. Rand, PhD
Assistant Professor of Business Management
Poole College of Management, North Carolina State University

Acknowledgments: This research was partially supported by a grant from the University of Michigan M-Cubed Project. We thank the members of the NIH/OBSSR-sponsored Network on Inequality, Complexity and Health for their suggestions and feedback.

Crime and Population Health

Crime is closely associated with problems in population health. Areas with high crime rates tend to have high infant mortality, low birth weights, preterm births, and drug and alcohol abuse, as well as an overriding anxiety fueled by fears of property and violent crime.

A large range of policy interventions has been implemented to decrease crime in the United States, including the war on drugs and harsher punishments such as three-strike laws and mandatory sentencing. Over 2.25 million people are in U.S. penal institutions, the highest per capita rate in the world. Moreover, minorities, especially young black men, have disproportionately experienced the rise in incarceration in the United States over the past three decades. More than half of African American men with less than a high school degree go to prison at some point in their lives, and African American males make up one-third of America's incarcerated male population. Activists and researchers have coined the phrase "school to prison pipeline" to describe the structural and socioeconomic problems and policies that have led to this result.

Yet, prison terms, often in brutal settings, have not been effective crime deterrents. For example, the Bureau of Justice Statistics reported in 2014 that 77 percent of those released from prison in 2005 were arrested again within five years.[1] Acknowledging the empirical evidence surrounding the ineffectiveness of overly harsh sentencing policies, President Obama launched a program to overhaul the criminal justice system and released a number of low-level nonviolent drug offenders in July 2015.[2] This is line with a growing national effort to cut the number of people in prison.[3]

Other policy interventions to reduce crime have included increasing the police force, expanding social services, and the "broken windows strategy," which focuses on eradicating small crimes like vandalism and toll-booth jumping to prevent escalation to worse offenses.[4]

Crime as a Complex System

The 1967 President's Commission on Law Enforcement and Administration of Justice[5] created a Science and Technology Task Force to show how systems models could be used to project the workload and operating costs of police, courts, and corrections, and to analyze the effects and costs of policies being proposed by the commission.

Systems approaches play a vital role in evaluating policies in the social, behavioral, biological, ecological, and health sciences. A systems approach views the phenomenon under study as a system with a number of components and connections between them that indicate how the components affect one another. Because of these connections, an intervention that focuses on one component has ramifications across the system, and may interact in surprising ways with other types of interventions. Without a systems approach, such ramifications can lead to negative unintended consequences.

For example, in the criminal justice system, long mandatory sentences for nonviolent offenses such as drug use have led to overcrowded prisons, necessitating the release of more violent offenders. They have also increased the number of long-term career recidivists, due in part to how difficult it is to find employment with a criminal record. Furthermore, the sudden removal of gang leaders has led to destabilization in some communities and has actually increased violence.

The failure to use systems thinking has ramifications in areas other than criminal justice policy. In the 1950s American farmers began using powerful chemicals such as DDT to protect their crops from destructive insects. However, they did not take the complex food webs of our ecosystem into account, in which birds relied on the insects for food. In 1962, Rachel Carson's book[6], *Silent Spring*, listed the environmental damages that resulted from overuse of DDT, and the spraying of DDT was eventually banned—but not before the Bald Eagle became an endangered species. In 1859, Thomas Austin brought 24 wild rabbits to Australia where he continued his hobby of rabbit hunting. Without natural predators, the rabbits took over, numbered in the millions by 1870, and devastated the Australian ecology. The indiscriminate use of antibiotics for infections has led to the evolution of drug-resistant strains of bacteria and concerns about the evolution of super-bugs for which there may be no available antidote.

This chapter is part of a long-term effort to study the spread of crime from a systems point of view—*in particular*, to understand the system-wide ramifications of policy interventions such as hiring more police, intensifying school-based prevention efforts, reforming prison life, encouraging or forbidding parolees to return to their home communities, and, of course, increasing or decreasing the harshness of sentencing.

The main thrust of such a systems approach is the construction and analysis of models that show how various components (or "compartments") of the system are linked to each other. We first describe the two models we have studied earlier,[7] models, which were simple enough to find explicit expressions for the endemic levels of crime and the thresholds that separate low-level crime from high-level crime, but too simple to incorporate workable empirical data. Before adding complexities to these models, we first clarify and correct the threshold formulations in the second model.[7] We extend these analytic models to include additional population dynamics and develop an expression for the threshold for this extended model. However, the thrust of this chapter is to begin constructing and analyzing agent-based models that are more reflective of the real world, allowing for the possibility of model calibration from real data, and the potential to inform policy. We build a series of agent-based models, eventually including several aspects of the role of age in the spread of crime. To increase confidence in model validation, we show that at each step the new agent-based model docks well with earlier versions and with the analytic models, in that if we turn off all the additions in the extended model, the results of the extended model agree with those of the simpler one.

The 3D Model

In our original paper (McMillon, Simon, and Morenoff [2014]), henceforth denoted as MSM[7]), we began our analysis with the simplest possible system—one with people in three populations (or compartments): the criminally active (C), law-abiding citizens (X), and the incarcerated (I) (figure 1). The Greek letters in figure 1 represent parameters for the connections or flows among these compartments. The parameters α_{11} and α_{10} are the rates of onset of initial participation in criminal activity, whether motivated by peer interactions (α_{11}) or not (α_{10}). The parameter α_{11} is analogous to the "effective contact rate" in infectious disease models, and indicates the extent to which having more contact with criminally active people increases one's risk of participating in crime. It relates to a number of criminological theories, premised on the idea that patterns of social interaction influence decisions to participate in crime. The parameter α_{10} represents transitions into criminal activity that are driven only by the propensity toward crime, independent of interactions. β is the rate at which the criminally active return directly to crime-free life (desistance that is unrelated to incarceration); γ is the rate at which the criminally active are incarcerated, which combines processes related to the police, courts, and correctional systems; and finally, δ and ε are the rates at which those incarcerated return to criminal activity (δ; recidivism) or crime-free life (ε; rehabilitation/re-entry) upon release from prison.

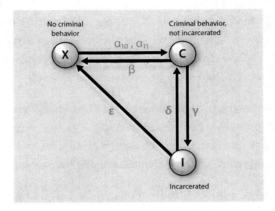

Figure 1. Simplest model of the spread of crime

The following system of differential equations captures the dynamics behind figure 1.

$$
\begin{aligned}
\frac{dX}{dt} &= \beta C - \alpha_{11} \frac{XC}{N-I} - \alpha_{10}X + \varepsilon I \\
\frac{dC}{dt} &= -\beta C + \alpha_{11} \frac{XC}{N-I} + \alpha_{10}X - \gamma C + \delta I \\
\frac{dI}{dt} &= \gamma C - I(\delta + \varepsilon) \\
X + C + I &= N
\end{aligned}
\tag{1}
$$

We begin with such a simple model in order to capture only the most fundamental aspects of criminal dynamics first. In this chapter, we gradually add complexities to make the model more realistic. This first model does not include aging, individual heterogeneities, a specific crime, or specifics about the criminal justice system.

One advantage of this simple system is that we can use mathematical analysis to understand relationships between the parameters, and the interactive roles they play in the long-run behavior of the system. We first assume that $\alpha_{10} = 0$, so that all new criminal activity is attributed to influence by other criminals. In this case, system (1) comes close to the well-studied models of the spread of infection: As previously indicated[7]:

$$
R_0 \equiv \frac{\alpha_{11}}{\beta + \gamma\left(\dfrac{\varepsilon}{\varepsilon + \delta}\right)}
\tag{2}
$$

is a threshold for system (1) in that:

- If R0 ≤ 1, then every solution of system (1) tends to a crime-free equilibrium with C = I = 0,

- If R0 > 1, then every solution of (1) tends to a unique endemic equilibrium with C > 0. In this latter case, the equilibrium "prevalence" of non-criminals on the street is

$$\frac{X}{N - I} = \frac{1}{R_0}. \tag{3}$$

Now we relax the assumption that people only turn to crime through peer influence. Suppose $\alpha_{10} > 0$, so that we allow law-abiding citizens to turn to crime independently of others. In this case there is no crime-free equilibrium. There are still two equilibria, high-crime and low-crime. If α_{10} is small enough, then the system goes to the low-crime equilibrium if the above R_0 is <1 and to the high-crime equilibrium if R_0 > 1. In both cases, it is possible to use the quadratic formula to calculate explicit expressions for the equilibrium values of X, C, and I.

The 5D Model

The first complexity we add to our system is to distinguish between criminally active people who have already spent time in prison (C_2), and those who have not (C_1). In doing so we add a state variable "R," representing those who have been (perhaps recently) released from prison are not criminally active, but have not yet assimilated back into society as law-abiding citizens. This also allows us to add prison term length to the model. With these additions, the model in figure 1 becomes the model in figure 2.

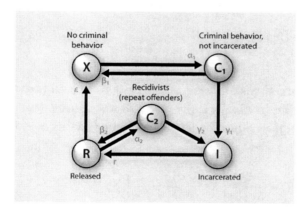

Figure 2. 5D model of the spread of crime

We decompose α_1 in figure 2 into α_{11} and α_{10} to capture the rate at which people first turn to criminal activity, either through peer influences (α_{11}) or on their own (α_{10}). Similarly, we decompose α_2—the rate at which those in the "R" state return to criminal activity—into α_{21} and α_{20}, representing recidivism due to influence from other criminally active people and recidivism independent of influence from others, respectively. Note that in this model recidivism is defined based on whether or not a criminal has been to prison before.

GROWING INEQUALITY

The desistance rate at which those in C_1 return to X is given by β_1. The parameter r represents the prison release rate; more intuitively, $1/r$ is the length of the prison term. The incarceration rates of those in C_1 and C_2 are given by γ_1 (the rate of "first-time imprisonment") and γ_2, respectively. In this extended model, the parameter ε is the rate at which people move from state R to state X. Like β_2, ε captures a desistance process among formerly incarcerated individuals, but unlike β_2, ε captures desistance for people who are not criminally active. The parameter ε also leads back to X, capturing pathways among people who are, for all intents and purposes, treated as non-criminals. For example, this could result from the formal expungement of a felony record. It is intended to capture the process of being released from bearing the mark of crime (rehabilitation) among those who have been to prison but are not criminally active. In contrast β_2, unlike ε, captures a desistance process among formerly incarcerated people who are criminally active, and leads back to R.

The corresponding differential equation system becomes:

$$\frac{dX}{dt} = \beta_1 C_1 - \alpha_{11}\frac{X(C_1+C_2)}{(N-I)} - \alpha_{10}X + \varepsilon R$$

$$\frac{dC_1}{dt} = -\beta_1 C_1 + \alpha_{11}\frac{X(C_1+C_2)}{(N-I)} + \alpha_{10}X - \gamma_1 C_1$$

$$\frac{dI}{dt} = \gamma_1 C_1 + \gamma_2 C_2 - rI$$

$$\frac{dR}{dt} = rI + \beta_2 C_2 - \alpha_{21}\frac{R(C_1+C_2)}{(N-I)} - \alpha_{20}R - \varepsilon R$$

$$\frac{dC_2}{dt} = -\beta_2 C_2 + \alpha_{21}\frac{R(C_1+C_2)}{(N-I)} + \alpha_{20}R - \gamma_2 C_2$$

$$X + C_1 + C_2 + R + I = N \qquad (4)$$

We build our analysis as before, first supposing that $\alpha_{10} = 0$, so that all first-time offenders turn to crime only through influence from the criminally active. We also first assume that $\alpha_{21} = 0$, so that all recidivism occurs without influence from the criminally active population. In this case, the threshold R_0' is:

$$R_0' \equiv \frac{\alpha_{11}}{\beta_1 + \gamma_1}\left(1 + \frac{\alpha_{20}\cdot\gamma_1}{(\gamma_2 + \beta_2)\cdot\varepsilon}\right). \qquad (5)$$

Once again, if $R_0' \leq 1$, the system converges to a crime-free equilibrium. If $R_0' > 1$, the system converges to an endemic equilibrium with C_1, C_2, and I all positive, and

$$\frac{X}{N-I} = \frac{1}{R_0'}. \qquad (6)$$

Policy Implications in MSM

As previously reported MSM,[7] the policy implications derived from the dynamical system (4) include:

- Increasing the rate of first-time imprisonment (increasing γ_1) could increase long-run crime if the formerly incarcerated are more likely to return to crime than to successfully rehabilitate (high α_2, low ε). For example, if prisons serve as schools of crime and employment is extremely difficult for those who were formerly incarcerated, then increasing the rate of first-time imprisonment is likely to contribute to the number of long-term recidivists.

- The equilibrium level of crime is independent of sentence length, at least in these simplified models.

- By expanding system (4) so that it differentiated between two and three-time recidivists, we found that a strict three-strikes policy leads to unreasonably high prison populations.

- The long-run levels of crime and incarceration are more sensitive to efforts to decrease the rate at which people turn to crime in the first place (prevention) than any other type of policy intervention in the system.

Correction to MSM

The goal of this chapter is to continue our systems approach to understanding the spread of crime. In particular, we continue the process of adding complexities to our models in order to make them more reflective of the real world. First, we need to clarify and correct one of the mathematical conclusions of MSM.

In MSM, we showed that (5) was a sharp threshold between the crime-free and endemic crime equilibria for system (4), when $\alpha_{10} = 0$ and $\alpha_{21} = 0$. The next step is to keep $\alpha_{10} = 0$, but allow α_{21} to be positive in system (4). In MSM we worked with the threshold candidate for this scenario:

$$R_0'' \equiv \frac{\alpha_{11}}{\beta_1 + \gamma_1}\left(1 + \frac{(\alpha_{20} + \alpha_{21})\cdot\gamma_1}{(\gamma_2 + \beta_2)\cdot\varepsilon}\right).$$

We showed in MSM that if $R_0'' < 1$, then system (4) with $\alpha_{10} = 0$ converges to a crime-free equilibrium. We suggested, without proof, that the converse is true, as it is for R_0 and R_0'. However, computer simulations have since shown that in fact system (4) with $\alpha_{10} = 0$, $\alpha_{21} > 0$, and $R_0'' > 1$ does sometimes converge to a crime-free equilibrium. In fact, as we will soon see, R_0' is a better threshold for the $\alpha_{21} > 0$ case than is R_0''. As we stated in MSM, when this system does converge to an endemic crime equilibrium, $X/(N - I)$ does not converge to $1/R_0''$.

Consider all proposed thresholds for the $\alpha_{21} > 0$ $\alpha_{10} = 0$ case. Clearly, $R_0' \leq R_0''$. There are three possible cases:

$$\text{Case 1: } R_0' < R_0'' < 1,$$

$$\text{Case 2: } 1 < R_0' < R_0'',$$

$$\text{Case 3: } R_0' < 1 < R_0''.$$

In case 1, we showed in MSM that all solutions converge to the crime-free equilibrium.

In case 2, we showed that if we decrease α_{21} to 0 and keep the other parameters the same, then the condition $1 < R_0'$ implies that the system goes to an endemic (crime-positive) solution. Now, if we increase α_{21} back to its original positive value, the long-run crime equilibrium will increase since including α_{21} gives an additional venue for the spread of crime. Mathematically, this is a result of Gronwall's Inequality: if $\mathbf{f(x)} > \mathbf{g(x)}$, then solutions of $d\mathbf{x}/dt = \mathbf{f(x)}$ are larger than solutions of $d\mathbf{x}/dt = \mathbf{g(x)}$ for each initial condition.

It follows that when $\alpha_{21} > 0$, case 1 implies a crime-free equilibrium, and case 2 implies an endemic crime equilibrium. Case 3 is much more difficult. We turn to computer simulations of system (4) using the Berkeley Madonna software, which can generate numerical solutions of complex differential equations that are not amenable to mathematical analysis.[8] In our simulations, we chose reasonable values for the parameters for our Madonna runs (table 1).

In table 1, runs 1–4 involved the $\alpha_{21} = 0$ case in which R_0' and R_0'' agree (cases 1 and 2). In these cases, $1/R_0''$ agrees with the equilibrium prevalence computed by Madonna in the last column of table 1.

Run 8 represents case 1. As predicted, the system converges to the crime-free equilibrium.

Runs 5, 6, 9, 10, 12 represent case 2. In all of these runs, the system converges to a positive-crime equilibrium, but, interestingly, the equilibrium $X / (N - I)$ is better approximated by $1/R_0'$ than by $1/R_0''$.

Case 3. Runs 7 and 11 represent case 3, with $R_0' < 1$ and $R_0'' > 1$. In both runs, the system converges to the crime-free equilibrium. From Runs 7 and 11 (and dozens of similar runs), whether or not R_0' is < 1 seems to be the more appropriate threshold for case 3.

In figure 3, we fixed all of the parameters to the values in Run 12 in table 1 with the exception of α_{20}. We let α_{20} increase from 0.02 to 0.05 and kept track of R_0' and R_0'' in the process. R_0'' remained above 1 throughout. However, when R_0' moved across the $R_0' = 1$ threshold at $\alpha_{20} \sim 0.033$, the equilibrium changed from crime-free to endemic crime. This further supports $R_0' = 1$ being the better threshold for case 3.

Now we present a mathematical argument for $R_0' = 1$ as the threshold for case 3. Let J denote the Jacobian derivative for system (4) at the crime-free equilibrium: a 4-by-4 matrix of the partial derivatives of the right-hand side of (4) evaluated at $X = 1$, $C_0 = C_1 = R = 0$, and $I = N - (X + C_1 - C_2 + R)$. For the $\alpha_{21} = 0$ case, in which R_0' is the threshold, the crime–free equilibrium is asymptotically stable, so all of the eigenvalues of J have a negative real part.

Now we repeat this procedure, allowing α_{21} to be positive. The corresponding Jacobian is still the same J,

Table 1

Initial Conditions for Runs 13-15, with X(0)/N=0.8, 0.5, and 0.1, Respectively

Run	Case	Alpha 11	Alpha 21	Alpha 20	Beta 1	Beta 2	Gamma 1	Gamma 2	Epsilon	r	R'_0 (without alpha21)		R''_0 (with alpha21)		Madonna
											R'_0	$1/R'_0$	R''_0	$1/R''_0$	$X/(N-I)$
1	2	0.42	0	0.10	0.17	0.22	0.15	0.18	0.070	0.20	2.016	0.496	2.016	0.496	0.496
2	2	0.30	0	0.10	0.17	0.22	0.15	0.18	0.070	0.20	1.440	0.695	1.440	0.695	0.695
3	1	0.20	0	0.10	0.17	0.22	0.15	0.18	0.070	0.20	0.960	N/A	0.960	N/A	1.000
4	1	0.12	0	0.10	0.17	0.22	0.15	0.18	0.070	0.20	0.576	N/A	0.576	N/A	1.000
5	2	0.42	0.10	0.10	0.17	0.22	0.15	0.18	0.070	0.20	2.016	0.496	2.719	0.368	0.458
6	2	0.30	0.10	0.10	0.17	0.22	0.15	0.18	0.070	0.20	1.440	0.695	1.942	0.515	0.661
7	3	0.20	0.10	0.10	0.17	0.22	0.15	0.18	0.070	0.20	0.960	N/A	1.295	0.772	1.000
8	1	0.12	0.10	0.10	0.17	0.22	0.15	0.18	0.070	0.20	0.576	N/A	0.777	N/A	1.000
9	2	0.31	0.10	0.10	0.20	0.02	0.01	0.20	0.015	0.01	1.924	0.520	2.370	0.422	0.481
10	2	0.31	0.10	0.00	0.2	0.02	0.01	0.20	0.015	0.01	1.476	0.677	1.920	0.521	0.634
11	3	0.28	0.15	0.00	0.20	0.10	0.10	0.20	0.100	0.10	0.933	N/A	1.400	0.714	1.000
12	2	0.27	0.05	0.05	0.20	0.10	0.10	0.20	0.100	0.10	1.050	0.952	1.200	0.833	0.949
13	3	0.28	0.91	0.00	0.20	0.10	0.10	0.20	0.100	0.10	3.764	0.266	0.933	N/A	0.615
14	3	0.28	0.91	0.00	0.20	0.10	0.10	0.20	0.100	0.10	3.764	0.266	0.933	N/A	0.615
15	3	0.28	0.91	0.00	0.20	0.10	0.10	0.2	0.100	0.10	3.764	0.266	0.933	N/A	1.000

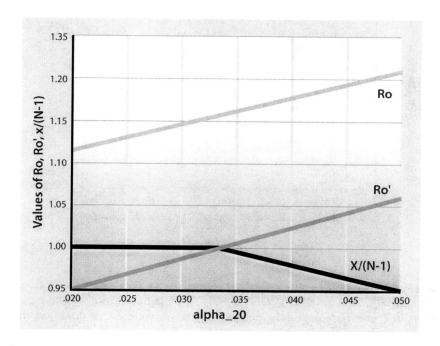

Figure 3. $R'_0 = 1$ may be a better threshold for case 3 than $R''_0 = 1$. As R'_0 crosses the 1.000 threshold, crime becomes endemic for run 11 in table 1, even with $\alpha_{21} > 0$

since α_{21} drops out of the Jacobian for the full system (4). When J has only eigenvalues with negative real part (i.e., when $R_0' < 1$), the crime-free equilibrium is at least locally asymptotically stable even when $\alpha_{21} > 0$.

To determine whether the crime-free equilibrium is still globally asymptotically stable, we studied the effect of parameter changes (figure 4). In particular, we varied α_{21} from 0 to 1 and kept the other parameter values as they were in Runs 13 to 15 in table 1. Since α_{21} is fixed at zero throughout these runs, R_0' is fixed (at $R_0' = R_0'' = 0.9333$). As α_{21} increases from 0 to 1, R_0'' increases from 0.9333 to 4.0444. As just shown, for most of this process, the system converges to the crime-free equilibrium. As α_{21} crosses 0.871, the system begins to converge to a positive crime equilibrium, at least starting with the initial fraction of criminals equal to 0.90. However, we know that the crime-free equilibrium is still locally asymptotically stable, and indeed, if the initial fraction of criminals is 0.10 instead of 0.90, Madonna shows the system tending to the crime-free equilibrium. In other words, for large α_{20} and for the other parameters (table 1), the system has two attracting equilibria, an uncommon phenomenon in contagion models.

In summary, in case 1 $(R_0' < R_0'' < 1)$, the system converges to the crime-free equilibrium. In case 2 $(1 < R_0' < R_0'')$, the system converges to an endemic crime equilibrium. However, in case 3 $(R_0' < 1 < R_0'')$, the crime-free equilibrium is locally asymptotically stable, and the vast majority of our Madonna runs converged to the crime-free equilibrium for any initial condition. For cases with large enough α_{21} and R_0'', while initial conditions near the crime-free equilibrium led to convergence to the crime-free equilibrium, other initial conditions led to convergence to an endemic crime equilibrium.

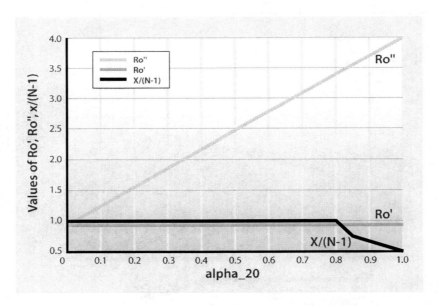

Figure 4. An example with two stable equilibria. In this version of run 13, α_{21} increases from 0 to 1, R_0' remains constant at 0.9333, and R_0'' increases from 0.9333 to 4.0444. The initial fraction of active criminals is 0.9. The system converges to the crime free equilibrium, until α_{21} increases beyond 0.8. At this point, there are two stable equilibria

Agent-Based Models

In MSM, we were able to add complexities to system (4), differentiating between criminally active people who have been to prison and those who have not, allowing us to shed light on the benefits of a systems approach to studying the spread of crime. However, these simple models do not include many critical aspects of the spread of crime. For example, they assume a generic crime and homogeneous agents, and do not include age structure, a nuanced criminal justice system, or an underlying community structure. With these simplifying assumptions, it is difficult to relate these models to actual crime data. To handle these important complexities, we needed to move from analytical models to agent-based models, which are especially powerful tools for modeling heterogeneities among individuals.

Agent-Based Models of Crime in the Literature

Agent-based modeling has not been a common approach in studies of crime and criminology. The 2014 *Encyclopedia of Criminology and Criminal Justice*[9] has three articles on their role in the study of crime, which provide background on how agent-based models work and how they are used. They challenge crime modelers to take advantage of agent-based models as "a technique that offers considerable promise to those who aim to build explanatory models of complex social systems."[10] Citing Epstein and Axtell,[11] Epstein,[12] Axelrod,[13] and Gilbert and Troitzsch[14] among others, they list the key characteristics of agent-based models:

- Autonomous agents in a bottom-up scenario.

- Heterogeneous agents and landscapes.

- Local interactions between agents in an explicit space.

- Bounded rationality in agents' choices.

They suggest that agent-based models would be valuable instruments to model the spatial and temporal clustering of crime, repeat victimization, repeat offending, spatial characteristics of crime trips, and the age-crime curve. As one example, they cite the generative models of Birks et al.[15], which use simulations to test specific criminological theories.

Citing Gilbert and Troitzsch,[15] Groff urges that "simulation models … start with simple models and then systematically add complexity to ensure that the dynamics are well understood before continuing,"[16] a caveat that lies at the heart of our approach. She cites Eck and Liu[17] and Groff and Birks[18] for overviews of agent-based models in the study of crime type, "including residential burglary, commercial robbery, fraud, heroin use, drug markets, and crime in general."

The third article[19] in the *Encyclopedia* summarizes papers that use agent-based models to study the spread of crime, including:

- Hayslett-McCall et al.,[20] which includes networks and social cohesion in their household burglary model.

- Malleson and Evans,[21] which models psychological motives that lead one to crime.

- Groff,[22] which models how the configuration of urban streets can influence the locations of street crime.

Each of these last two add geographic realism to their models by including a geographical information system (GIS).

Malleson et al.[19] conclude their survey article by pointing out that most agent-based models "concentrate on one particular aspect of the system." It is the central goal of our project to use agent-based models and compartmental models to understand how the system fits together and how interventions in one area can have important ripples in other areas, spurred on by the conviction that the whole is truly more than the sum of its parts.

Step 1: Agent-based Models with Homogenous Agents, Stochastic System Dynamics

We constructed the first agent-based model (ABM1), as a bridging exercise between compartmental system (4) and later agent-based models in which each agent has its own identity and underlying characteristics (such as age, sex, and SES). In this first step, agents are homogeneous actors without individual identities. They are divided into the five classes of system (4): law-abiding citizens (X), the criminally active population that has not yet been incarcerated (C_1), the incarcerated (I), parolees (R), and the formerly incarcerated criminally active (C_2). We use the same transition parameters as in system (4). For each time step, law-abiding citizens will turn to criminal activity with probability $\{\alpha_{10} + [\alpha_{11} * (C_1 + C_2)/(N - I)]\}$, criminals in C_1 will reform with probability β_1 and become incarcerated with probability γ_1, etc. Of course, this model is only weakly agent-based, there are individuals but they act on population-level dynamics—and mirrors closely the compartmental model (4). An important contribution in this first step in agent-based modeling is to add stochasticity to the deterministic dynamics of system (4).

We used the Netlogo software[23] to build and analyze our agent-based models. The Netlogo program is available at http://www.lsa.umich.edu/cscs/research/onlineresources.

As expected, for nearly all of our runs, the Netlogo program mirrored closely the Madonna results, but in a stochastic manner. For 10 runs with the same parameter values, the average long-run proportion of non-incarcerated individuals who are law-abiding citizens ($X / (N - I)$) was consistent with that found by the deterministic program Madonna.

However, in the runs with α_{21} over 0.9, we found interesting divergences. Runs 13–15 used the same parameters (table 1) but different initial conditions; Run 13 started with $X(0) = 0.9$ and $C_1(0) = 0.1$, Run 14 had $X(0) = C_1(0) = 0.5$, and Run 15 had $X(0) = 0.1$ and $C_1(0) = 0.9$.

The Madonna runs showed that Run 13 converged to the crime-free equilibrium and thus started in its basin of attraction. Madonna runs 14 and 15 converged to $X / (N - I) = 0.6154$ and thus started in its basin of attraction.

The more stochastically oriented Netlogo run 13 also converged to the crime-free equilibrium, but its Run 14 stayed near the endemic crime equilibrium for a few thousand steps before eventually converging to the crime-free equilibrium (unlike the Madonna runs). The Netlogo versions of Run 15 eventually converged to the crime-free equilibrium, but sometimes the system stayed close to the endemic crime equilibrium ($X/(N - I) \sim 0.6154$) for thousands of steps—once for over 16,000 steps. These last runs indicate that the set of initial conditions that lead to the positive-crime equilibrium (with $X/(N - I) \sim 0.6154$) is not as robust as that of the crime-free equilibrium, since stochasticity can drive the system back to the crime-free equilibrium.

This illustrates another benefit of agent-based models. Only by running agent-based simulations with high α_{21} and watching them converge to the crime-free equilibrium, unlike the deterministic Madonna model, did we realize the existence of two stable equilibria for some parameters in system (4).

Step 2: Agent-based Models With Heterogeneous Agents By Age

The next step in our modular process of building agent-based versions of system (4) is to allow individual-level dynamics that mirror system (4). Once individuals have identities that interact on an individual level, we can also study the roles that characteristics such as age and SES play in the spread of crime.

We first focus on age. As *The Encyclopedia of Criminality and Criminal Justice* [9] points out:

> "One of the most consistent findings across studies on offending in different countries is the age-crime curve.[24,25] The relationship between age and crime is of an asymmetrical bell shape, showing that the prevalence of offending (the percentage of offenders in a population) tends to increase from late childhood, peaks in the teenage years (around ages 15 to 19), and then declines from the early 20s, often with a long tail."[26]

Figure 5 shows the predicted probability of offending by age for all crime, as compiled and smoothed by Sampson and Laub,[27] with separate curves for those with higher-risk childhoods versus those with lower-risk childhoods.

Our second agent-based model (ABM2) includes ages and friendship networks in a number of ways. Most importantly, each agent is a distinct individual with an age that increases with each computer tick (Netlogo's unit of time). At various ages, these agents have differing proclivities to engage in criminal activity. In particular, the transition parameters into criminal activity (α_{10}, α_{11}, α_{20}, and α_{21}) vary with age, and can be set by sliders in ABM2. To achieve this, ABM2 uses a bell-shaped or tent-shaped function that peaks at a chosen age and multiplies the alphas of ABM1.

Next, in ABM2 individuals are more likely to be lured into crime by people whose age is within a certain range of their own age. This range is set by a slider. In ABM1, an agent can be initiated into criminal activity by any criminal, and age plays no role.

Finally, ABM2 includes the option of setting up a network of friendships in which contagion into crime is most likely to occur. Any of these of three options would be extremely complicated, if not impossible, to include in a deterministic differential equation model.

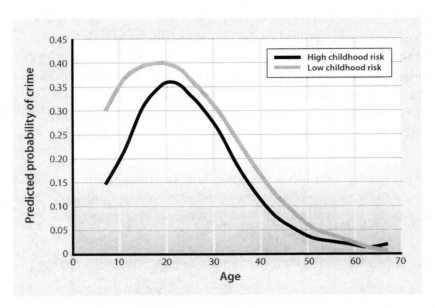

Figure 5. Predicted probability of committing a crime by age, adapted from Sampson and Laub.[27]

Details of Model ABM2

Once the model begins running, a certain number of agents are created: a number determined by the global constant **people**, which is set to a default value of 1,000. Each individual is then initialized into one of the five classes (X, C_1, C_2, I, or R). The proportion of agents assigned to each class is determined by the sliders **initial_criminals, initial_prisoners, initial_parolees,** and **initial_recidivists**.

One key difference between ABM1 and ABM2 is the **peer-effects** slider, which can be set to **global, age,** or **network**. If it is set to **global**, the model runs without age effects and reflects ABM1, but with individual-level dynamics. An agent that is currently a law-abiding citizen (X) will become a criminal (move to C_1) with a probability $\alpha_{10} + [\alpha_{11} * (C_1+C_2)/(N − I)]$. An agent that is currently a criminal becomes a law-abiding citizen with probability β_1 or a prisoner with probability γ_1. An agent that is currently a prisoner gets released from prison and goes to the R class with probability r. An agent that is currently in the R class becomes a law-abiding citizen with probability ε or becomes a recidivist (in C_2) with probability $\alpha_{20} + [\alpha_{21} * (C_1 + C_2)/(N − I)]$. An agent that is currently a recidivist becomes a prisoner with probability γ_2 or returns to the R class with probability β_2.

If the **peer-effects** slider is set to **age**, then each agent has an age between minimum age (min-age) and maximum age (max-age) as one of its characteristics, and this affects the inter-agent dynamics. Ages are assigned randomly at the onset of each run and increase with each tick. When an agent reaches max-age, the agent "dies" (leaves the program) and is replaced by a min-age agent in the law-abiding citizen class X.

When **peer-effects** is set to **age** there are two possible cases. In the first case, the **risk-growth** button is set to **none**. In the second case, it is set to either a normal or tent distribution.

When the risk-growth slider is set to **none**, an agent's actions nearly follow the same rules as in the **global** setting. The important difference here is that the agent's "**my_pce**," or peer-criminal effect variable [(C1 + C2)/(N − I)] only includes non-incarcerated agents who are criminally active but whose age is within **age-threshold** ticks of the current agent's age. Here, age only affects the dynamics insofar as people are influenced into criminal activity by their peers, that is, by agents who are close to them in age.

When the **risk-growth** slider is set to **tent** or **normal**, the alpha transition rates are also affected by age. Each alpha is multiplied by a real-valued function f(x) of age (x) whose graph is either a tent- or bell-shaped map. The area under the graph of f is one and the support of f is the interval between min-age and max-age. For clarity, suppose the age at which the maximum value of f occurs is called the peak-risk. For the sake of flexibility, the program uses a slider to choose the fraction (**mean-peak-risk**) between 0 and 1 of the "lifespan" at which peak-risk occurs:

mean-peak-risk = [(peak-risk) minus (min-age)]/[(max-age) minus (min-age)].

The value of f is called **risk-multiplier**. Altogether, in this case, the probability that a law-abiding citizen gets lured into crime is given by:

risk-multiplier * alpha_10 + risk-multiplier * alpha_11 * my_pce.

Finally, the **peer-effects** slider can be set to **network**. In this case, one establishes a network among the agents so that those agents in C_1 and C_2 who are also in the agent's network have a much higher chance of luring the agent into criminal activity than those outside the agent's network. This option should be especially valuable when we study specific community structures or the effects of gangs, but we have not yet explored it in our simulations.

Docking Our Models

These agent-based models can seem ad hoc and complex. To ensure that they remain relevant and informative as we add these complexities, we check that each new expanded model docks well with the previous version. We indicated above that ABM1 docks well with our analytical model (4). The next step is to check that ABM2 docks well with model (4), and ABM1 when ABM2 is in the global setting (age turned off). Tables 2A and 2B illustrate that it does indeed dock well, even though the dynamics in ABM2, which focuses on agents as individuals, differs considerably from the population-level dynamics of ABM1 and system (4) (table 2).

Adding Population Dynamics to System (4)

Docking ABM2 with ABM1 and system (4) was trickier when we begin to incorporate age effects into ABM2. After all, age plays no role in system (4). We began by altering system (4) by including birth and death rates so that agents at least have a life span distribution. To keep population size constant, we kept the birth and death rates equal to each other. Note that "initiation rate" is a more suitable phrase than "birth rate," since we are not concerned with agents at extremely young ages, who have a negligible risk of

Table 2A

System (4), ABM1 and ABM2/global (μ = 0): Parameters Values for 18 Runs

Run	ABM1 $X/(N-I)$	ABM2 Global $X/(N-I)$	ABM2 Age Threshold at max	Analytic R_0'	Analytic $X/(N-I)$ $1/R_0'$	Madonna Threshold R_0
1	0.12	0.12	0.12	8.55	0.1170	8.55
2	0.13	0.13	0.13	7.77	0.1287	7.77
3	0.15	0.15	0.16	6.73	0.1486	6.73
4	0.22	0.22	0.21	4.52	0.2212	4.52
5	0.33	0.33	0.33	3.06	0.3268	3.06
6	0.50	0.5	0.51	1.98	0.5051	1.98
7	0.58	0.58	0.58	1.72	0.5814	1.72
8	0.61	0.61	0.60	1.65	0.6061	1.65
9	0.70	0.70	0.68	1.42	0.7042	1.42
10	0.76	0.74	0.76	1.31	0.7634	1.31
11	0.84	0.80	0.82	1.19	0.8403	1.19
12	0.96	0.92	0.95	1.04	0.9615	1.04
13	1.00	1.00	1.00	0.90	N/A	0.90
14	1.00	1.00	1.00	0.81	N/A	0.81
15	1.00	1.00	1.00	0.71	N/A	0.71
16	1.00	1.00	1.00	0.71	N/A	1.17
17	0.85	0.85	0.86	1.11	N/A	1.84
18	0.68	0.70	0.68	1.11	N/A	2.56

criminal involvement. Similarly, "termination rate" is more suitable than "death rate." For simplicity, we continued to use more straightforward terms and the Greek letter mu (μ) to represent this common birth rate and death rate. We assumed that individuals enter the model as law-abiding citizens with the same probability (μ) of dying in each of the five states. This transforms system (4) to system (6):

$$\frac{dX}{dt} = +\beta_1 C_1 - \alpha_{11} \frac{X(C_1 + C_2)}{N - I} - \alpha_{10} X + \varepsilon R + \mu N - \mu X$$

$$\frac{dC_1}{dt} = -\beta_1 C_1 + \alpha_{11} \frac{X(C_1 + C_2)}{N - I} + \alpha_{10} X - \gamma C_1 - \mu C_1$$

216

$$\frac{dI}{dt} = +\gamma_1 C_1 + \gamma_2 C_2 - rI - \mu I$$

$$\frac{dR}{dt} = +rI + \beta_2 C_2 - \alpha_{21}\frac{R(C_1 + C_2)}{N - I} - \alpha_{20}R - \varepsilon R - \mu R \qquad (6)$$

$$\frac{dC_2}{dt} = -\beta_2 C_2 + \alpha_{21}\frac{R(C_1 + C_2)}{N - I} + \alpha_{20}R - \gamma_2 C_2 - \mu C_2$$

$$N = X + C_1 + C_2 + R + I.$$

In MSM, we analyzed equation-based dynamical systems of the spread of crime by computing: 1) a threshold that separates global convergence to a crime-free equilibrium from global convergence to an equilibrium with endemic crime, and 2) an explicit formula for the prevalence of crime in the latter case. In laymen's terms, what does it take to beat crime, and how much crime is there if we can't beat it? We do the same for system (6). In MSM we first assumed $\alpha_{10} = 0$, in which case there is a crime-free equilibrium, and then relaxed that assumption, noting that when $\alpha_{10} > 0$ the crime-free equilibrium bifurcates to a low-crime equilibrium and the endemic crime equilibrium bifurcates to a higher-crime equilibrium. Furthermore, as we indicated at the beginning of this paper, when $\alpha_{21} > 0$ the analysis becomes extremely complicated, with relatively little gain in insight. In carrying out tasks 1) and 2) for system (6), for the sake of simplicity and insight, we first assume $\alpha_{10} = 0$ and $\alpha_{21} = 0$ in our first derivations—in words, criminal activity among those who have never been incarcerated is linked only to interactions with others, but interactions play no role in recidivism (among those who have previously been incarcerated).

In MSM, we used a Lyapunov function technique to compute the threshold for (4). We use a similar technique to compute the following threshold for (6):

$$(7)$$

$$R_0 = \frac{\alpha_{11}}{\beta_1 + \gamma_1 + \mu}\left(1 + \frac{\alpha_{20}\gamma_1}{B}\right), \quad \text{where}$$

$$B \equiv \mu\alpha_{20}\left(1 + \frac{\gamma_2 + \mu}{r}\right) + (\varepsilon + \mu)(\gamma_2 + \beta_2 + \mu)\left(1 + \frac{\mu}{r}\right).$$

For the case $\alpha_{10} = \alpha_{21} = 0$, system (6) converges to the crime-free equilibrium (from any initial condition) if and only if $R_0 \leq 1$. If $R_0 > 1$, the system converges to an endemic crime equilibrium with the equilibrium prevalence of law-abiding citizens equal to one over R_0:

$$\frac{X}{N - I} = \frac{1}{R_0}. \qquad (8)$$

The proofs of (7) and (8) follow the pattern in MSM; for completeness, we sketch the proof of (7) in the Appendix to this paper.

Table 2B

**System (4), ABM1 and ABM2/global (μ = 0): Noncriminal Prevalence, X/(N − I)
for the 18 Runs, Computed Four Different Ways**

Run	ABM1 X/(N − I)	ABM2 Global X/(N − I)	ABM2 Age Threshold at max	Analytic R'_0	Analytic X/(N − I) $1/R'_0$	Madonna Threshold R_0
1	0.12	0.12	0.12	8.55	0.1170	8.55
2	0.13	0.13	0.13	7.77	0.1287	7.77
3	0.15	0.15	0.16	6.73	0.1486	6.73
4	0.22	0.22	0.21	4.52	0.2212	4.52
5	0.33	0.33	0.33	3.06	0.3268	3.06
6	0.50	0.5	0.51	1.98	0.5051	1.98
7	0.58	0.58	0.58	1.72	0.5814	1.72
8	0.61	0.61	0.60	1.65	0.6061	1.65
9	0.70	0.70	0.68	1.42	0.7042	1.42
10	0.76	0.74	0.76	1.31	0.7634	1.31
11	0.84	0.80	0.82	1.19	0.8403	1.19
12	0.96	0.92	0.95	1.04	0.9615	1.04
13	1.00	1.00	1.00	0.90	N/A	0.90
14	1.00	1.00	1.00	0.81	N/A	0.81
15	1.00	1.00	1.00	0.71	N/A	0.71
16	1.00	1.00	1.00	0.71	N/A	1.17
17	0.85	0.85	0.86	1.11	N/A	1.84
18	0.68	0.70	0.68	1.11	N/A	2.56

Two observations about (7) and (8): first, when μ = 0, (7) reverts to (5) above. However, unlike (5), the threshold R_0 and the endemic level of crime now depend on the length of the prison term $1/r$. This seems more realistic than the situation in (5). However, note that the dependence involves only r/μ. The long-run equilibrium (7, 8) is affected by the prison term length only relative to the expected "life span" of susceptibility to criminal involvement.

The next step in this process is to include μ > 0 in the dynamics of ABM1 and ABM2 in the global setting mode. Table 3 shows that the results of both the population-level ABM1 and the individual-level ABM2

Table 3

Comparison of System (6), ABM1 and ABM2/global with $\mu > 0$

Run #	Alpha 11	Beta 1	Gamma 1	Epsilon	Rho	Gamma 2	Alpha 20	Beta 2	Alpha 21	Mu	R0'''	1/R0 '''	Madonna X/(N-I)	ABM 1 X/(N-I)	ABM 2 Global
1	0.50	0.00	0.09	0.11	0.09	0.17	0.36	0.04	0.00	0.27	1.42	0.70	0.70	0.69	0.70
2	0.50	0.00	0.18	0.11	0.09	0.17	0.36	0.04	0.00	0.27	1.17	0.86	0.86	0.85	0.86
3	0.50	0.00	0.18	0.11	0.09	0.17	0.36	0.04	0.00	0.20	1.42	0.70	0.70	0.71	0.70
4	0.50	0.05	0.18	0.11	0.09	0.17	0.36	0.04	0.00	0.10	1.86	0.54	0.54	0.55	0.55
5	0.50	0.05	0.09	0.11	0.09	0.09	0.36	0.04	0.00	0.10	2.40	0.42	0.42	0.42	0.42
6	0.50	0.05	0.09	0.03	0.09	0.09	0.45	0.04	0.00	0.10	2.50	0.40	0.40	0.41	0.41
7	0.50	0.05	0.09	0.03	0.09	0.09	0.45	0.04	0.00	0.04	4.62	0.22	0.22	0.22	0.21
8	0.50	0.05	0.09	0.03	0.09	0.09	0.45	0.04	0.00	0.01	11.92	0.08	0.08	0.09	0.09
9	0.16	0.05	0.09	0.03	0.09	0.09	0.45	0.04	0.00	0.05	1.27	0.79	0.79	0.81	0.80
10	0.17	0.05	0.09	0.03	0.09	0.09	0.45	0.04	0.00	0.06	1.19	0.84	0.83	0.84	0.84
11	0.18	0.06	0.09	0.03	0.09	0.09	0.45	0.04	0.00	0.07	1.09	0.92	0.92	1.00	1.00
12	0.18	0.06	0.09	0.03	0.09	0.09	0.45	0.04	0.34	0.07	1.09	0.92	0.92	1.00	1.00
13	0.31	0.06	0.09	0.03	0.09	0.09	0.45	0.04	0.34	0.07	1.87	0.53	0.52	0.53	0.53
14	0.42	0.17	0.15	0.07	0.20	0.18	0.10	0.22	0.10	0.00	2.09	0.50	0.46	0.45	0.45
15	0.28	0.20	0.10	0.10	0.10	0.20	0.00	0.10	0.15	0.00	0.93	1.07	1.00	1.00	1.00
16	0.27	0.20	0.10	0.10	0.10	0.20	0.05	0.10	0.05	0.00	1.05	0.95	0.95	1.00	1.00
17	0.31	0.06	0.09	0.03	0.09	0.09	0.00	0.04	0.91	0.07	1.41	0.71	0.54	0.54	0.55

dock well with the results of analytic model (6) in this case. The third and fourth columns from the right in table 3 show that for $\mu > 0$ equality (8) works perfectly for $\alpha_{21} = 0$ and fairly well for $0 < \alpha_{21} < 0.5$. Comparing the last three columns of table 3 we see that that the global settings of ABM1 and ABM2 closely agree with the analytic value of $X / (N - I)$; we cannot expect exact agreement due to the stochastic nature of ABM1 and ABM2.

Having established that ABM2 in the global setting is consistent with our analytical expectations, we can begin to compare it with ABM2 in the age setting. In the ABM2 age setting, we first set **age – threshold** to its maximum value, so that a criminally active agent of any age can lure an agent of any age into crime (which is consistent with the global setting). Recall that at each tick in age setting of ABM2/, an agent of age **max-age** dies and is replaced by a **min-age** agent in the law-abiding citizen class (X). We therefore expect that the effective rate at which agents of any class are replaced by new **min-age** agents in the law-abiding citizen class is

1 / (max-age – min-age).

Accordingly, we hypothesize that ABM2 in the age setting should dock well with ABM2 in the global setting, with μ in the latter set in accordance with max-age and min-age from ABM2 in the former:

$\mu = 1$ / (max-age – min-age).

We further expect that the results should agree more as the distance between max-age and min-age increases, due to discrete-size effects. Our simulations suggest that these expectations do hold. Table 4 shows that for min-age = 0, increasing max-age increases the agreement between ABM2/global and ABM2/age.

Table 4

ABM2/global Docks Well with ABM2/age for Increasing Values of Age-threshold

Max_age	ABM2/age No RiskGrowth Age_threshold = max Max_age from Col 1 X/(N − I)	μ for ABM2/global μ = 1/max_age	ABM2/global with μ from Col 3 X/N− I)
20	0.62	0.050	0.52
30	0.46	0.033	0.41
40	0.36	0.025	0.33
50	0.31	0.020	0.29
60	0.27	0.017	0.26

Note: In ABM2/age, risk growth is set to "none," min-age to 0, max-age takes on the values in column 1, and age-threshold = max-age. In ABM2/global, birth/death rate μ is set to 1/(max-age), as in column 3. Other parameters are set at: $\alpha_{10} = 0$, $\alpha_{11} = 0.26$, $\alpha_{20} = 0.36$, $\alpha_{21} = 0$, $\beta_1 = 0.06$, $\gamma_1 = 0.09$, $\varepsilon = 0.03$, $\rho = 0.09$, $\gamma_2 = 0.09$. Column 2 shows endemic X/(N − I) for ABM2/age, column 4 shows endemic X/(N − I) for ABM2/global

Findings from ABM2

Our work gradually adding complexities and docking with previous models has culminated with an agent-based model that we can confidently use to relax many of our simplifying assumptions, investigate whether old insights still hold, and search for new insights that we could not have reached in more simplified versions. Our simulations suggest not only that all of our old insights still hold, but also that there are new insights to be gained.

For example, we show that increasing the rate of first-time imprisonment γ_1 can actually increase the long-run prevalence of crime when recidivism ($\alpha_{20} + \alpha_{21}$) is large compared with successful rehabilitation (ε). We show that this relationship holds when many of our assumptions are completely relaxed: all parameters are positive including α_{10} and α_{21}, so that people can turn to crime both through interactions with criminals and without such interactions. We also relax **age-threshold** so that a law-abiding agent can only be influenced into criminal behavior by criminals close to the agent's age. In figure 6, we plot the long-run proportion of law-abiding citizens among those not in prison (the fraction X/(N – I) of law-abiding citizens on the street) against the rate of first-time imprisonment (γ_1) using three different curves, with each curve corresponding to a different ratio of recidivism ($\alpha_{20} + \alpha_{21}$) to rehabilitation ($\varepsilon$).

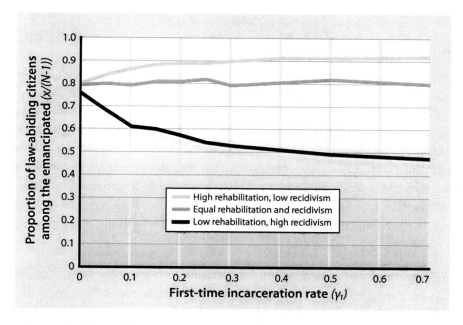

Figure 6. Dependence of effects of first-time incarceration on recidivism and rehabilitation. The effects of increasing the rate of first-time imprisonment (γ_1) depends on recidivism ($\alpha_{20} + \alpha_{21}$) and rehabilitation ($\varepsilon$). The highest curve shows that for low recidivism ($\alpha_{20} = 0.05$, $\alpha_{21} = 0.1$) and high rehabilitation ($\varepsilon = 0.5$), increasing γ_1 weakly increases the proportion of law-abiding citizens (X/(N – I)). The middle curve shows that when recidivism ($\alpha_{20} = 0.05$, $\alpha_{21} = 0.1$) and rehabilitation ($\varepsilon = 0.15$) are about the same, increasing γ_1 has a negligible effect on (X/(N – I)). Finally, the lower curve shows that when recidivism ($\alpha_{20} = 0.48$, $\alpha_{21} = 0.1$) is large relative to rehabilitation ($\varepsilon = 0.01$), increasing γ_1 actually decreases X/(N – I), increasing the prevalence of crime. Parameter values are as follows: $\alpha_{10} = 0.01$, $\alpha_{11} = 0.19$, $\beta_1 = 0.16$, r = 0.09, $\gamma_2 = 0.01$, $\beta_2 = 0.01$, min-age = 0, max-age = 60, age-threshold = 20, and mean-peak-risk = 0.28

This is another example of the importance of systems thinking. It may seem intuitive that increasing incarceration rates should always decrease crime in the long run. But in a community in which recidivism is much more likely than successful rehabilitation, increasing the rate of first-time imprisonment does little more than contribute to the total population of long-term career recidivists, increasing both crime and mass incarceration. These conditions could be created, for example, if prisons serve as "schools of crime" (making incarcerated people more likely to re-offend), or if quality employment is extremely difficult to come by for people who have been to prison.

With the complete agent-based model, and even with the same assumption relaxations, we gained additional insights. When we set the **risk-multiplier** so that the relationship between age and susceptibility to criminal behavior follows that of a tent or bell-shaped distribution, we found that increasing the **mean-peak-risk** decreases the long-run prevalence of crime. In other words just by delaying the time in a person's life that they are most likely to turn to crime, we can decrease crime in the long-run. This implies that even when alumni turn to crime later in life, prevention programs in schools help reduce long-run crime if they are able to delay its onset.

Future work will include incorporating aging into our analytic equations (7) and compute the corresponding R_0 and endemic levels. We expect these to be rather unwieldy expressions.

Moving Toward Data-Driven Simulations

The long-term goal of this collaboration is to construct, analyze, and apply dynamic models of the spread of crime and mass incarceration to facilitate systems approaches for interventions. Many policies are proposed and used in efforts to control crime, such as increasing police presence and strength, increasing the probability and severity of incarceration, strengthening social programs, and varying options for resettling those recently released from prison. As we mentioned earlier, the 1967 President's Commission on Law Enforcement and Administration of Justice presented a list of 200 policies that would make a difference in the war on crime. Many of these interventions have serious ripple effects across society that are infrequently addressed. We hope that building a comprehensive model of the whole system—a "flight simulator," if you will—will lead to more effective comparisons of different interventions and a deeper understanding of long- run consequences.

To build such a systems model, we will need reliable estimates of the model parameters. Our first models (MSM) provided general insights but were too simple and abstract to relate to empirical data. We hope that the complexities we have incorporated in the agent-based models described in this paper—especially the age effects—will bring us closer to data analysis and parameter estimation.

To this end, we have begun analyzing a rich data set, the Longitudinal Cohort Study that was part of the Project on Human Development in Chicago Neighborhoods[28] This study kept track of six age-defined cohorts in 1994 (ages 3, 6, 9, 12, 15, and 18). It included a self-report of offending in which respondents explained which violent and/or nonviolent crimes they had participated in during the previous year. The responses were recorded for three waves between 1994 and 2000; only cohorts 9–18 participated in all three waves. The study also included a year-by-year history of the respondents' arrests. We intend to use this study in modified versions of our model not only to estimate parameters, but also to investigate how covariates and interventions can empirically influence those parameters to reduce long-run crime and mass incarceration. We will also investigate how differences in covariates such as race and SES generate differences in each parameter, and how these differences accumulate to generate large disparities as one moves through the system. In doing so we can also consider the best types of interventions to reduce long-run disparities reflected in the school-to-prison pipeline from a systems perspective.

References

1. Durose MR, Cooper AD, Snyder HN. *Recidivism of Prisoners Released in 30 States in 2005: Patterns from 2005 to 2010.* Bureau of Justice Statistics. April 2014.

2. Davis JH, Harris G. Obama Commutes Sentences for 46 Drug Offenders. *New York Times.* http://www.nytimes.com/2015/07/14/us/obama-commutes-sentences-for-46-drug-offenders.html?_r=0. Accessed July 13, 2015.

3. Williams T. Police Leaders Join Call to Cut Prison Rosters. *New York Times.* http://www.nytimes.com/2015/10/21/us/police-leaders-join-call-to-cut-prison-rosters.html. Accessed October 20, 2015.

4. Gladwell M. *The Tipping Point: How Little Things Can Make a Big Difference.* Boston, MA: Little Brown; 2000.

5. President's Commission on Law Enforcement and Administration of Justice. *The Challenge of Crime in a Free Society.* 1967.

6. Carson R. *Silent Spring.* Boston, MA: Houghton Mifflin; 1962.

7. McMillon D, Simon C, Morenoff J. Modeling the underlying dynamics of the spread of crime. *PLoS One.* 2014;9(4):e88923.

8. Macey R, Oster G. 1993. Berkeley Madonna. Berkeley, CA: University of California, Berkeley. http://www.berkeleymadonna.com/.

9. Bruinsma GJ, Weisburd D, eds. *Encyclopedia of Criminology and Criminal Justice.* New York, NY: Springer; 2014.

10. Birks D, Elffers H. Agent-based assessments of criminological theory. In: Bruinsma GJ, Weisburd D, eds. *Encyclopedia of Criminology and Criminal Justice.* New York, NY: Springer-Verlag; 2014.

11. Epstein J, Axtell R. *Growing Artificial Societies: Social Science from the Bottom Up.* Cambridge, MA: MIT Press; 1996.

12. Epstein J. Agent-based computational models and generative social science. *Complexity.* 1999;4(5):41–60.

13. Axelrod R. *The Complexity of Cooperation: Agent-based Models of Competition and Collaboration.* Princeton, NJ: Princeton University Press; 1997.

14. Gilbert N, Troitzsch K. *Simulation for the Social Scientist.* 2nd ed. London, UK: Open University Press; 2005.

15. Birks D, Townsley M, Stewart A. Generative models of crime: using simulation to test criminological theory. *Criminology.* 2012;50(1):221–254.

16. Groff ER. Agent-based modeling for understanding patterns of crime. In: Bruinsma GJ, Weisburd D, eds. *Encyclopedia of Criminology and Criminal Justice.* New York, NY: Springer-Verlag; 2014.

17. Eck J, Liu L. Contrasting simulated and empirical experiments in crime prevention. *J Exp Criminol.* 2008;4:195–213.

18. Groff ER, Birks D. Simulating crime prevention strategies: a look at the possibilities. *J Policy Pract.* 2008;1:1–10.

19. Malleson N, See L, Evans A, Heppenstall A. Implementing comprehensive offender behaviour in a realistic agent-based model of burglary. *Simulation.* October 2010. http://sim.sagepub.com/content/early/2010/10/20/0037549710384124.

20. Hayslett-McCall K, Qui F, Curtin KM, Chastain B, Schubert J, Carver V. The simulation of the journey to residential burglary. In: Liu L, Eck J, eds. *Artificial Crime Analysis Systems: Using Computer Simulations and Geographic Information Systems.* Hershey, PA: Information Science Reference; 2008.

21. Malleson N, Evans A. Agent-based models to predict crime at places. In: Bruinsma GJ, Weisburd D, eds. *Encyclopedia of Criminology and Criminal Justice.* New York, NY: Springer-Verlag; 2014.

22. Groff ER. Simulation for theory testing and experimentation: an example using routine activity theory and street robbery. *J Quant Criminol.* 2007;23(2):75–103.

23. Wilensky, U. 1999. NetLogo. Evanston, IL: Center for Connected Learning and Computer-Based Modeling, Northwestern University. http://ccl.northwestern.edu/netlogo/.

24. Farrington DP. Age and crime. *Crime and Justice: An Annual Review of Research.* 1986;7:189–250.

25. Tremblay RE, Nagin DS. The developmental origins of physical aggression in humans. In: Tremblay RE, Hartup WW, Archer J, eds. *Developmental Origins of Aggression.* New York: Guilford Press; 2005:83–106.

26. Loeber R, Farrington DP. Age-crime curve and its relevance for policy and interventions. In: Bruinsma GJ, Weisburd D, eds. *Encyclopedia of Criminology and Criminal Justice.* New York, NY: Springer-Verlag; 2014.

27. Sampson RJ, Laub JH. A life-course view of the development of crime. *Ann Am Acad Pol Soc Sci.* 2005;602:12–45.

28. Sampson RJ, Morenoff JD, Raudenbush S. Social anatomy of racial and ethnic disparities in violence. *Am J Public Health.* 2005;95:224–232.

APPENDIX: CALCULATION OF THRESHOLD FOR SYSTEM (7)

In this Appendix, we show that, for R_0 given by expression (8), $R_0 \leq 1$ is necessary and sufficient condition for all solutions of system (7) to converge to the no-crime equilibrium,

$$X = N, \quad C_1 = C_2 = I = R = 0.$$

for the case where $\alpha_{10} = 0$ and $\alpha_{21} = 0$. First, noting that population size is conserved, we work with the last four equations in system (7), replacing X by $N - C_1 - C_2 - R - I$. Call this reduced four-equation system (7a).

We follow the Lyapunov Function approach used in MSM. We begin by constructing a (linear) function

$$V(C_1, I, R, C_2) = C_1 + A_1 I + A_2 R + A_3 C_2.$$

with positive coefficients A_1, A_2, A_3, so that (0,0,0,0) is the minimum of V in the positive orthant.

Our condition that "all solutions go to (0,0,0,0)" becomes equivalent to the condition that "for any solution $(C_1(t), I(t), R(t), C_2(t))$ of system (7a), $V(C_1(t), I(t), R(t), C_2(t))$ is a decreasing function of time t," which is equivalent to the condition that the time derivative of t $\rightarrow V(C_1(t), I(t), R(t), C_2(t))$ is negative. After a bit of rearranging, this time derivative is:

$$\dot{V} = \frac{dC_1}{dt} + A_1 \frac{dI}{dt} + A_2 \frac{dR}{dt} + A_3 \frac{dC_2}{dt}$$
$$= C_1 \left[\alpha_{11} \frac{X}{N-I} - (\beta_1 + \gamma_1 + \mu) + A_1\gamma_1 \right]$$
$$+ I \left[A_2 r - A_1(r+\mu) \right]$$
$$+ R \left[A_3\alpha_{20} - A_2(\alpha_{20} + \varepsilon + \mu) \right]$$
$$+ C_2 \left[\alpha_{11} \frac{X}{N-I} + A_1\gamma_1 + A_2\beta_2 - A_3(\beta_2 + \gamma_2 + \mu) \right],$$

(1.1)

The question is: when can we choose non-negative coefficients A_1, A_2, A_3 so that (1.1) is negative? We start by making the middle two bracketed expressions equal to zero by choosing:

$$A_2 = A_1 \left(\frac{r+\mu}{r} \right),$$
$$A_3 = A_2 \left(\frac{\alpha_{20} + \varepsilon + \mu}{\alpha_{20}} \right) = A_1 \left(\frac{r+\mu}{r} \right)\left(\frac{\alpha_{20} + \varepsilon + \mu}{\alpha_{20}} \right).$$

(1.2)

Using the fact that $X/(N-I) \leq 1$, the first bracketed term in (1.1) will be negative if:

$$\alpha_{11} + A_1\gamma_1 \leq (\beta_1 + \gamma_1 + \mu),$$

or

$$A_1 \leq \frac{(\beta_1 + \gamma_1 + \mu) - \alpha_{11}}{\gamma_1}. \tag{1.3}$$

Similarly, the fourth bracketed term in (1.1) will be negative if:

$$\alpha_{11} + A_1\gamma_1 + A_2\beta_2 \leq A_3(\beta_2 + \gamma_2 + \mu),$$

or using (1.2):

$$\alpha_{11} + A_1\gamma_1 + A_1\left(\frac{r+\mu}{r}\right)\beta_2 \leq A_1\left(\frac{r+\mu}{r}\right)\left(\frac{\alpha_{20} + \varepsilon + \mu}{\alpha_{20}}\right)(\beta_2 + \gamma_2 + \mu). \tag{1.4}$$

With a bit of algebra, (1.4) can be written as:

$$\alpha_{11} \leq A_1 \cdot \left[(\beta_2 + \gamma_2 + \mu)\left(\frac{\varepsilon + \mu}{\alpha_{20}}\right)\left(1 + \frac{\mu}{r}\right) + \mu\left(1 + \frac{\gamma_2 + \mu}{r}\right) \right], \tag{1.5}$$

or as:

$$\frac{\alpha_{11}\alpha_{20}}{\left((\beta_2 + \gamma_2 + \mu)(\varepsilon + \mu)\left(1 + \frac{\mu}{r}\right) + \mu\alpha_{20}\left(1 + \frac{\gamma_2 + \mu}{r}\right) \right)} \leq A_1. \tag{1.6}$$

Denote the denominator of (1.6) by B as we do in (8). Combining (1.3) and (1.6), we conclude that we can find non-negative coefficients A_1, A_2, A_3 so that the derivative of V along solutions of (7a) is negative, provided we can find A_1 with the property:

$$\frac{\alpha_{11}\alpha_{20}}{B} \leq A_1 \leq \frac{(\beta_1 + \gamma_1 + \mu) - \alpha_{11}}{\gamma_1}. \tag{1.7}$$

But we can find an A_1 satisfying (1.7) if and only if:

$$\frac{\alpha_{11}\alpha_{20}\gamma_1}{B} \le (\beta + \gamma + \mu) - \alpha_{11}, \tag{1.8}$$

or, after more algebra, if and only if:

$$\frac{\alpha_{11}}{(\beta_1 + \gamma_1 + \mu)} \cdot \left(1 + \frac{\alpha_{20}\gamma_1}{B}\right) \le 1. \tag{1.9}$$

Let's summarize. If (1.9) holds, we can find (positive) A_1 so that (1.7) holds. If we then define A_2 and A_3 by (1.2), we have found positive coefficients A_1, A_2, A_3 so that the derivative of V along solutions of (7a) is negative, that is, from any starting point, solutions of system (7a) move across lower and lower levels of V to the minimum of V at the origin. In this case, the no-crime equilibrium of system (7) is globally asymptotically stable.

On the other hand, if (1.9), and therefore (1.8), do not hold, then for any $A_1 > 0$ and with A_2 and A_3 defined by (1.2), for X(0) close to 1—that is for starting points near the no-crime equilibrium—solutions of (7) will move to higher level sets of V, that is, away from the no-crime equilibrium. In this case, the no-crime equilibrium is unstable, and a bit of algebra as in MSM leads to the conclusion that the only other equilibrium has:

$$\frac{X^*}{N - I^*} = \frac{1}{\dfrac{\alpha_{11}}{(\beta_1 + \gamma_1 + \mu)} \cdot \left(1 + \dfrac{\alpha_{20}\gamma_1}{B}\right)}.$$

CHAPTER 11

BEYOND DRILL AND FILL: MODELING THE IMPACTS OF RISK-BASED CARE ON ORAL HEALTH DISPARITIES

Kurt Kreuger, MSc
Doctoral student in Computer Science
University of Saskatchewan

Robin Flint MacBride, MPH
Doctoral Student in Health Policy and Management
University of California, Los Angeles

Nathaniel A. Osgood, PhD
Associate Professor, Department of Computer Science
Associate Faculty, Department of Community Health & Epidemiology
University of Saskatchewan

Acknowledgments: We are indebted to the members of the NIH-funded Network on Inequality, Complexity and Health for valuable discussion. This work was funded by the Canadian Foundation for Innovation.

The oral health of the U.S. population as a whole has substantially improved in the last 50–60 years,[1] but profound disparities persist.[2] In 2000, the U.S. Surgeon General raised awareness of a "silent epidemic of oral diseases" disproportionately affecting poor children, the elderly, and members of racial and ethnic minority groups.[2] A large component of this burden arises from caries (tooth decay), a prevalent, multifactorial, chronic-yet-preventable disease. In the United States, such oral health disparities are both a symptom and a cause of an equally profound set of disparities in patient-provider trust and care-seeking behavior. These disparities reflect special vulnerabilities among children exacerbated by the predominant reliance on surgical solutions to address caries and aspects of the care experience.

Achieving oral health equity and improved health outcomes require an understanding of the underlying dynamics leading to oral health disparities. However, it is difficult to interpret empirical data and design interventions, due to the interplay between diverse factors, such as childhood vulnerabilities, the complex dynamics of trust, and patient interaction with the dental care system. Dynamic modeling can help to address this complexity and support opportunities for high and rapid gains from judiciously chosen child-focused interventions.

Caries Disease and Disparities

Caries is the most common disease of childhood. It is five times more common than asthma,[1] and the largest unmet health care need for children.[3] It is both an infectious and chronic bacterial infection, commonly acquired through transmission of *Streptococci mutans* from mothers to their infants.[4,5] Preventive and restorative treatment of the mother can prevent or delay a child's acquisition of the harmful caries-causing bacteria. Children who are exposed and infected at a younger age tend to develop much more aggressive caries,[6] and early childhood caries is the greatest risk factor for caries in permanent teeth.[6-8] This progressive nature of the disease is manifested in escalating prevalence rates across life stages, with a majority of 6- to 8-year-old children showing decay. Two-thirds have caries by adolescence,[9] with considerably higher rates among adults.[10] These rates are consistently lower for white and non-poor Americans, and consistently higher for lower income and minority persons. Rates of untreated decay exhibit the same gaping disparities;[9-11] in short, those who need care the most get it the least.

In addition to the biological transmission of caries, there is also an important "social contagion" aspect to the disease's progression. Lifestyle risk factors from the family related to dental hygiene and eating habits are shared throughout social networks. Also, fairly unique to dental care is the how a parent's history of negative care experiences can affect their likelihood of seeking care themselves and for their children.[12-14] Those with higher dental anxiety are more likely to go to the dentist when they have symptoms or pain, and are less likely to follow recommended schedules of ongoing dental care. Individuals with dental fear are also almost three times as likely to have poor oral health compared to those with no dental fear.[13] Negative experiences are not only a result of pain, but also of how patients (and/or their parents) experience office staff and providers. Mofidi et al.[14] found that perceived discriminatory behavior related to being a Medicaid recipient, and the time a provider dedicates to addressing the patient's oral health concerns, can have important effects on delays in care-seeking.

Caring for Disease: A Risk-based Approach

Current evidence suggests that the traditional surgical approach to caring for caries—both an infectious and chronic disease—does little to alter its course. Evidence supports a global movement toward minimally invasive dentistry, embracing risk-based care pathways to prevent disease and preserve tooth structure rather than focus on the number of surgical restorative procedures.[15] This changes the focus from a "drill and fill" approach to one that encourages preventive care and changing lifestyle risk factors in a manner tailored to a patient's circumstances, susceptibility, and disease status. Despite clear evidence supporting risk assessment procedures and care modalities, the profession has been slow to promote and train in these new models of care.

Without effective approaches to influence behavior, surgical treatment will persist as the prevailing model of care[16] Motivational interviewing (MI), an alternative to traditional health education, is a patient-centered conversational counseling technique that replaces advice-giving and direct persuasion with a patient-centered conversation aimed at evoking the person's intrinsic motivation and commitment to change.[17,18] MI has yielded promising results for patient activation,[16,19] but the jury remains out regarding dentists' ability to effectively integrate this technique to influence lifestyle risk behaviors related to oral health. It may be that engaging patients in a meaningful and respectful way and/or restructuring the schedule for patient follow up visits—so that higher-need patients receive more opportunities for prevention as well as relationship-building with their providers—elevates the patient's trust level and future care-seeking behavior, reversing behaviors that would otherwise result in significant health disparities and burdens for providers. Understanding the complex interconnections between the dynamics of trust and care-seeking, SES and social networks, and disease status are significant to the success of this approach to care and the study of disparities.

Trust and Disparities

Trust is an important dimension of the care experience. It has received increased attention in the literature over the last few decades, and evidence suggests that it plays an important role in health disparities. Lower trust has been associated with the underuse of health services,[20] reduced treatment adherence, and inhibited care-seeking for needed services, leading to increased health care costs.[21] Furthermore, trust has been associated with positive patient health outcomes, such as a more participatory patient role, improved chronic disease management, increased use of preventive services, and higher satisfaction with care.[22,23] Trust also increases the likelihood of recommending treatment to others.[24] All of these are important for managing and achieving good oral health.

A significant amount of research explores the role of trust in health care, but few experiments have been conducted to study interventions that successfully increase trust.[22,23,25] The complexity of studying trust is reflected in its many conceptualizations across disciplines. Trust is often conceptualized as either interpersonal trust or social trust. It may include domains such as fidelity, competence, honesty, confidentiality, and global trust. Trust is related to satisfaction, but studies indicate it is conceptually distinct from it: satisfaction looks back, while trust looks forward. It has an expectation component as well as a strong emotional component. Factors such as experiences, sense of shared values, mutual understanding, caring attitude, and good communication skills are strongly related to patient trust.[26]

As indicated earlier, anxiety associated with dental care can influence the care-seeking of a person and those connected to them, such as a child or family members. Trust also increases the likelihood of recommending treatment to others.[24] It is a significant predictor of having a dental provider independent of education, income, and race/ethnicity.[27] Patient trust of a provider was recently found to be an important precursor to patient activation, which in turn was associated with a higher likelihood of patient engagement in a variety of self-management behaviors.[28] When racial differences were removed, the racial gap in health outcomes was also narrowed.[28,29]

New Lens on Oral Health Disparities

Various conceptual frameworks have been employed to better understand the complex interconnected factors associated with health disparities, and the nature of pathways resulting in them.[30,31] This understanding often leads to recommendations for addressing inequalities in upstream causal factors through long-term social policies. While these changes are possible, the feasibility for meaningful changes in the short-term may be limited.[28]

The model presented in this chapter takes a different approach to understanding and explaining oral health disparities. Complex adaptive systems suggests that systems and structures emerge from the behavior of individuals, which in turn can themselves serve to constrain that behavior. Better understanding the underlying processes driving the emergence of disparities may help clarify the interplay between associated factors and identify feasible and high-leverage strategies that could change population health dynamics both in the short and long term.

Why Complex Systems Methods?

The oral health ecosystem and the disparities associated with it exhibit classic hallmarks of complex systems, especially feedbacks, whereby downstream elements can affect those upstream. For example, a decline in trust can precipitate a vicious cycle in which reduced frequency of care-seeking leads to lower opportunities for cleaning and prophylactic fluoride applications, all elevating the risk of serious oral health issues, making visits more costly and painful, thereby further eroding the sense of trust. Other feedbacks include those associated with the communication of pathogens, norms, and provider trust over peer networks and between generations.

Delays are another pronounced feature of complex systems in the oral health and health care area; they make the identification of effective intervention and implementation strategies in this area substantially more difficult. Diverse delays mediate oral health dynamics, including those associated with the progression of tooth decay, care-seeking, trust building, communication of bacteria and risk, and protective behavior norms in the earliest years. At a smaller scale, delays in a provider's workflow can materially worsen the patient experience, adversely affecting trust. Such systemic delays can have profound and complex effects on the benefits of intervention, in terms of quality of life, health-service delivery, and cost.

Oral health and health care also exhibit pronounced *heterogeneity*, marked by many different types of actors who differ not only in SES, but also in vulnerability and agency, due in part to differing ages and families. How these variations within the population affect oral health disparities is of key interest.

Nonlinearities, when change at one point leads to disproportionate change elsewhere, is present in the oral health and health care system. Tipping points, when a series of small changes suddenly cause larger systemic changes, and lock-in effects, where a system state becomes "locked in" due more to its prevalence than an inherent benefit, can be seen with the vicious cycle involving loss of trust and subsequent delays in care-seeking. Likewise, the gains secured by combining two interventions may be different than (and either large or smaller than) the sum of the gains secured by each intervention by itself, and interventions often exhibit pronounced differences in gains at different scales.

Such features of complex systems are not merely of intellectual interest, but pose major practical challenges for both understanding and successfully intervening in the oral health arena. The challenges associated with understanding intervention trade-offs are particularly notable in oral health because of the diversity of intervention options. These interventions can vary from changes to provider processes—such as the risk-based methods examined here—to community-based efforts focused on reducing risk exposures (e.g., to refined sugars) or to enhancing personal protective behaviors such as flossing and tooth brushing.

Methods

Our model incorporates factors known to be associated with health and oral health disparities and posits causal mechanisms for interactions. Dynamic models of health disparities often focus on upstream factors affecting the health trajectories of population members and omit the representation of care pathways. But for oral health as well as many other health areas, care pathways can have great influence on disease prevention and development, including impacts on trust levels, and the risky and protective behaviors of patients and their families. Our model focuses on specific aspects of the dental care process that hold promise for preventing disease and engaging patients in self-management: scheduling appointment intervals based on risk level and effective counseling time aimed at activating patients to manage their own or their child's oral health. We modeled ways that care pathways interact with the disease and care experience to affect trust levels, which, along with SES, influence care-seeking behaviors and the effectiveness of the care pathway, thereby creating disparities in care and health.

Simulation Model Design

Our model examines care-seeking behavior, including the impacts of SES and trust level. We have two agent types: clinics, which offer treatment options, and people who get sick and seek care. People have states associated with a variety of behaviors. For our purposes, the most significant state classifications are associated with care-seeking, infection, and lesion development. We also track an individual's status with respect to fluoride protection (on a graduated scale) and their health risk (for risk-based interventions). To capture intergenerational effects, we also included factors related to reproduction and birth.

In the context of the models presented in this book, our model is an example of a hybrid model on account of its representation of clinic dynamics. The flow of patients through clinics is captured using a discrete event simulation (DES) approach rather than via standard agent-based mechanisms. Discrete event simulation models are widely used in modeling health-services delivery processes due to their expressiveness in characterizing resource-constrained workflows and their capacity to capture the reasoning around impacts on waiting times, counts, and throughput of changes in resource allocation (e.g., the effect on patient flow of adding an additional dental hygienist), and of facility layout. The analysis presented here simply relies upon discrete event simulation as a means of concisely and conveniently capturing the logic of care encounters. However, its use not only spares the need to create much more complex—and error prone—logic, but also offers tremendous flexibility in the examination of future health-service delivery concerns.

State Classifications

Care Seeking Behavior

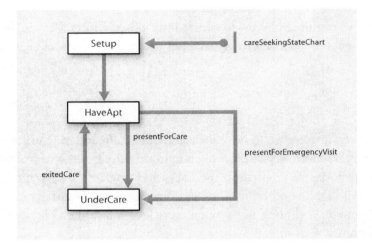

Figure 1. Care-seeking state chart

Figure 1 shows a state chart used to control the individual's care-seeking behavior. State charts describe the set of allowable states of an agent. Transitions between those states, governed by rules, constitute actions by which that person changes states over time. This state chart shows the basic cycle of people moving between the "UnderCare" (receiving treatment) and "HaveApt" (have scheduled appointments) states, (*Setup* only serves to initialize certain values). Each care-seeking individual in the model has an appointment type (restorative versus checkup) and an appointment time with the dental clinic. For prescheduled appointments, the subsequent appointment type and time are determined during the previous appointment in the clinic, and generally depend on their disease state at that time. When presenting to the clinic, the disease state of each person affects which treatment path they follow. Once an individual leaves the clinic following a restorative visit, we assume that they leave with no lesions regardless of their disease state when entering. However, the scheduled appointment time of each person's visit is not the only factor guiding the timing of their return to the clinic: in addition to SES (SES), their trust of the clinic also plays a role and is the more detailed calculation (see figure 2).

Socioeconomic status: While SES is traditionally conceptualized as being composed of many factors, we conceptualized it here as a simple, scalar factor affecting the time in which people present for care. When enabled in the model, each agent is assigned a SES level at the outset, which can range from 0.01 to 1. To determine the time until presentation for a prescheduled appointment, the scheduled appointment time is then divided by the SES level. This formulation reflects the fact that a wealthy individual would have few limitations to making their appointment, but an individual with a very low SES might not have the financial means to present for care frequently, might be working more than one job to cover expenses, or might have any other number of restrictions on their ability to present, even if they completely trust their clinic. Therefore, the wealthier individual would be likely to come closer to the appointed time, whereas a poorer

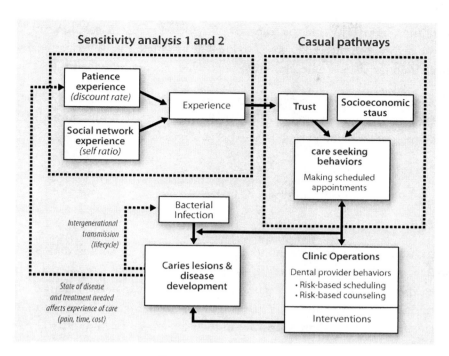

Figure 2. Return-time logic

individual would be compelled by life circumstances to come at a later time—a tendency that we posit to hold even for emergency care-seeking.

Trust: Like the SES level, trust affects the model by modifying the scheduled return time. While a person's SES is fixed throughout the simulation, their trust value evolves dynamically. Trust is represented as a number between 0.1 and 1, which then divides the return time: if someone completely trusts the clinic, they will return only as often as the clinic tells them to, whereas someone who completely distrusts the clinic will return 10 times less often (e.g., 60 months later instead of 6 months).

Trust evolves over time based on a dynamic, clinic-specific experience variable. After each visit, the person calculates an experience score for that visit, which is then used to update their overall experience value for the clinic (figure 2).

Experience is a function of two factors, the amount of time providers spend developing strong relationships each patient (respect time); and the *severity* of the treated condition (e.g., from a significant surgical procedure rather than a simple cleaning). Respect time may include conversations with the patient about their challenges related to oral care, care-seeking, and personal protective behavior, as well as any general interaction that enhances the respect they feel. Respect time can only increase the experience score; if no time is spent, it has no effect on that trust level. However, condition severity can decrease the experience score. With three severity types tracked in the model (cleaning only, and treatments for some lesions and advanced lesions) we associated a corresponding neutral, moderately negative, or significantly negative severity score. For the sake of simplicity, this impact of treatment type on experience lumps together aspects of discomfort, financial cost, inconvenience, and so on. Experience for a given clinical encounter is calculated as $\beta_R R - \beta_S S$, where R is respect time, S is severity, and the respective β values are relative weighting coefficients chosen so that individuals regularly presenting and exposed to fluoride experience no severity penalty, and individuals even with advanced lesions can have a neutral experience when offered sufficient respect time.

A person's experience value is updated with each successive visit. A discount rate λ is applied to factor in a person's earlier experiences in the presence of successive new ones. A running weighted total number of experiences, $\bar{X}$, is kept, and updated at each new experience, as follows:

$$\bar{n}_t = \bar{n}_{t-1} \exp(-\lambda\Delta t) + 1$$

$$X_t = X_{t-1} \exp(-\lambda\Delta t) + 100 \tanh(X_{new}/100)$$

$$\bar{X}_t = X_t / \bar{n}_t$$

where $\bar{n}$ is the (discounted) count of data points, X_t is the (discounted) sum of data points, Δt is the time since the last update, and the subscripts t and $t-1$ indicate the current time step and the previous one, respectively. Since experience is in principle unbounded, we used the hyperbolic tangent to bound the new experience value to between -100 and 100. Trust is then calculated from the function depicted in figure 3A. At 0 experience, the agents are slightly positive in their trust assessment (with a level 0.6).

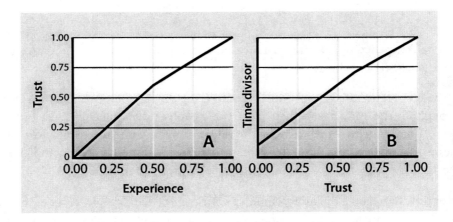

Figure 3. (A) Relationship between an individual's experience and the resulting trust value. (B) Relationship between an individual's trust and the resulting divisor used to determine the return time of that individual

Finally, a time divisor is calculated from trust that divides the clinic-specified return time. Trust (a number from 0 to 1) is mapped to the time divisor (a number between 0.1 and 1) [$f(t)$] (figure 3B); this requires all people to present to the clinic at some point in their lives. $f(t)$ maintains the same piecewise linear form as trust (figure 3A and B).

Beyond simply having each person gather experiences and modify their trust accordingly, the impact of trust is spread along a social network: agents have access to the experiences of their neighbors in the network and can use those experiences as they would their own. The self-ratio indicates how much an agent weights their own experience versus the experiences of their neighbors when determining a consensus effective trust level, determined as follows:

$$E_{effective} = E_{personal}\ SelfRatio + E_{neighbor\ average}\ (1 - SelfRatio)$$

Life-cycle State Chart

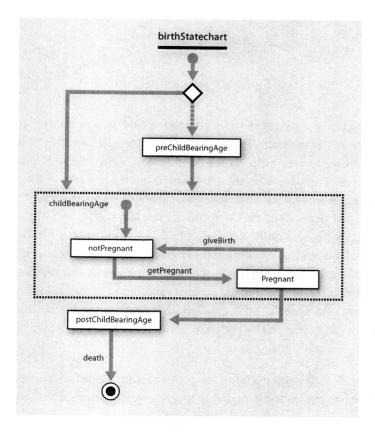

Figure 4. Life-cycle state chart

One goals of this model is to look at the intergenerational forces involved in the formation or maintenance of health disparities. To probe this phenomenon, we modeled how agents are born, inherit their SES, are influenced by the trust and health condition of their mother in their future infection risk and care-seeking, and then reach the stage of having a child themselves. Agents in our model each have a life-cycle state chart (figure 4), which provides this functionality. To simplify the assumptions and model scope, the model includes only female agents. To capture the reproductive life cycle, our agents are in "pre-childbearing age" for their first 18 years. Upon their 18th birthday, each becomes an adult and within an average of 5 years gives birth to another agent. After giving birth to a single child, agents transition to "post-childbearing age," where they remain for 35 years. Following those 35 years, they remove themselves from the population through death.

Infection and Progression

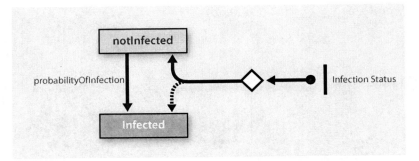

Figure 5. Infection state chart

The simple two-state infection state chart (figure 5) represents an agent's dichotomous infection state. Aside from the initialization transitions enabling a proportion (90 percent, reflective of current adult prevalence[10]) of agents to be created with an initial infection status, there is only one transition: from "not infected" to "infected." Everyone is given a base infection hazard rate of roughly 3 percent per year, and infection is life-long. Reflecting the transmissible nature of caries from mother to child, we made a child's infection hazard rate dependent on the mother's disease status, with the child's infection hazard multiplied by a successively higher coefficient (1.4, 1.8, 2.3, 4.0, 6.0) as the mother proceeds from uninfected to infected with advanced lesions. This reflects research that mothers with higher levels of caries bacteria tend to have children with higher levels of bacteria.[5] However, this effect only lasts until the child is 12 years old, at which point their progression hazard reverts to a standardized rate, representing lower contact between the mouths of older children and mother and among older children and adults. While the infection risk of the child is affected by the mother's oral health, the disease state of an infected child evolves endogenously.

Agents in the "not infected" state remain in the "no lesions" state of the lesion status state chart (figure 6). Once infected, the agent progresses to successively more severe disease states (from "white spot lesions," the earliest sign of a caries is a non-cavitated carious lesion appearing as chalky white spots on the surface of the tooth indicates demineralization of enamel, to cavitated lesions: "some lesions," or "advanced lesions") based on the lesion development hazard. This hazard is calculated by a base hazard rate of 0.5 per year, with terms added for relative fluoride exposure and the person's SES (optional). A final term raises this hazard rate if the person is a child, reflecting the fact that primary teeth have thinner enamel, which can demineralize and develop cavities at a faster rate. In line with treatment of hazards in survival analysis, the hazard is calculated as (p), where

$$p = \ln(0.5) - 0.1 \times relativeFluorideLevel + 2(1 - SES) + 1.5I_{child}$$

and I_{child} is an indicator function that is 1 for children, and 0 otherwise. Finally, taking into account the accelerating nature of disease progression, for each of the three disease transitions (no lesions to white spot, white spot to some lesions, and some lesions to advanced) the base hazard rate was multiplied by a coefficient (1, 2, and 3, respectively).

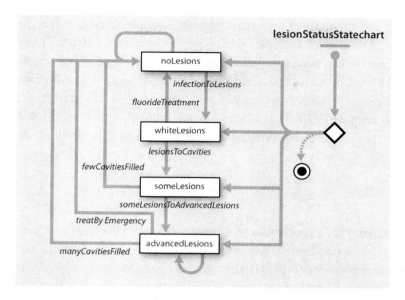

Figure 6. Oral disease progression state chart

Treatment is provided according to the patient's disease state: fluoride for no lesions or white spot lesions, restorative treatment otherwise. These restorative treatments always transition the patient to the no lesions state. In the model, restorative treatments are more painful to the patient, so there is an experience cost with this outcome.

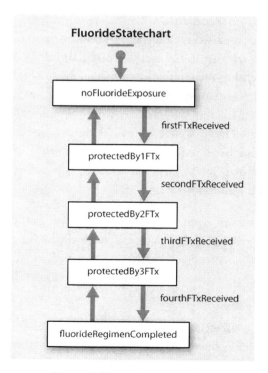

Figure 7. Protection state chart

239

A final state chart captures the simple progression between levels of fluoride protection and fluoride status (figure 7). Each fluoride treatment increases protection by one level. With a fluoride-decay hazard (33 percent per year) the patient can regress to lesser protection levels. Each successive state in this state chart elevates the fluoride protection term, lessening the lesion development hazard (from least protective to most, the "relative fluoride level" is 0, 2, 4, 6, and 8). This state chart is also used in intervention conditions that require classifying each patient as high risk or not, a classification that affects the care pathways delivered. Agents that reach the final state become low risk. If they fall back to either of the first two states, they become high risk again.

Clinic Operation

The clinic is characterized with a simple discrete event model. Agents have two possible treatment paths depending on their condition and scenario settings: "restorative" and "checkup," with the latter used for both prescheduled checkup visits and dental emergencies. The checkup path gives them a fluoride treatment (increasing their fluoride state chart level). If they have no lesions, or only white spot lesions, they leave the clinic with no lesions, an increased fluoride level and an appointment for another checkup in 6 months. If they have lesions (some or advanced), they still receive fluoride and increase their fluoride level, but when leaving the clinic, they are booked 1 week later for a restorative visit. An agent presenting for a restorative visit will exit the clinic with no lesions. They do not receive another fluoride treatment.

To examine model behavior and understand its sensitivity to parameter assumptions, we ran the model under alternative scenarios (table 1), each with different assumptions (highlighted in the table in grey). To ease scenario understanding, and in accordance with standard modeling practice, we selected a baseline scenario as a point of reference against which alternative scenarios could be compared. For all scenarios, the model was run for 200 years with an initial starting population of 2,305. Given the open population and the average life span, at the end of the simulation between 5,500 and 6,000 agents were present, none of whom were part of the initial population. Initial agent SES levels were drawn uniformly from 0.01 to 1. A square space was used to visualize the effects of income segregation, where a person's x coordinate corresponded to the SES level scaled by the space width (500 units). The y coordinate was random. Agents were further placed into a social network where agents within a range of 20 units from each other were connected. We examined the following standardized outputs: clinic visit count versus trust, lesion days versus trust, trust versus SES, and lesion days versus SES.

Scenario 1. Effect of causal pathways. Scenarios within this group examined the impact of pathways by which trust and SES operate. When trust or SES pathways were allowed to influence care-seeking behavior, they shaped model evolution. When these pathways were disabled, trust continued to be calculated and spread socially and SES still determined the x coordinate of each agent, but they did not influence clinic return time.

Scenario 2. Sensitivity analysis 1, effect of experience discount rate. This first sensitivity analysis varied the contribution of patient experience over the baseline scenario by adjusting the discount rate (λ). We examined three extremes: a case in which older experiences were valued fully as much new experiences ($\lambda = 0$), a case in which older experiences were discounted quickly ($\lambda = 4$/year), and a middling case ($\lambda = 1/[5$ years$]$).

Table 1

Description of Scenarios Examined

Scenario		Pathways		Sensitivity Parameters		Intervention	
Scenario group	Scenario designation	TTrust	SSES	Experience discount rate, (λ)	SSelf ratio	Counseling	Scheduling
Baseline	Baseline	Yes	Yes	0.2/Year	.5	No	No
1 - Causal pathways	1a (baseline)	Yes	Yes	0.2/year	.5	No	No
	1b	No	No	0.2/year	.5	No	No
	1c	Yes	No	0.2/year	.5	No	No
	1d	No	Yes	0.2/year	.5	No	No
2 - Sensitivity analyses 1	2a	Yes	Yes	0	.5	No	No
	2b (baseline)	Yes	Yes	0.2/year	.5	No	No
	2c	Yes	Yes	1/year	.5	No	No
	3d	Yes	Yes	4/year	.5	No	No
3 - Sensitivity analyses 2	3a	Yes	Yes	0.2/year	0	No	No
	3b (baseline)	Yes	Yes	0.2/year	.5	No	No
	3c	Yes	Yes	0.2/year	1	No	No
4 - Interventions	4a (baseline)	Yes	Yes	0.2/year	.5	No	No
	4b	Yes	Yes	0.2/year	.5	Yes	No
	4c	Yes	Yes	0.2/year	.5	No	Yes
	4d	Yes	Yes	0.2/year	.5	Yes	Yes

Scenario 3. Sensitivity analysis 2, effects of varying social network influence. This scenario focused on understanding the impact of different levels of social influence (defined by the self ratio) on a person's trust levels. This was realized by changing the self ratio, by which a person looked to their own experience versus the experience of network connections when determining their trust levels. Three extreme cases were examined: cases where an individual (1) purely trusted the experiences of those around them, (2) trusted only their own experience, and (3) considered both.

Scenario 4. Interventions. This scenario explored the impact of implementing two elements of a risk-based approach to care for high-risk patients: counseling, which increased the experience quality of each visit; and scheduling, which reduced the interval between visits.

Findings

Results are displayed using two diagrammatic mechanisms showing the state of the population at $t = 200$ years: 2D histograms, which are like classic histograms instead using bins with length and width, and color density indicating relative data records in that bin; and bar charts, which aggregate the results of 30 separate realizations and including standard deviation error bars. Because the current level of trust can change over the course of a year (particularly for those exhibiting low levels of care-seeking), for analyses involving trust that involve outcomes accumulated over the life-course (e.g., lesion days), we sought to emphasize regularities by comparing such outcomes against trust averaged over the life course rather than the instantaneous trust value at the final time. In the 2D histogram plots, stochastics played a visually minor role between simulation realizations, as evidenced by figure 8, which displays population-wide some and advanced lesion days, respectively, for 100 successive runs.

Baseline Scenario

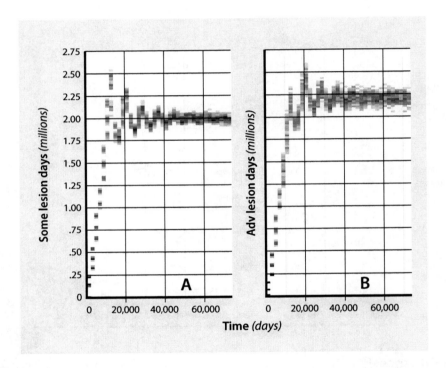

Figure 8. (A) Some and (B) advanced lesion days of population on a 2D histogram; the variation is small, indicating that stochastics have little impact

Figure 9 shows a marked gradient associated with accumulated lesion days (whether for some, or advanced lesions) with respect to the average trust level of a person over their lifetime. This gradient reflects many factors. For agents with high SES, the accumulated number of lesion days tends to be low due to the virtuous cycle of regular care-seeking, which both confers protective fluoride applications and helps identify incipient problems before they develop into serious issues, thereby supporting better experiences and higher levels of trust. For agents with low SES the opposite vicious cycle applies, where most individuals are in the severe state and spend less time with only some lesions due to much less frequent care.

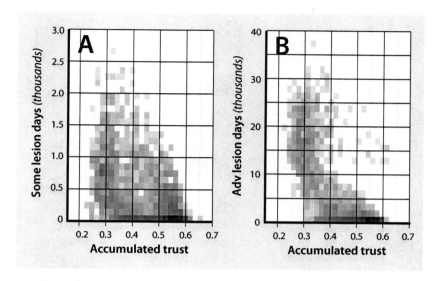

Figure 9. (A) Advanced and (B) some lesion days versus accumulated trust level for baseline

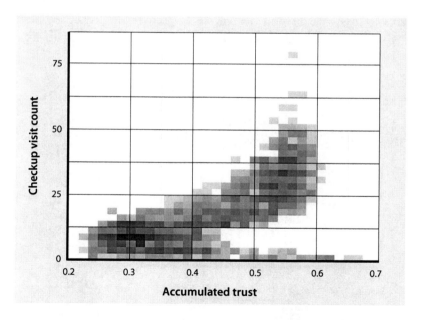

Figure 10. Checkup visit counts versus accumulated trust for baseline

This pattern also reflects two pronounced gradients for care-seeking over trust. The first demonstrates the predominance of higher levels of care-seeking among those with higher levels of life-course trust (figure 10). Figure 11, which shows restorative instead of checkup visits, shows a generally reversed trend.

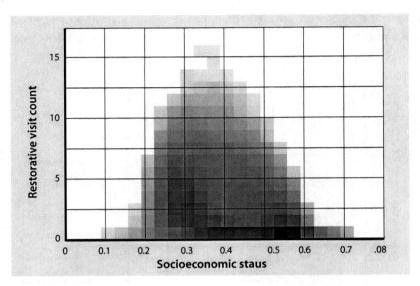

Figure 11. Restorative visit count versus accumulated trust for baseline

Lower-trust individuals have more restorative visits due to delaying treatments, thereby experiencing worse health outcomes when visits are made. In figure 10, however, a unique bifurcation is apparent at roughly trust level 0.4. The minority of people in the lower level "arm" visit rarely. Further simulation verifies that these people are unable to seek care due to their low SES. While having relatively high trust of the dental care system (unspoiled by adverse experiences), they exhibit little care-seeking due to other constraints.

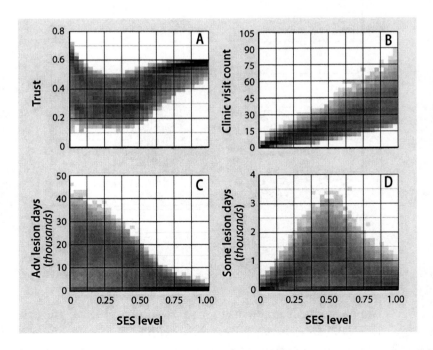

Figure 12. (A) Trust, (B) clinic visits, (C) advanced lesions, and (D) some lesions versus SES level for baseline

While the comments above related to patterns over trust, the next set of baseline results demonstrate notable but interlinked patterns over SES. Figure 12A shows a non-monotonic relationship between trust and SES. As a general rule, trust level increases with SES, reflecting an elevated level of care-seeking with SES (figure 12B), and a correspondingly lower burden of advanced lesions (figure 12C). However, in lower regions of the socioeconomic-status spectrum, this relationship is muted, and even reversed. Among the most impoverished, care-seeking behavior is comparatively rare, and instantaneous trust levels tend to fall into two categories, reflective of different possible care-seeking outcomes. Figure 12D demonstrates a more textured relationship between moderate-severity lesion days and SES. This function is lower both at high end of the SES spectrum (supporting the virtuous cycle) and at the low (where presence of moderate-severity lesions often just progress quickly to advanced lesions).

Scenario 1. Effect of causal pathways. In scenario group 1, we examined the effect of assuming operation of different combinations of causal pathways (figure 13). Because SES is imposed exogenously (rather than being determined by other elements of the model), assuming no SES influence leads to no discernable associations between SES and other model variables. By contrast, even when it exerts no impact, trust is determined endogenously within the model; it is affected by experiences from care-seeking and via social networks. In short, it represents both a symptom and a cause. As a result, even assuming no impact of trust elsewhere in the model, a person's trust still exhibits notable associations with their other characteristics, such as accumulated lesion days, as well as their SES.

Scenario 2. Effect of experience discount rate. In scenario group 2, we examined the impact of varying the assumption concerning discount rate of previous experiences (figure 14). Within this scenario group, we examined the effect of assuming four different experience discount rates: λ, a situation in which new experiences are strongly weighted ($\lambda = 4/year$, i.e., experiences from 3 months ago are discounted by a factor of e compared to a new experience); two scenarios in which experiences from 1 and 5 years ago are discounted by the same factor; and an extreme scenario in which older and recent experiences are weighted identically (i.e., $\lambda = 0$).

The most notable outcome from the high discount factor concerns the trust versus SES level graph (lower right plot on figure 14), which exhibits two distinct arms, individuals of medium and lower SES. Through further simulation, it is drawn out that each arm consists almost exclusively of the most recent visit type (lower arm with restorative treatments, upper with checkup). Due to their reduced clinic visit rate, by the time that lower SES individuals present for care, earlier experiences tend to be more heavily discounted. As a result, in the absence of interventions, lower SES individuals tend to be vulnerable to more variable perceptions of trust with respect to oral care than are higher income individuals, whose trust reflects a long series of encounters.

Scenario 3. Effects of varying social network influence. In scenario group 3 (figure 15), and partly inspired by Esfahbod et al.,[32] we examined the effect of assuming different levels of social influence. Despite income segregation and network proximity with respect to SES, with the extreme of social influence (self ratio = 0), the system tends toward more consolidated consensus outcomes. The trust versus SES graph is correspondingly tighter. By contrast, with more emphasis on individual experience, the relationship becomes far less defined. As in the baseline, for the case of no network influence, there is a distinct bifurcation in the lowest

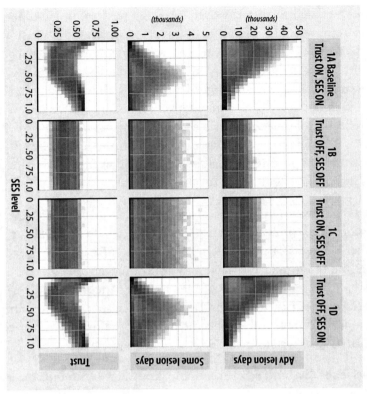

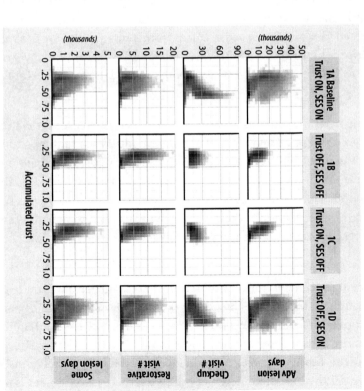

Figure 13. Scenario testing of (A) SES level and (B) accumulated trust in group 1

SES ranges. The individuals at the extremes of the low SES end of the bifurcation will have visited a clinic fewer than five times throughout their life. With no input from their neighbors, individuals are required to decide on a trust value based on limited information, resulting in either the vicious cycle between low trust and reduced care-seeking, or to quite higher and sometimes naive levels of trust associated with a corresponding lack of recent adverse outcomes. Despite these differences, many outcomes are surprisingly robust.

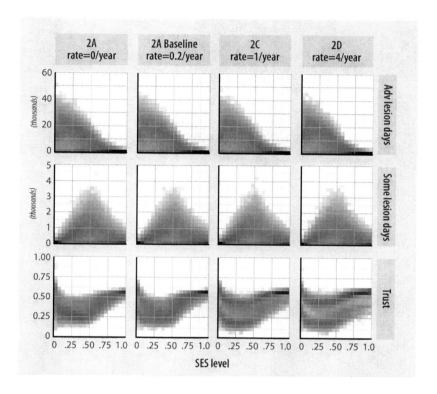

Figure 14. Scenario testing of SES level in group 2

Scenario 4. Intervention outcomes. Figures 16 and 17 show results from scenario group 4, which studies the impact of two intervention pathways relative to baseline. Figures 18 and 19 were made from 30 realizations showing data aggregated over SES category (separated into three quantiles).

Under the counseling-only intervention, trust among individuals with the lowest SES is significantly increased (figure 16), though no significant simultaneous improvement is apparent in advanced-lesion days. The comparison between baseline and counseling-only implies that the group associated with higher advanced-lesion days simply increases in trust value without decreasing the disease burden (figure 17). This is due to the extremely low SES value, which profoundly limits the impact of changing trust. These individuals whose trust has been elevated by the intervention desire oral care, but are limited by their life circumstances. The individuals most affected in trust have few checkup visits, and only a moderate number of restorative visits (figure 17).

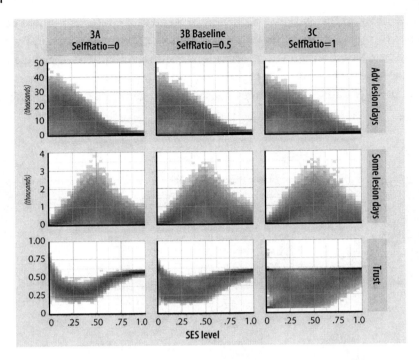

Figure 15. Scenario testing of SES level in group 3

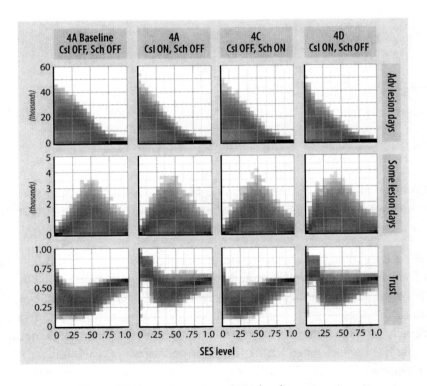

Figure 16. Scenario testing of SES level in group 4

Apart from verifying the above conclusions, figure 18 exhibits dramatic nonlinear effects when interventions occur in tandem. For the lowest SES (third quantile), each intervention alone does little to alter the overall advanced-lesion disease burden. When they occur together, however, the disease burden decreases nearly 15 percent relative to the baseline ($p < 0.001$). Concurrently, the prevalence of some (as opposed to advanced) lesions increases substantially, indicating that these interventions are not clearing the disease, but only lessening its burden. Increasing trust alone does not affect the ability of individuals to seek care. Scheduling alone (directly reducing the time between visits) also does little to affect their desire to present for care.

At the same time, drawing on both interventions has synergistic effects. Unexpectedly, risk-based scheduling alone modestly lowered the trust level for those approximately in the bottom quartile of SES level (figure 16). Presumably, this was associated with people who present for care just enough to experience adverse outcomes on a regular basis, but not enough to serve as an effective preventive strategy.

Overall, the greatest impact of each intervention was seen with moderate SES individuals, those who require significant care yet have the means to secure it (figure 18). Counseling alone reduced the severe disease burden by nearly 30 percent, with an only slightly higher reduction when combined with scheduling. The limiting factor for these individuals appears to be their relationship with care clinics, in contrast to the lower SES population who are quite limited by material ability. For individuals with high SES, counseling was slightly more effective at eliciting behavior change for similar reasons as with the moderate SES group. In all cases, both interventions in tandem reduce disease burden more than any single intervention.

For all intervention scenarios, higher SES levels correlated with more checkup visits (figure 19). In the baseline, however, individuals of low SES actually present for fewer restorative visits than their counterparts of moderate SES. This is again due to the material barriers to care-seeking among individuals of the lowest SES. When any intervention occurs, the largest change for individuals of low SES is in the number of restorative visits; visit types are determined solely by their health state, indicating generally lower health conditions in this population. Even under strongly positive intervention conditions, there are clear limits to the health improvement imposed by SES.

Implications

This approach is associated with a number of limitations. Like all dynamic models, our characterization simplifies a complex external reality. While highlighting possible hypotheses and key uncertainties that may stimulate insights about the external world, the results are conditional on model assumptions. The goal is to stimulate more focused enquiry, but requires additional examination before firm translations can be made in the real world.

Many quantitative assumptions were made concerning model parameters. This research sought to assemble evidence regarding diverse forces fundamental to trust and oral health carehealth care, including disease acceleration, SES impacts on risk and care-seeking behavior, mother-to-child infection, components of the disease progression hazard, and fluoride treatment and protection. Each is associated with parameter values that must be specified. Some of these values were drawn from literature, but the available evidence

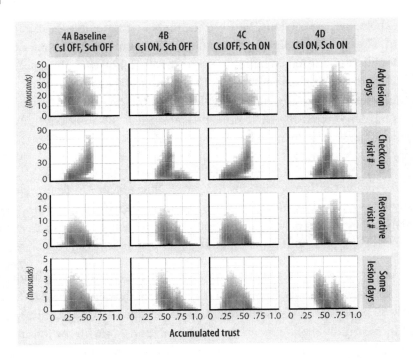

Figure 17. Scenario testing of accumulated trust in group 4

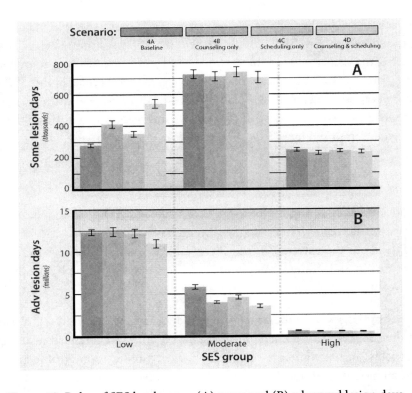

Figure 18. Roles of SES level versus (A) some and (B) advanced lesion days

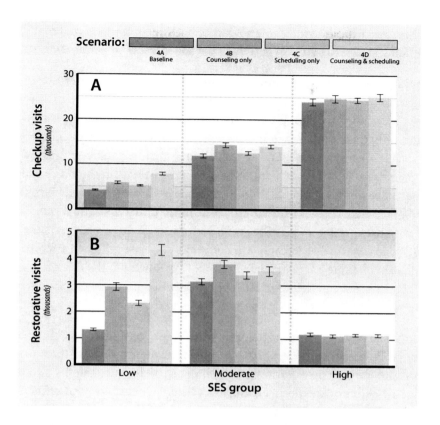

Figure 19. Role of SES level versus (A) checkup and (B) restorative visits

is limited; as is often the case, these limitations were particularly acutely for factors involving vulnerable populations. For example, most studies track the equivalent of some lesion days, but not the rate of prevalence of white spot lesions across the SES spectrum, and understanding of how SES affects the frequency of presenting for care under different disease severities is limited. Nonetheless, this simulation model exhibits quite complex behavior that can be compared with substantial empirical evidence, and informal calibration—adjusting parameter values to best align model results with empirical evidence—helped secure plausible model dynamics. We also relied heavily on sensitivity analysis to alert us to assumptions that strongly influenced the model results. While this helped identify particularly important uncertainties, more thorough sensitivity analyses are required, which will help inform the data collection and calibration feedback cycle.

Our findings highlight opportunities and priorities at many levels. They suggest the central importance of conceptualizing trust as both a symptom and a cause, and recognizing and designing interventions that take into account the associated feedbacks. This dual role of trust is reflected in the persistence of many dominant patterns, even when trust is disabled as a driving factor (scenario D, figure 13), and it plays a key role in understanding the effects of potential interventions. At face value, the interventions studied appear to differ fundamentally with respect to their impacts on trust: while counseling seeks to directly elevate trust levels among those at risk, scheduling interventions instead work to bring at-risk individuals in more often. Because trust serves as both symptom and cause, both interventions materially affect trust levels, with scheduling reducing severe negative experiences via more frequent care-seeking.

Our simulated interventions demonstrate how trust and care-seeking are intertwined in a "chicken and egg" scenario. While risk-based care models can confer strong benefits to those presenting for care—even occasionally—they fall far short of helping individuals of very low SES with minimal care-seeking. Given the hurdles that such individuals often face in seeking care (financial, logistic, employment, cultural, to name a few), to the degree that they present for care at all they are likely to do so only rarely, and frequently only for dental emergencies when they are likely to have much adversity in their care experience. Even with counseling, that experience in the model is at best likely to be neutral as far as changing trust is concerned, and to be unlikely to precipitate regular care-seeking. The limited success of interventions in elevating oral health among these low-presenting, low-socioeconomic-status individuals suggests the urgent need to investigate the effects of pairing risk-based care with community-based outreach and other efforts designed to help such individuals overcome barriers related to SES (e.g., lowering the financial, transportation, and child-care barriers). Our model can help evaluate the efficacy of paired intervention strategies, but would benefit greatly from more-detailed depictions of barriers related to SES.

The area of pediatric oral health remains particularly fruitful for continued modeling, because it can shed light on the need for child-focused interventions that yield pronounced short-term oral health gains and secure benefits across the life course. Additional modeling can yield new insights into underlying risk dynamics, such as reducing childhood exposure to sugar-sweetened beverages and refined sugars; enhancing protective behaviors such as tooth brushing; and examining the likely impacts of clinical encounters on such behaviors. Because dental behaviors are strongly influenced by parental attitudes and the quality of care encounters, they can be readily examined using a slight variant of the current modeling framework. Another priority is to refine the model's representations of aspects of the clinical experience, such as the quantification of pain relief and the discomfort patients experience outside the clinic.

We have laid out a methodological approach that seeks—for the first time, to our knowledge—to use a complex systems lens to examine the dynamics of trust within the dental health arena. Trust is a key link between the social determinants of health and the care pathways that shape outcomes through the life course in diverse areas of health. Building theories about the role of trust can provide important insights into intervention trade-offs. With this contribution, we hope to inspire complex models that can serve for theory building in this important area by, for example, providing testable predictions, and aid in the evaluation of possible intervention strategies.

References

1. US Department of Health and Human Services. *Oral Health in America: A Report of the Surgeon General.* Rockville, MD: Institute of Dental and Craniofacial Research, National Institutes of Health; 2000.

2. US Department of Health and Human Services. *A National Call to Action to Promote Oral Health.* Rockville, MD: Public Health Service, Centers for Disease Control and Prevention, National Institutes of Health, National Institute of Dental and Craniofacial Research; May 2003. NIH Publication No. 03-5303.

3. Newacheck PW, Hughes DC, Hung YY, Wong S, Stoddard JJ. The unmet health needs of America's children. *Pediatrics.* 2000;105(4):989–997.

4. Li Y, Caufield PW. The fidelity of initial acquisition of *Mutans streptococci* by infants from their mothers. *J Dent Res.* 1995;74(2):681–685.

5. Dye BA, Vargas CM, Lee JJ, Magder L, Tinanoff N. Assessing the relationship between children's oral health status and that of their mothers. *J Am Dent Assoc.* 2011;142(2):173–183.

6. Fisher-Owens S. Broadening perspectives on pediatric oral health care provision: social determinants of health and behavioral management. *Pediatr Dent.* 2014;36(2):115–120.

7. Li Y, Wang W. Predicting caries in permanent teeth from caries in primary teeth: an eight-year cohort study. *J Dent Res.* 2002;81(8):561–566.

8. Wen A, Goldberg D, Marrs CF, et al. Caries resistance as a function of age in an initially caries-free population. *J Dent Res.* 2012;91(7):671–675.

9. Dye B, Thornton-Evans G, Li X, Iafolla T. Dental caries and sealant prevalence in children and adolescents in the United States, 2011–2012. *NCHS Data Brief.* 2015;(191):1–8.

10. Dye BA, Thornton-Evans G, Li X, Iafolla T. Dental caries and tooth loss in adults in the United States, 2011–2012. *NCHS Data Brief.* 2015;197.

11. Dye BA, Li X, Beltran-Aguilar ED. Selected oral health indicators in the United States, 2005–2008. *NCHS Data Brief.* 2012;(96):1–8.

12. Milsom KM, Tickle M, Humphris GM, Blinkhorn AS. The relationship between anxiety and dental treatment experience in 5-year-old children. *Br Dent J.* 2003;194:503–506.

13. Armfield JM, Stewart JF, Spencer AJ. The vicious cycle of dental fear: exploring the interplay between oral health, service utilization and dental fear. *BMC Oral Health.* 2007;7:1.

14. Mofidi M, Rozier RG, King RS. Problems with access to dental care for Medicaid-insured children: what caregivers think. *Am J Public Health.* 2002;92(1):53–58.

15. Tellez M, Gomez J, Kaur S, Pretty IA, Ellwood R, Ismail AI. Non-surgical management methods of noncavitated carious lesions. *Community Dent Oral Epidemiol.* 2013;41(1):79–96.

16. Weinstein P, Harrison R, Benton T. Motivating mothers to prevent caries: confirming the beneficial effect of counseling. *J Am Dent Assoc.* 2006;137(6):789–793.

17. Miller WR, Rollnick S. *Motivational Interviewing: Helping People Change.* 3rd ed. Guildford Press; 2013.

18. Freudenthal JJ, Bowen, DM. Motivational interviewing to decrease parental risk-related behaviors for early childhood caries. *J Am Dent Hyg Assoc.* 2010;84(1):29–34.

19. Borrelli B, Tooley EM, Scott-Sheldon LA. Motivational interviewing for parent-child health interventions: a systematic review and meta-analysis. *Pediatr Dent.* 2015;37(3):254–265.

20. LaVeist TA, Isaac LA, Williams KP. Mistrust of health care organizations is associated with underutilization of health services. *Health Serv Res.* 2009;44(6):2093–2105.

21. Thom DH, Hall MA, Pawlson LG. Measuring patients' trust in physicians when assessing quality of care. *Health Aff.* 2004;23(4):124–132.

22. Ozawa S, Sripad P. How do you measure trust in the health system? A systematic review of the literature. *Soc Sci Med.* 2013;91:10–14.

23. Murray B, McCrone S. An integrative review of promoting trust in the patient-primary care provider relationship. *J Adv Nurs.* 2015;71(1):3–23.

24. Hall MA, Zheng B, Dugan E, et al. Measuring patients' trust in their primary care providers. *Med Care Res Rev.* 2002;59(3):293–318.

25. Pearson SD, Raeke LH. Patients' trust in physicians: many theories, few measures, and little data. *J Gen Intern Med.* 2000;15(7):509–513.

26. Yamalik N. Dentist-patient relationship and quality care 2. Trust. *Int Dent J.* 2005;55(3):168–170.

27. Graham MA, Logan HL, Tomar SL. Is trust a predictor of having a dental home? *J Am Dent Assoc.* 2004;135(11):1550–1558.

28. Hibbard JH, Greene J, Becker ER, et al. Racial/ethnic disparities and consumer activation in health. *Health Aff.* 2008;27(5):1442–1453.

29. Hibbard JH, Mahoney ER, Stock R, Tusler M. Do increases in patient activation result in improved self-management behaviors? *Health Serv Res.* 2007;42:1443–1463.

30. Fisher-Owens SA, Gansky SA, Platt LJ, et al. Influences on children's oral health: a conceptual model. *Pediatrics.* 2007;120(3):e510–e520.

31. Patrick DL, Lee RSY, Nucci M, Grembowski D, Jolles CZ, Milgrom P. Reducing oral health disparities: a focus on social and cultural determinants. *BMC Oral Health.* 2006;6(Suppl 1):S4.

32. Esfahbod B, Kreuger K, Osgood ND. Gaming the social system: a game theoretic examination of social influence in risk behavior. *Social Computing, Behavioral-Cultural Modeling, and Prediction;* 2015:206–301.

CHAPTER 12

THE RELATIVE IMPORTANCE OF SOCIOECONOMIC STATUS AND OTHER MAJOR FACTORS FOR POPULATION HEALTH: ESTIMATES USING THE HEALTHPATHS AGENT-BASED MICROSIMULATION MODEL

Michael Wolfson, PhD
Canada Research Chair in Population Health Modeling/Populomics
School of Epidemiology, Public Health and Preventive Medicine, Faculty of Medicine
University of Ottawa

Geoff Rowe, PhD
Demographer, Retired
Statistics Canada

Acknowledgments: This research was developed as part of the NIH-funded Network on Inequality, Complexity and Health (NICH) led by George Kaplan. We are deeply indebted to NICH colleagues for many valuable discussions, and to Steve Gribble for software wizardry.

The epidemiological literature is replete with studies showing many and diverse impacts on individuals' health. As, in the case of smoking and obesity, these are typically described as "risk factors." Less narrow analyses in the spirit of social epidemiology and population health refer to broader health determinants, especially the pervasive observation that the higher one's SES (as measured by income or education), the better one's health (as measured by mortality rates or self-reported health status). The extensive corpus of work on the global burden of disease[1] represents an ambitious effort to integrate data on a very broad range of conventionally defined diseases and risk factors, though they omit broader health determinants, including poverty. Aside from this work on global burden of disease, it remains a challenge to undertake empirically based analyses that, in a coherent manner, assesses the relative quantitative importance of a diverse range of factors that could be known to influence health, in an integrated and simultaneous manner.

Furthermore, research on various risk factors and health determinants generally ignores an obvious source of complexity, that they each not only affect health but also affect one another; risk factors and health determinants *co-evolve* with one another as well as with health. For example, both physical activity and body mass index (BMI) have been shown to affect health. But physical activity can reduce higher BMI, while high BMI can predispose individuals against physical activity. Single regression equations, even if multivariate, cannot capture these kinds of dynamic interactions. To continue this example, health, physical activity, and BMI co-evolve over the life course, in a mutually interacting manner via both contemporaneous and lagged causal influences. Moreover, from the perspective of understanding health inequalities, conventional risk factors such as smoking and obesity are socially patterned. They are not only correlated with SES at a point in time, but their evolution over the life course is also patterned by the co-evolution of individuals' SES. These kinds of dynamics, interactions, and feedbacks are the hallmarks of a complex system.

Another problem in assessing the ways health determinants affect health is the conceptual framework within which health is defined. The dominant measure of health is biomedically defined disease, along with biomarkers such as hypertension and cholesterol levels. However, such biomarkers are often completely asymptomatic, while clinically defined diseases such as arthritis and angina can range from asymptomatic to extremely disabling. Since our objective is to assess impacts on population health in terms meaningful to individuals, this analysis focuses on individuals' capacity to function in day-to-day life, in turn based on health domains such as mobility, vision, and pain. (When individuals are asked how they think about health, they mention functional health status more often than disease.[2])

Another significant problem is the ways that risk factors and broader health determinants are analyzed. The challenge arises because conventional risk factors such as smoking and obesity interact and co-evolve with broader health determinants like SES in what Rose et al.[3] and Marmot[4] call "the causes of the causes." The reality is that these relationships form a complex system, a set of relationships with feedbacks, non-linearities, delayed effects, and reciprocal causation. Standard epidemiological concepts such as population-attributable fractions (as conventionally measured), and categorical attribution (as used in the global burden of disease),[1] fail to reflect these complex systems aspects.

Why Complex Systems Methods

In this chapter, we take on the ambitious task of developing a dynamic multivariate approach to estimating and then drawing out the implications of co-evolving trajectories of health status, in conjunction with a diverse set of health-related individual characteristics. We do so by tightly coupling an extensive process of statistical estimation, based on a richly multivariate longitudinal data set, Statistics Canada's National Population Health Survey (NPHS),[5] with a specially designed agent-based microsimulation model, HealthPaths.

This HealthPaths analysis is an example of a complex systems method. In this case, and as discussed in chapter 2, the HealthPaths model lies at an intermediate point along the spectrum between simple agent-based models and more detailed microsimulation models. Historically, these two kinds of models are polar opposites in terms of size, empirical grounding, and character of agents' behavior. Still, both involve computer simulation software where the units of observation and analysis are evolving individual agents from which population features over time (e.g., totals, averages, proportions, and distributions) are derived by aggregation and tabulation. The HealthPaths model described here builds on the strengths of both poles of microsimulation model development.

Most importantly for understanding the relative importance of risk factors and broader health determinants, the complex systems methodology represented by HealthPaths uniquely enables critical aspects like population heterogeneity, co-evolution, nonparametric specifications of quantitative relationships, and lagged effects to be explicitly incorporated.

The following section describes the statistical analysis used to generate the needed empirical results. We then use the HealthPaths model to simulate a series of counterfactual scenarios designed to assess the relative quantitative importance of a diverse set of health determinants. In a manner somewhat similar to "knocking out" a gene in an animal model, the counterfactuals set each factor in turn to its best value for everyone. For example, instead of observed patterns of smoking, everyone is posited to be a nonsmoker throughout their lives; that is, the role of smoking is "knocked out." The HealthPaths model is then used to simulate what a measure of population health would be in the counterfactual world without that factor's adverse health effects. This analysis is a significant extension of Wolfson and Rowe,[6] with an expanded set of covariates and more sophisticated statistical estimations.

Measuring Population Health

The most widely used measure of population health by far is life expectancy (LE). However, this measure makes absolutely no distinction between years of life lived in full health, and those lived with serious illness and functional limitations. Health-adjusted life expectancy (HALE) is the most widely accepted indicator of population health that takes health status while living into account.[7-9] In this analysis, we focus on both: LE due to its ubiquity, and HALE since it is a far better indicator of population health.

LE and HALE are typically estimated using life-table methods. These are semi-aggregate approaches, where individuals are considered within groups (e.g., by age and sex), and within each group they are assumed to be homogeneous, rather individuals are obviously heterogeneous and multidimensional. The alternative approach is explicitly microanalytic, in which individuals rather than population subgroups are the units of analysis. However, such microanalytic approaches necessarily have much more detail and involve much more computation. In order to embody such realistic heterogeneity, we used a microsimulation model as the core analytical method rather than the spreadsheet methods more typically used for conventional life tables, and for Sullivan-style estimates of HALE.[7]

As widely measured, LE is based on a hypothetical birth cohort where individuals, no matter their age, are exposed to a given year's vector of age-specific mortality rates. The resulting survival curve is the implicit distribution of life lengths of this hypothetical (and steady state) birth cohort, whose mortality exposure is constant at the rates observed in a given year. The average age at death for this cohort is the average of the life lengths, which is then conventional LE.

In our microanalytic approach using HealthPaths, the life lengths are explicit; each one is simulated individually. Further, we can generalize the Sullivan life-table approach[7] so that estimates of HALE are also microanalytic by using both health status while alive and life length (age at death) to construct a composite lifetime or life-course measure for each individual, called health-adjusted life length (HALL). Instead of simply counting the number of years of life (LL), we weight each year (or succession of time intervals of life if health status evolves in continuous rather than discrete time) by the unit-interval index of health status, based on measures like the McMaster Health Utility Index (HUI)[10] or EuroQuol EQ-5D,[11] both multidimensional generic functional health status measures. We then take the sum (or integral if we are in continuous time). The result for each simulated individual is their HALL.

Life-table measures like LE and HALE are typically based on rates and averages observed over a year, as if the cohort were aging outside of calendar time and going through its entire life cycle in a given short period of time. Hence, these are commonly referred to as *period* life-table results. (The main alternative, true *cohort* life-table results, is much more demanding in terms of data, requiring both detailed historical data plus detailed projections of mortality and health status.)

Our measures of population health (LE and HALE), however, are conceptually intermediate between standard period and cohort life-table estimates. We construct "thick" period cohort estimates of LE and HALE, where we assume steady state, or more accurately constant transition probabilities as in period life-table analyses. These probabilities are based on dynamic relationships estimated over 14 years of repeated longitudinal observations, not simply the rates observed in a given year.

Statistical Analysis

The HealthPaths model involves two distinct but tightly coupled phases: statistical estimation and then microsimulation modeling. The statistical analysis is intensively based on the NPHS,[1] focusing on the variables shown in table 1, with an added mortality follow-up.

The empirical relationships for both phases of the analysis—statistical estimation and then microsimulation—form a network (figure 1),[2] where each "blob" (circle or rectangle) represents a measure of each of the indicated constructs, and each arrow represents a "causal pathway," or more concretely, coefficients representing (in epidemiological parlance) effect sizes. The factors shown (SES, smoking, family, and others) illustrate the evolution over the life course of these posited risk factors and health determinants.

Health status, in contrast, is shown as a rectangle, in order to indicate that this construct is actually a composite, an eight-dimensional vector of health states in each of the domains forming the McMaster Health Utility Index[10]: vision, hearing, speech, mobility, dexterity, pain, cognition, and emotion. Each of these

---

1   The NPHS started in 1994 with interviews every two years. The sample included the institutionalized population and has been augmented with mortality follow-up. By the end of the period considered in this analysis, 2008, the sample size was about 14,000. All survey responses are self-reported. The content is mostly conventional (e.g., socio-demographics), a chronic disease checklist, major risk factors, and health care utilization. However, there was some more exploratory content, for example, Antonovsky's Sense of Coherence,[20] Pearlin/Schoolers' Sense of Mastery,[21] and the McMaster Health Utilities Index (HUI).[10]

2   All figures used with permission from Wolfson 2016 (https://goo.gl/4M5iuP). Colors are visible in the online versions.

Table 1

Risk Factors/events and Helath States Included

Ordinal Variables		Binary Variables
Vision		Employed this year
Hearing		Family member
Speech	Functional	Institutional resident
Mobility	health	High school graduate
Dexterity	summarized	Community college
Emotion	by HUI	University graduate
Cognition		Mortality
Pain		
Income decile		**Quantitative Variables**
Leisure activity		Body mass index
Daily activity		Sense of Mastery
Smoking		Sense of Coherence
		Years daily smoking

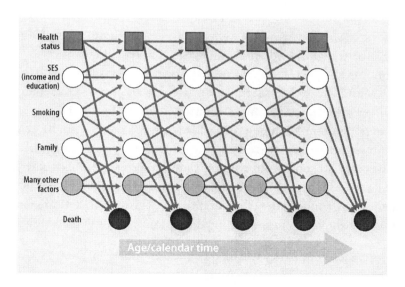

Figure 1. System of recursive equations. The sequence of circles for SES represents educational attainment and income decile; those for smoking show current, former, never, or occasional on a daily basis; and those for family show whether living alone or not. "Many other factors" represents all others not shown. Death represents exact time of death. Not all possible arrows are shown. All other variables have been included in the statistical analysis

domains is measured as an ordered categorical variable with five or six levels. Additionally, there is a valuation or scoring function that maps the full vector of eight ordered categorical variables into a scalar index in the unit interval where 1 is full health and 0 is dead.

For each of these factors or variables, the sequence of circles or rectangles indicates their evolution over one individual's life course, and arrows indicate potential causal pathways. In order for the diagram not to be too cluttered, only a few of these arrows are actually shown. For example, while at each period there are arrows from SES to health, to smoking, and to SES in the following time period, and to death during the intervening interval, no arrow is shown from smoking or from the "many other factors" to family, for example, though empirically there is likely some relationship.

While all the possible arrows indicating causal pathways are not drawn in figure 1 (to avoid clutter), our theory is that everything can potentially affect everything else; individuals' characteristics all co-evolve, though we have made the simplifying assumption that these effects always involve at least a one-year lag. Thus, each variable must be a dependent variable in one regression equation, and it is given the chance to be an independent variable in the equations estimated for all the other co-evolving state variables, both by itself and combined with other variables via a set of interaction terms.

While figure 1 shows only arrows for one period lags (a conventional first-order Markov assumption), the statistical analysis of the NPHS data allowed up to two period lags (second-order Markov). The result is a coherent and complete network of recursive equations. Since every equation in this network of recursive relationships is estimated from the same NPHS data, the equations are coherent both in terms of variable definitions, and their measurement and error structures.

Given the conceptual framework in figure 1, in effect a system of simultaneous equations describing the stochastic co-evolution for any given individual of all the variables shown in table 1, a unique approach to statistical estimation was afforded by the existence of bootstrap weights in the main data set used, the National Population Health Survey.[5] In order to allow users to account for the complex, multistage, clustered design of the NPHS sample, each individual observation in the NPHS data was given a set of 500 bootstrap sample weights. Ordinarily, these are used to estimate more-accurate sampling errors for any given statistic derived from the sample. These sampling errors are typically larger than those derived under the assumption that the data had come from a simple random sample.[3] For example, the sampling error of a number in one cell of a cross tabulation, or of a coefficient in a regression, can be simply generated (albeit via intensive computation) by running the tabulation or the regression 500 times, once using each vector of bootstrap weights, and then *post facto* computing the variance of the 500 resulting estimates.

In this analysis, we used these bootstrap weights in a highly novel fashion, as described in Rowe and Binder.[12] Not only have we used the bootstrap weights to determine the variances of the estimated coefficients in each of the regressions in the system of equations outlined above, but also to estimate a form of specification error and ultimately the variances of our simulations. Each regression equation in the

---

3   The ratio of the variance of the bootstrap replicates to the simple random sample variance is termed the "design effect" of the complex sample, and for the NPHS is generally well over two. NPHS users have been provided these bootstrap weights to enable straightforward and correct variance estimation.

coherent network of relationships was estimated 40 times, once with each of 40 bootstrap weights (sampled from the set of 500 available). Further, the fitting was done using the elastic net method with penalized likelihoods to estimate a range of candidate equations, and then using out-of-sample prediction error to choose from among those candidate equations.[4]

The overall regression specification is illustrated in figure 2. Since waves of the NPHS were every two years, the equations to predict the values at time t for a given age (a) and sex (s) were based on the observed values at times $t - 2$ and $t - 4$. The set of coherently estimated transition dynamics relationships forms the first phase of the analysis. Including interaction terms, there were typically about 200 right-hand-side variables available in each regression. These regressions were done by single year of age.[5]

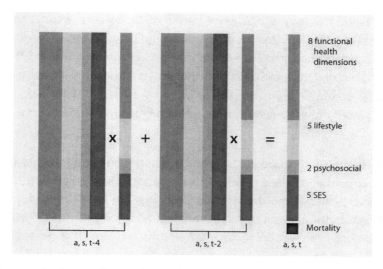

Figure 2. Estimated network of co-evolving relationships; a = age (years), s = sex; t = calendar time (years, n.b. survey waves were every second year.)

One way to think about this statistical analysis of the NPHS data is that we mapped a sample of observed fragments of individuals' health and covariate life-course trajectories onto a set of transition probability densities, each of which is a function of the included covariates. In effect, these can be considered a set of stochastic "laws of motion" for the multivariate dynamics of health status and its correlates for the

---

4 Each bootstrap weight vector provides a convenient partition of the sample into two parts: one part that can be used for estimation (the part with nonzero weights) and one part that can be used to compute out-of-sample prediction error (the part with identically zero weights). This estimation via cross-validation and minimizing out-of-sample prediction error prevents over-fitting.[12] In general, just over one-third of the sample has a zero weight in each bootstrap. The set of bootstrap weights also provides the basis for estimating coefficient variances that include not only sampling error but also model selection variance, using the elastic net (a mixture of ridge and lasso[23] via GLMNET.[24] Further, as will be seen below, the simulations themselves have been bootstrapped to quantify variance in simulation outputs by means of replicate simulations, using one set of equations estimated from each of the separate bootstrap samples for each simulation. In this way, both sampling error and specification error variances can be explicitly propagated and incorporated in estimating the variances of the HealthPaths simulation results, a *de facto* probabilistic sensitivity analysis.

5 To mitigate sample-size concerns, a kernel including adjacent ages was used in each regression.

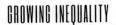

Canadian population, with explicit account taken of both sampling and estimation errors.

HealthPaths Agent-Based Microsimulation Model

This richly empirical, quantified, and stochastic description of individuals' life-course dynamics was next used to construct a Monte Carlo microsimulation model, HealthPaths. This microsimulation starts by creating one fully synthetic individual biography, then repeating this process millions of times to generate a representative population sample.

To synthesize one biography, an individual is first "born" (*in silico* in the memory of the computer) by being endowed with the values for all their state variables (specifically all those in table 1), including their correlation structure. "Birth" occurs at age 20, since the NPHS data were not sufficient to support estimates of transition dynamics below this age. The set of equations indicated in figure 2 is then applied recursively to generate all the individual's state space/covariate values as events occur, in particular changes in state such as becoming a smoker, or deteriorating in one or other functional health status dimension. The given individual's synthetic biography is then completed, event by event, in as realistic a manner as possible, using many random number draws to determine whether a given transition occurs, until the individual is simulated to die.

This second-order Markov assumption is a compromise. On the one hand, higher order terms (i.e., variable values lagged three or more periods) would likely be statistically significant.[13] Still, it is a notable improvement on analyses that assume the relevant processes are only first-order Markov. Further, the second-order Markov assumption, given the eight waves of NHPS data from 1994 to 2008 that have been used, enables more than one observation of three time-period sequences three-tuples) of events for each individual. For example, and individual will have data for the three periods (1994, 1996, and 1998), and then again for 1996, 1998 and 2000. Having these multiple sequences allows direct estimation of individual heterogeneity terms.

Note, however, that figure 1 is misleading in our context because it gives the impression that the simulation uses discrete time. The estimation necessarily used discrete times, since the NPHS had observations every two years. But the simulation is considerably more sophisticated since it uses continuous time. Correspondingly, instead of the model generating changes in status (e.g., changes in the values of any of the state variables in table 1) that occur, for example, only at fixed annual time intervals, the simulation proceeds by generating event histories with discrete events such as an improvement or decline in health status that can occur at any time t, where t is a continuous variable. As a result, the statistical analysis forms a bridge between the discrete time data from the NPHS and the continuous-time microsimulation modeling of HealthPaths.[6]

Given a complete set of empirically based stochastic descriptions of an individual's state transition dynamics—used to generate a single individual's synthetic but realistic biography—the next step is simply

---

6   This structure implies that HealthPaths is a discrete event simulation model, albeit embedded in continuous time. But in this case, the term has a different meaning than that in chapter 2 when describing the class of discrete event simulation models.

to repeat this process many times in order to generate a complete representative sample of the Canadian population. We focused on individuals in a hypothetical 1976 birth cohort,[7] and generated representative population samples of millions of individuals in order to assure Monte Carlo error would be negligible. (The sampling variability of LE was explicitly examined to verify this.)

Finally, the eight functional health status variables are aggregated using the McMaster HUI weighting function to produce—for each individual during the (continuous time) interval between state changes—a summary health status index with values in the [0, 1] interval. The sum (actually integral, given the model's use of continuous time) of this summary health index provides each individual's entry into the distribution of health-adjusted life lengths (HALLs). The sample of HALLs, our main individual-level measure of health, is then averaged to construct our summary population health indicator, HALE, which is microanalytic and based on full individual or micro-level life-course trajectories. This method contrasts with the semi-aggregate Sullivan[7] life-table method (for example, as generalized by McIntosh et al.[14] to estimate SES gradients in HALE), which assumes both that individuals are homogeneous within age, sex, and income groups, and that health status and mortality are conditionally independent given age, sex, and income group.

Our HealthPaths simulation results embody a critical assumption about causality. There is no guarantee that the statistical relationships estimated from the observed data—as population representative, multivariate, and dynamic as they are—accurately represent causality. Indeed, given the myriad known factors and causal pathways that have not been included, the system of equations embodied in HealthPaths is certainly incomplete, and therefore wrong. However, our estimated relationships do provide a strong and potentially illuminating basis for drawing out their joint implications on the assumption that they are causal. Our simulation results should therefore be considered suggestive.

Comparing Simulations and Observations

Figure 3 shows the observed NPHS and HealthPaths simulated average age-specific mortality hazards for each sex. The vertical dispersion of dots at each age derives from the 40 bootstrap weight vectors used in the NPHS observations and the corresponding replicate simulations. For example, this dispersion is much wider for the NPHS observations at younger ages, due to the relatively few numbers of deaths at these ages.

Figure 4 shows a corresponding display of health scores by age, comparing the NPHS data to the HealthPaths simulations. At each age and sex, there are 40 dark dots, showing the actual NPHS data for each of the 40 bootstrap weights, and 40 light dots showing the set of corresponding simulated values. And each of the 80 dots at each age and sex in turn gives the average of the HUI scores for the hundreds or thousands of individuals observed in the data, and for the millions of simulated individuals, respectively. In this case, the wider dispersion of HUI scores observed with the NPHS data at higher ages is due to the relatively small sample sizes. The simulated HUI scores are key constituents in the simulation of HALE.

---

7   The cohort starts with an observed multivariate joint distribution of the state variables in table 1 for 20 year olds in 1996 (i.e., born in 1976). The trajectories of all their state variables are then simulated based on the regressions from the NPHS that used data from 1994 to 2008. For this reason, the simulation can be thought of as generating a "thick" period birth cohort, one whose transition dynamics derive from data spanning 14 years.

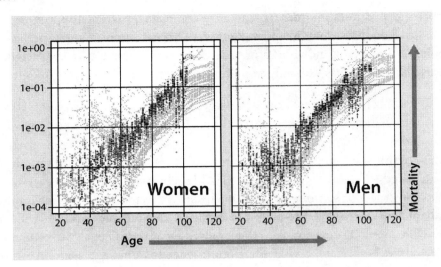

Figure 3. Observed (1900–1976 birth cohorts—dark dots) and simulated (1976 birth cohort—light dots) for mortality hazards

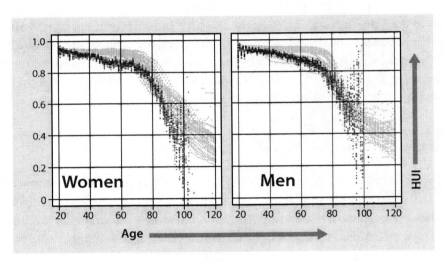

Figure 4. Observed (1900–1976 birth cohorts—dark dots) and simulated (1976 birth cohort—light dots) for average Health Utility Index (HUI) values

For both mortality (figure 3) and health status (figure 4), there are necessarily important conceptual differences between the two cohorts: The observed NPHS data represent a mix of overlapping and mostly older birth cohorts, while the HealthPaths simulations show a hypothetical 1976 ("thick" period) birth cohort with 1994–2008 characteristics and transition dynamics.[8] The slower decline in average HUI in the

---

8 We refer to this as a "thick" period cohort in order to distinguish it from conventional demographic period life tables where the transition rates are typically annual. Annual transition rates, in this case, represent a "thin" time interval compared to the "thick" 14-year time interval used in HealthPaths to estimate transition probabilities (actually, conditional transition probability functions).

HealthPaths simulated results (in the middle age range in figure 4), for example, compared to the NPHS observations, is related to the fact that the NPHS data reflect the health status of earlier birth cohorts. As a result, such differences between observed and simulated results should not be surprising.

These differences show up most starkly for nonsmoking rates (figure 5). Specifically, as observed in the NPHS, older women were far less likely to smoke than women projected to smoke in the simulated 1976 birth cohort. On the other hand, for men, observed smoking rates for older cohorts were much higher than for the simulated 1976 "thick" birth cohort.

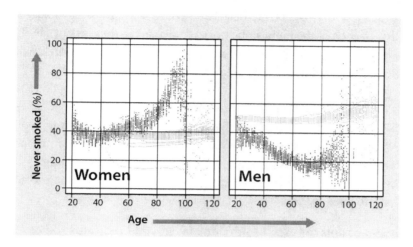

Figure 5. Observed (1900–1976 birth cohorts—dark dots) and simulated (1976 birth cohort—light dots) for nonsmoking rates

Smoking is a significant risk factor for both LE and HALE. However, as will be shown below, it is not the factor with the largest impact on overall population health of those considered. Even though the difference between the observed and simulated nonsmoking rates is stark (figure 5), it is not necessarily the main reason for the differences between observed and simulated mortality hazards (figure 3) or average HUI values (figure 4).

Constructing Counterfactuals

Given all the myriad estimated dynamic relationships from the NPHS, and the HealthPaths microsimulation model designed to embody these estimates and to draw out their implications, this *in silico* lab apparatus is ready for experiments. The statistical estimation process has effectively provided a posited "web of causality,"[15,16] albeit a complex one, with numerous lagged and cross dependencies. The core of the analysis of the relative importance of various health risk factors, characteristics, and broader determinants now uses this *in silico* lab apparatus, HealthPaths, to simulate a series of carefully constructed counterfactual scenarios.

The previous section presented several results from the baseline simulation scenario (involving 40 replicate simulations). A counterfactual scenario is one where part of the network of posited causal pathways (figure 1) is altered, and the HealthPaths simulation is re-run. Specifically, we have constructed counterfactual scenarios by altering one or other of the estimated connections among the co-evolving factors, such as eliminating smoking or socioeconomic inequalities. These counterfactual changes apply from "birth" (actually age 20) throughout each of the lives of millions of individuals simulated, not only at the beginning of each life.

Figure 6 introduces this kind of counterfactual simulation by showing the impacts of simply eliminating functional health-status limitations, one at a time, for each of the eight underlying health domains of the McMaster HUI. Whatever the baseline simulation entailed, by virtue of the inputs to the dynamics of a given domain such as mobility, in the counterfactual scenario that domain is repeatedly reset, over the entire lifetime, to full mobility. In each of the panels, the horizontal axis is a measure of the change in either LE in years or HALE in weighted years, due to eliminating the adverse effects on individuals' overall functional health status for particular health domains (as defined for the McMaster HUI).

In each of the panels in figure 6, these health domains were independently ordered from smallest (top) to largest (bottom) health impact, as measured by the median of 40 bootstrap replicate estimates. For example, in figure 6A, vision has the smallest median impact while the median impact of mobility on LE for women was the largest, with impacts over the 40 bootstrap replicates ranging from just above zero to almost 5 years. Correspondingly, in figure 6D vision has the largest median impact on HALE for men and ranges from just under 2 to over 3 years.

The horizontal dispersion of dots for each health domain, sex, and indicator (LE or HALE) clearly shows substantial uncertainty in these results, since each of the dots is the difference in the indicator for one pair of replicate simulations (in turn based on one of the 40 replicate estimations from the NPHS). Specifically, each dot indicates the difference in years between the counterfactual and the baseline simulated LE or HALE. It is important to note that the uncertainty indicated by the dispersion in each row of 40 dots derives from both conventional uncertainty in the coefficient estimates plus that associated with the specification of each equation (i.e., which variables have nonzero coefficients at all). Perhaps not surprisingly, the uncertainty was greater for HALE (figure 6B and 6D) than for LE (figure 6A and 6C).

These functional health domains have a much larger impact on HALE than on LE, since they are often burdens throughout long periods of life without necessarily being quickly fatal, or even fatal at all. Pain and cognition are particularly notable because they show the greatest discrepancies between impacts on LE (relatively small) and on HALE (quite large). Yet these health problems tend to garner much less attention than heart disease and cancer because they are not visible as major factors in the NPHS mortality data. This is the key reason we focus on HALE and HALLs rather than exclusively on LE and LLs: to obtain a more complete picture of the burdens of various health problems.

Given that the average range of a sample of size 40 has nearly the same width as a 95% confidence interval, we conclude that almost all of the scenarios show effects significantly greater than zero. Apart from that, the dominant feature of these distributions is the degree of overlap, indicating that definitive conclusions about the relative quantitative importance of these eight functional health domains cannot be drawn.

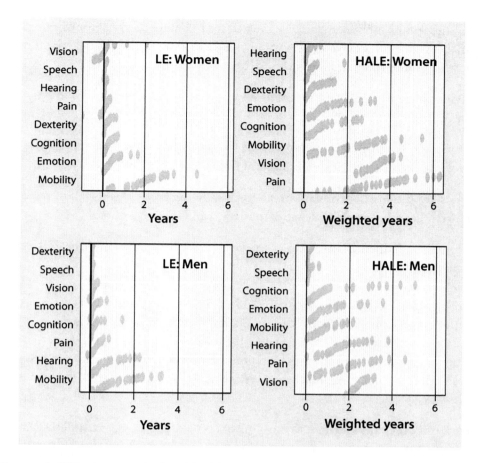

Figure 6. Changes in life expectancy (LE) and health-adjusted life expectancy (HALE) for eight components of the Health Utility Index (HUI) of functional health status. Note the different horizontal axis ranges for LE (up to 6 years) and HALE (up to 8 "weighted years"). Results shown for 1,280 counterfactual simulations (eight health domains × male and female × LE and HALE × 40 replicates), each compared with the corresponding baseline from among the 160 (male and female × LE and HALE × 40 replicates) simulations run

Finally, we turn to a fuller use of HealthPaths' capacity to simulate counterfactuals (figure 7). All of these counterfactuals involve taking one risk factor or health determinant and then, no matter what the estimated equations entail, continually resetting that variable to its best value. In the cases of four factors—BMI, smoking, family membership and employment—the variables are used directly. For example, in the smoking counterfactual, no matter what else is simulated to happen in each and every individual's life course, their entire life course is simulated as if they were always a nonsmoker. In the case of BMI, whatever its value would have been, the value is continually reset to a BMI of 27. We appreciate that according to WHO guidelines, this is actually in the overweight category. But there is important evidence that health risks may actually be minimized at a BMI of around 27.[17–19] For family membership and employment, which are both dichotomous, whatever value is implied by the estimated transition functions, these variables were always reset to "in a family" and "employed," respectively.

In order to keep the results more compact, we created four composite variables from those included in the statistical analysis of the NPHS (table 1): SES, physical function, psycho-social condition, and sensory function. In these cases, the counterfactuals were defined as follows:

- SES: Individuals are treated as if they are always university graduates and in the top income decile, the top categories.

- Physical function: Individuals are always in the top (healthiest) categories for all of leisure and daily nonleisure time physical activity, mobility, and dexterity.

- Psychosocial conditions: Individuals are always in the top categories for all of Antonovsky's sense of coherence,[20] Pearlin/Schooler's sense of mastery,[21] and the HUI emotion and cognition domains.

- Sensory function: Individuals are always in the top categories for all of the HUI vision, hearing, speech, and pain domains.

Figure 7 parallels figure 6, but this time eliminates, one at a time, any adverse effects of each of these eight risk or composite factors. For parsimony, the results are shown for men and women combined. Each row in each chart shows the impacts—measured by the difference between the counterfactual simulation where everything for that factor is fine, to the baseline—for each of the eight risk factors, characteristics, and broader health determinants. Again, the curves are actually scatters of dots for each of 40 bootstrap replicates.

The factors were again ordered, from least to most impact on years of LE and HALE, respectively, based on the median of the replicates. Using the LE ranking, the counterfactual with the smallest impact was the one where everyone is always a never-smoker, year in and year out, no matter what else is happening to their other covariates. This result may appear surprising, but recall that it is based on the smoking rates of the simulated 1976 birth cohort, which are much better for men, though getting worse, especially for younger women (figure 5). Even though this never-smoked counterfactual had the smallest impact on LE, it still increased LE by about one year, and HALE by about a half year.

Perhaps surprisingly, a counterfactual where everyone is always somewhat overweight, with a BMI of 27, was actually protective compared to the observed distribution of BMIs where individuals range from underweight to obese. This "BMI always equal to 27" counterfactual added about one year to LE and about a half-year to HALE. In the baseline simulation there were many individuals with BMIs above 27, but there were even more with lower BMIs. This finding suggests that normal BMI (according to the WHO, in the 20–25 range) may actually be harmful for both LE and HALE. While this result runs counter to predominant current thinking and public commentary, it is in line with our own more-detailed probing of this result using the NPHS data (Rowe and Wolfson, unpublished), and with several excellent published results in the epidemiological literature.[17–19]

Another way to account for this possibly surprising result in this HealthPaths analysis is that, in contrast to a large majority of the literature on the impacts of obesity, many other covariates, in a time-varying mode, have been explicitly taken into account, hence reducing possible bias from omitted variables. As a result,

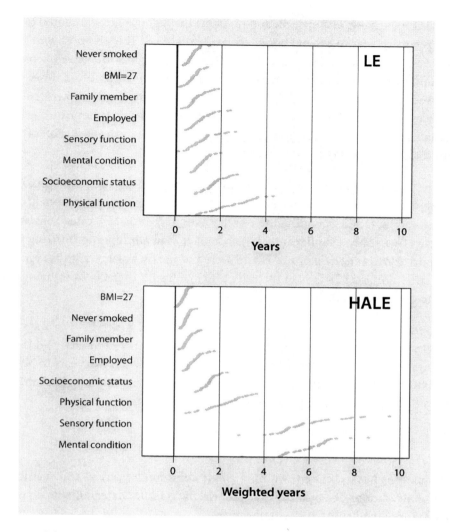

Figure 7. Changes in life expectancy (LE) and health-adjusted life expectancy (HALE) for various risk factors, characteristics and broader health determinants

our analysis of BMI may be analogous to that of Stringhini et al.[22] when re-analyzing the Whitehall data. In that case, when time-varying covariates were included, the estimated effects of civil service level on the SES gradient were substantially reduced.

We also found that living in a household with at least one other family member all one's life was somewhat more protective compared to the observed patterns of household composition, where many individuals spend considerable portions of their lives living alone. Likewise, being employed all one's life was even more protective; in our simulation, this added more than a year to both LE and HALE. The rank order of these risk factors and broader health determinants was not much changed in terms of their impacts on HALE as compared to LE.

For the four other factors, the rank order changes were more pronounced. Having full sensory function (full capacity for vision, hearing, and speech, and no pain) throughout life, compared to the baseline scenario, added a bit over one year to LE, but about six years to HALE. The situation with psychosocial conditions (the emotion and cognition domains of the McMaster HUI, plus the sense of coherence and sense of mastery) was similar, with the impact on HALE again being on the order of six times that on LE. These discrepancies between impacts on LE and HALE are dramatic. They clearly show substantial reductions in the rank importance of a range of major and more conventional risk factors and health determinants (e.g., BMI and smoking) when only mortality results are considered, to the exclusion of typically nonfatal functional health status and psychological characteristics.

For SES, the counterfactual posits that no matter what else is happening, each individual is always considered to be in the top income decile and to have completed postsecondary education. This scenario where everyone has equal and high SES, spending their entire lives in the top SES categories, increased both LE and HALE by almost two years, a significantly larger impact than eliminating smoking in this hypothetical population cohort. However, the gains in HALE were not nearly as large as those for sensory function and psychosocial condition, so SES falls in the rank order of health impacts from being the second most important for LE to the upper-middle range for HALE.

Finally, the counterfactual where everyone always has full physical function (is always physically active and has full mobility and dexterity in the HUI functional health status domains) had the greatest impact of all the (sometimes composite) covariates examined, adding more than two years to both LE and HALE. Despite the emphasis in popular media and public health research on smoking and obesity, these results showed much larger impacts related to physical function.

Implications

This HealthPaths analysis has examined, within a single common empirical and methodological framework, the relative contributions of a number of health risk factors and determinants on population health, with both methodological and substantive implications.

Methodologically, this analysis brought together detailed statistical data analysis with a form of agent-based computer simulation modeling (microsimulation) in order to address questions related to health inequality that intrinsically involve complex systems features, including heterogeneity, multivariate co-evolution, feedbacks, and lagged effects. HealthPaths transcended conventional epidemiological methods (such as single equation analyses and simple formulae for population attributable fractions); rather, it explored a coherent network of empirically based dynamic relationships, those whose structure was constrained as little as possible by *a priori* assumptions such as functional forms, or concerns about parsimony.

The analysis also explicitly accounted for uncertainties in the data analysis, including all of sampling, estimation, and specification errors, by making novel use of the NPHS bootstrap weights. Methodologically, it is a concrete proof of concept that many prevalent simplifying assumptions in epidemiological (and related demographic) analyses can be effectively transcended.

The analysis focused on Health-Adjusted Life Expectancy (HALE) as the summary measure of population health. HealthPaths also shifted the focus from biomedically defined diseases to functional health status—domains such as vision, mobility and pain. As a result, this analysis has demonstrated the much greater salience of HALE compared to the far more widely used Life Expectancy (LE). For example, the impacts of mobility and sensory limitations were far larger when measured using HALE than LE.

Substantively, our HealthPaths analysis has found that:

- In terms of health inequalities, SES differences had roughly twice the impact on HALE as smoking (based on recent rather than historical smoking rates).

- The adverse health impacts of smoking on LE and HALE were far larger than those associated with BMI; indeed, our HealthPaths analysis suggested that moderate overweight (BMI = 27 for everyone) would actually be protective.

Socioeconomic inequalities as a factor in determining HALE, at about 2 years, are large when compared to smoking and overweight, even though these are given by far more emphasis in public health initiatives. On the other hand, socioeconomic inequalities are small compared to the impacts of pain and sensory function, and of psychosocial conditions. These results are provocative. They suggest the need for much more attention to the health burdens of chronic pain, compared to the public health risks associated with obesity. Our HealthPaths analysis has demonstrated a novel approach to estimating such comparative population health impacts. However, considerable work remains to corroborate or contradict our conclusions, such as by including more health risk factors and drawing on other data sets. Nonetheless, our conclusions are sufficiently dramatic that they should give pause to much current thinking on relative health priorities.

References

1. Lim SS, Vos T, Flaxman AD, et al. A comparative risk assessment of burden of disease and injury attributable to 67 risk factors and risk factor clusters in 21 regions, 1990–2010: a systematic analysis for the Global Burden of Disease Study 2010. *Lancet.* 2012;380:2224–2260.

2. van Dalen H, Williams A, Gudex C. Lay people's evaluations of health: are there variations between different subgroups? *J Epidemiol Community Health.* 1994;48:248–253.

3. Rose G. *The Strategy of Preventive Medicine.* Oxford, UK: Oxford University Press; 1992.

4. Marmot M. Social determinants of health inequalities. *Lancet.* 2005;365:1099–1104.

5. Beaudet M, Chen J, Perez C, Ross N, Wilkins K. *National Population Health Survey Overview 1996–97.* Statistics Canada Health Statistics Division. 82M0009XCB.

6. Wolfson M, Rowe G. HealthPaths: Using functional health trajectories to quantify the relative importance of selected health determinants. *Demogr Res.* 2014;31:941–974.

7. Sullivan DF. A single index of mortality and morbidity. *HSMHA Health Rep.* 1971;86:347–354.

8. Wolfson MC. Health-adjusted life expectancy. *Health Rep.* 1996;8(1):41–45.

9. World Health Statistics. Geneva, Switzerland: World Health Organization; 2014. www.who.int.

10. Feeny D, Furlong W, Torrance GW, et al. Multiattribute and single-attribute utility functions for the health utilities index mark 3 system. *Med Care.* 2002;40:113–128.

11. Kind P, Brooks R, Rabin R, eds. *EQ-5D Concepts and Methods: A Developmental History.* Netherlands: Springer; 2005.

12. Rowe G, Binder D. Can survey bootstrap replicates be used for crossvalidation. In: *JSM Proceedings.* 2008:1430–1437.

13. Wolfson M, Rowe G, Gentleman JF, Tomiak M. Career earnings and death: a longitudinal analysis of older Canadian men. *J Gerontol.* 1993;48:S167–S179.

14. McIntosh CN, Finès P, Wilkins R, Wolfson MC. Income disparities in health-adjusted life expectancy for Canadian adults, 1991 to 2001. *Health Rep.* 1009;20:55.

15. MacMahon B, Pugh TF, Ipsen J, et al. Epidemiologie Methods. *Epidemiol Methods.* 1960.

16. Krieger N. Epidemiology and the web of causation: Has anyone seen the spider? *Soc Sci Med.* 1994;39:887–903.

17. Flegal KM, Graubard BI, Williamson DF, Gail MH. Excess deaths associated with underweight, overweight, and obesity. *JAMA.* 2005;293:1861–1867.

18. Flegal KM, Kit BK, Orpana H, Graubard BI. Association of all-cause mortality with overweight and obesity using standard body mass index categories: a systematic review and meta-analysis. *JAMA.* 2013;309:71–82.

19. Tomiyama AJ, Hunger JM, Nguyen-Cuu J, Wells C. Misclassification of cardiometabolic health when using body mass index categories in NHANES 2005–2012. *Int J Obes.* 2016;40(5):883–886.

20. Antonovsky A. The structure and properties of the sense of coherence scale. *Soc Sci Med.* 1993;36:725–733.

21. Pearlin LI, Schooler C. The structure of coping. *J Health Soc Behav.* 1978;19:2–21.

22. Stringhini S, Sabia S, Shipley M, et al. Association of socioeconomic position with health behaviors and mortality. *JAMA.* 2010;303:1159–1166.

23. Zou H, Hastie T. Regularization and variable selection via the elastic net. *J R Stat Soc Ser B Stat Methodol.* 2005;67:301–320.

24. Friedman J, Hastie T, Tibshirani R. Regularization paths for generalized linear models via coordinate descent. *J Stat Softw.* 2010;33(1):1–22.

CHAPTER 13

AGENT-BASED MODELS AND HEALTH-ORIENTED MOBILE TECHNOLOGIES

Sara McPhee-Knowles
Policy Analyst
Government of Yukon

Nathaniel Osgood
Departments of Computer Science and Community Health & Epidemiology
University of Saskatchewan

Chapter 2 noted the important role that the complex systems approach of dynamic modeling—and particularly agent-based modeling and variants—can play in stimulating insights into the character of and interventions to alleviate health disparities. We examine the relationship between dynamic models and elements of Big Data—the rapidly rising flood of electronically sourced data that is available from diverse sources, such as sensors incorporated in consumer electronic devices or embedded in building control systems or the environment, electronic communications such as text messaging (SMS); and email or social media platforms such as Twitter, blogs, Facebook, and point-of-sale data. This chapter provides an overview of the relationship between Big Data and dynamic models, and provides an agent-based case study to further illustrate the opportunities for insight provided by this fusion of methods.

The Rise of Big Data

Over the past three decades, society's communications and behaviors have increasingly taken place through, or have been mediated by, information technology. Early processes during this time reflected contact with discrete and fragmented computational and communications technologies, such as personal computers, phone networks and their associated technologies, and niche communities using bulletin board systems and other online resources. The advent of the World Wide Web in the early 1990s and its widespread adoption in the developed world in the mid-to-late 1990s supported electronic presence and communication for hundreds of millions of people. The availability and subsequent immersion in these technologies rose rapidly throughout the world during the first decade of the new millennium. However, contact with such technologies was most commonly limited to times in which active computer use was taking place.

GROWING INEQUALITY

The 1990s also saw the rise of pervasive and increasingly interconnected information technology systems in diverse environments, including the health care arena. There was also a new push toward using data collected for operational reasons, such as billing information or prescriptions filled, for decision-making insight. Organizations increasingly united databases that had been fragmented in different regions into data warehouses, enterprise resource planning systems, and supplier interfaces. Governments at the municipal and federal levels increasingly utilized electronic infrastructure for monitoring traffic, measuring pollutant levels, quantifying transportation system use, and collecting data on the population level.

Outside of institutional environments, the widespread appearance of mobile technologies at the end of the twentieth century and early twenty-first century brought about a sea change in individual uses of technology. Personal digital assistants and cell phones that permitted ongoing interaction between the personal, communication, and digital worlds supported increasing rates of online use. The advent of smart phones in the 2000s supported a new level of online presence, which follows up individuals through their lives. As an exceptionally popular class of mobile technologies, smart phones are of particular note because they allow ongoing online location-aware presence through services such as Facebook, Foursquare, and other apps and facilitate communication via social media, blogs, and customizable feeds on services such as Twitter, Pinterest, and Tumblr. These service and communication tools naturally gave rise to the availability of, and automatic accessibility to, dramatically enlarged amounts of information regarding health and health-related behavior. The messages themselves, as well as Facebook status updates, tweets, and blog and Tumblr posts, communicate additional information on relationship dynamics, feelings and attitudes, potential symptoms of illness, sentiments toward current events, and more.

Smart phones are also distinguished by their capacity to serve as formidable tools for collecting information regarding health behavior, primarily via smart phone apps. All the functions of smart phones that users value, such as the capacity to connect to Wi-Fi, provide location coordinates, take pictures, record videos, and so on, are made possible by a variety of sensors built into phones. Such sensors can be repurposed to capture aspects of health behavior that are traditionally burdensome to measure, such as location, physical activity, and communications behavior. Smart phones can also analyze data and collect information from diverse, third-party sensors, such as watches that measure heart rates, heart-rate variability, and galvanic skin response.

In addition, smart phones can issue small questionnaires termed "ecological momentary assessments." These survey instruments—which can be triggered by context such as location or sedentary activity or triggered at fixed or random times—can readily sample a person's immediate situation via self-report, such as enquiring about barriers to physical activity after sensing long bouts of sedentary behavior, or motivations for coming to certain spaces. Smartphones can also be used for "crowdsourcing"—the proactive reporting of information volunteered by participants. For instance, via buttons or other elements in an app, device holders can report information of as diverse as subclinical symptoms, food being ingested (with photos or via food diary apps), cravings, ideation, or the self-administration of medicine or use of medical devices. All these features provide new and exciting data sources that can provide new insights into health.

Hallmarks of Big Data

A tremendous amount of electronically sourced data is currently available to inform health insights. The characteristics of this electronically sourced data—the digital evidence known as Big Data—can be described in general terms as follows.

Volume: The data derived from electronic data sources are often voluminous. As an example, consider the iEpi[1] system, a flexible epidemiologic monitoring system that can collect study-specific sensor, ecological momentary assessment responses and crowdsourced data from apps on iPhones and Android smart phones. iEpi commonly records between 20 and 100 MB per day of data per participant, depending on the study.

Velocity: Velocity refers to the data arriving with high temporal resolution. For example, in the iEpi system (and the earlier and more study-specific "Flunet" system, built around wireless sensors), data on factors such as contact patterns and locations were collected in intervals at minute-level resolution.[2,3]

Veracity: The data gained through mobile devices are often more reliable than those secured by traditional instruments. In some cases, this reflects the fact that mobile data are drawn from physical measurements. Often such measurements, particularly when taken in combination, are more objective and truthful quantifications of physical activity, sedentary behavior, and social and physical environment than self-reported measurements. However, enhanced veracity not only applies to sensor data, but also reflects that self-reports by phone are often delivered more closely to the times or events of interest (the meal that was eaten, or the self-administration of medicine, for example), and in turn are less likely to be affected by recall bias. The elevated veracity associated with such data also reflects the key ability to "triangulate" from multiple lines of evidence (see below), each ambiguous, but collectively far less so.

Variety. The data from multiple sensors, surveys and crowdsourced data are cross-linked, such that the analysis of behavior over time can be studied on the basis of temporally aligned evidence from multiple sensors and self-reporting mechanisms. The capacity to engage in such triangulation often greatly sharpens the insights that can be secured from the data.

By themselves, any of these four characteristics might seem modest; their collective implications are profound in the context of health. The sheer volume and diversity of evidence, taken together with its intensively longitudinal character and greater capacity for accurate management of many behaviors, substantially elevates the quality of the health-behavior evidence base.

Big Data Enhances Simulation Modeling

Big Data can be exceptionally valuable when used in conjunction with simulation models: it can greatly inform and enhance the value of simulation modeling, while simulation modeling synergistically enhances the value of Big Data.

Simulation models can serve as powerful learning tools, or (more specifically) "learning prostheses." By helping us to reason consistently about the implications of our assumptions, simulations models—when combined with evidence—can serve as powerful tools to aid learning more deeply, quickly and robustly. Even when used in a stylized fashion, with little data available, models can confer great insights, as the case study presented here demonstrates. The designation of such models as "learning prostheses" reflects the fact that, like medical prosthesis, they help enhance our ability to function by compensating for our limitations—in this case, our ability to think with clarity and consistency through the quantitative implications of our assumptions.

However, stakeholders frequently pursue models in order to obtain quantitative results, such as understanding detailed trade-offs between proposed policies. The reliable use of models to secure such quantitative trade-offs requires considerable data. While dynamic models serve as operationalizations of theory, a common limitation of such models is that the level of detail articulated in the model frequently outstrips the empirical evidence available to inform the proposed theory. This gap can be particularly acute for components of health behavior in which traditional methods of data collection are burdensome, unreliable, or impossible. Examples of such health behaviors include nutritional intake, contact patterns, mobility and physical activity.

In such situations, mobile-based data collection—including sensor data, ecological momentary assessment, or crowdsourcing—may be able to confer the greatest advantages. "Microdata" collected from mobile devices and the detail inferred from such data can help to ground a model in empirical data, which is often longitudinal and at fine time scales. Examples of relevance for the model considered below would include visitation to food vendors and food consumption many times a day (with supporting minute-level sensor data helping to flag likely such visits and occurrences of food consumption, to trigger questionnaires), self-reports of illness via the device, EMA-based statements of risk perception. For studies of communicable disease or social and environmental influence on norms data utilized in the modeling might include minute-level contact patterns, and location. For studies seeking to understand effects of housing vouchers on obesity, the data might include measures drawn from minute-level data on physical activity and sedentary behavior (as measured via accelerometry), and location (to capture exposure to the built environment and visit to markets, convenience stores and other food vendors), and (several times during each day) reports of nutritional intake via the smart phone and documented by images from the smart phone camera, statements of perceptions of safety and barriers to physical activity.

These types of data can be particularly valuable for individual-based models (which follow the trajectories of individual agents) in myriad ways that cross-sectional data would not. Mobile data can provide evidence regarding the dynamic interactions of diverse factors (such as location, social context, sedentary behavior, vehicular use, and communications behavior) over time, with particularly powerful potential for informing theories about such processes. Such variety can be helpful for validating models. In this approach, some evidence (e.g., time series for particular intervals) can be temporarily put aside when parameterizing and calibrating a model. In a step known as cross-validation, such evidence can then be compared against the resulting model predictions, lending additional veracity and weight to the evidence.

Mobile data collection can be linked with models in several ways, including:

- Simulation model calibration: Computational statistical methods, such as the particle filtering (sequential Monte Carlo methods) and particle Markov Chain Monte Carlo (MCMC) methods, may make use of incoming empirical data that recurrently re-grounds the model in new observations.

- Parameter estimation: Parameters such as the hazard rates associated with state transitions (such as for vehicular use or travel outside) or the frequencies of particular events (such as tobacco use, blood sugar testing, and suicidal ideation) can be estimated.

- Dynamic hypotheses: Microdata can help to formulate dynamic hypotheses that are interpreted within model structure. In the absence of other empirical data to ground the model, such microdata can be very helpful in generating the hypotheses operationalized in the model.

Electronically sourced data can also play a critical role in validating models. Specifically, models can be used to anticipate the results of counter factual interventions (or emergent natural experiments, such as the introduction of a new regulatory regime or economic crisis) with the results then tested against evidence gathered empirically. By virtue of its longitudinal character, high temporal resolution, and cross-linked variety, electronically gathered data can help us to confirm the model's anticipated impacts across multiple pathways simultaneously.

This evidence base drawn from mobile data can aid learning in two key ways. First, such mobile data can shed light on how individual behavior and exposures are altered by an intervention, for example by identifying which particular causal pathways were successfully changed, and which were not—for example, identifying a case in which an intervention designed to reduce obesity successfully elevates moderate to vigorous physical activity, but fails to alter sedentary behavior in the intervention group, or where a housing voucher program enhances the quality of foods purchased and eaten, but fails to alter the level of use of recreational facilities in the voucher recipients. Such learning can foster ideas for how to improve the effectiveness of interventions. Second, by checking dynamics anticipated from running a model, mobile data can aid in model-based learning, by identifying inconsistencies between the implications of the computational model (and thus typically the underlying mental models) and the empirical data. This often plays out by more quickly identifying model omissions, inaccuracies, and oversimplifications. Identifying such problems does not represent a failure of the model, but rather demonstrates the success of the modeling process.

Simulation Modeling Enhances Big Data

The simulation model can greatly enhance the value and significance of electronically sourced data. By grounding causal models—those that operationally capture a theory of the system—in understanding of human behavioral patterns, we can anticipate future trends in ways that would not be possible with collected data alone. By articulating the posited causal structure of a system, models can help inform reasoning about the implications of counterfactuals (situations that have not yet been observed, such as outcomes of a novel intervention being considered) in ways that are not possible using observed associations and relationships alone. Simulation models add value to the data collected.

Simulation models can also aid in formulating and testing theory regarding the processes underlying observed patterns. For example, electronically sourced evidence could suggest unexpected temporal patterns linking sedentary behavior and physical activity, or the use of e-cigarettes and traditional tobacco use. On its own terms, such evidence provides no direct indication of the causal structure driving such patterns. A simulation model can aid in reasoning about the consistency of theories and observed evidence.

For elements of the collected data that occur with lower temporal resolution, a simulation model capturing a theory of the underlying processes can further allow for "filling in the gaps" in the observed data. Models can also help identify the duration and frequency of sampling required to arrive at reliable inferences.[2]

While they can confer great insights, electronically mediated data do have limitations. For example, regardless of its veracity, such data can exhibit substantial "noise" or random variability. In the classic case of data collected from global positioning systems (GPSs), even in cases of excellent GPS reception, the data stream can exhibit considerable variability (with standard deviations of 10 or 15 meters) due to atmospheric variability and other factors. Dynamic models aid in conditioning and filtering the measured data by limiting the effects of sensor noise and capturing temporal regularities. Machine learning approaches such as the particle filter and particle MCMC that recurrently reground a model state and/or parameters based on observations can be particularly powerful, helping compensate for limitations in both incoming data and the model.

Reflecting the synergy between dynamic models and electronically sourced data at both the high and low levels, simulation models can not only benefit from electronically sourced data, but can also enhance the value and utility of such data.

Case Study: Models, Big Data, and Foodborne Illness

The increased interest in crowdsourcing and mobile technology has resulted in novel research that complements existing public health surveillance. For example, in the case of foodborne illness, where traditionally collected data such as food surveys are prone to recall bias, it can be difficult to get a true sense of the number of people affected by an outbreak or in a particular year. Data on the full extent of foodborne illness are incomplete because many cases are so mild and those affected do not seek medical treatment; and of those who do, cases are not always confirmed through laboratory testing and reported to the appropriate health department.[4,5] Another uncertainty is attributing diseases to specific foods.[6] However, eating in restaurants is a well-established risk factor for foodborne illness.[7]

Although many cases are mild, the impacts of foodborne illness are serious. Each year, there are an estimated 47.8 million foodborne illnesses in the United States, resulting in 127,839 hospitalizations and 3,037 deaths, but the estimates are based on rough extrapolations. The vast majority of these cases (80 percent) are caused by unspecified agents.[8] In similarly rough estimates, the Public Health Agency of Canada estimates that approximately 4 million people, or one in eight Canadians, become sick each year.[9] The uncertainty associated with foodborne illness and estimating its associated costs impede the development of effective interventions and prevention policies. New methods have the potential to change that.

In applying mobile technology and crowdsourcing to the study of foodborne illness, researchers have linked tweets to GPS tags from mobile phones indicating restaurants, and then correlated the data with health department inspections.[10] Another project used reviews on the website Yelp to find unreported cases where customers experienced foodborne illness in New York City. In partnership with the New York Department of Health and Mental Hygiene, Yelp reviews were triangulated with 311 reports on restaurants, and, in some cases, further investigation was initiated. Three outbreaks were identified that had not previously been reported.[11] Although this study was successful, the authors also noted that it was extremely labor intensive with the potential to overwhelm local health departments.

In 2014, IBM built a system designed to help food retailers and public-health officials detect likely sources of food contamination to assist with foodborne illness investigations. The system uses the location of supermarket food items sold each week to identify likely sources for an outbreak, using as few as 10 case reports. By integrating existing retail and public-health data, investigators can see maps, distributions of potential foods, clinical cases, and lab reports. Additional reports feed into an algorithm, which predicts the probability that suspected food products causing an illness outbreak.[12]

Although mobile health technology is a growing field with numerous applications for gathering health data, designing such research studies is time-consuming, expensive, and difficult. To avoid these pitfalls, we sought to use an agent-based model, a simulation methodology that allows for many interacting agents to reveal emergent properties of systems,[13] to investigate the potential for the crowdsourcing of study design and develop a proof of concept. Agent-based modeling has grown in popularity in the social and health sciences for its ability to simulate outcomes and test alternative scenarios. We employed an agent-based model to evaluate the use of mobile technology to crowdsource data on foodborne illness and evaluate the impact of a possible intervention that would leverage this technology.

Health Disparities and Foodborne Illness

Although data on foodborne illness are incomplete due to the limitations of existing surveillance methods, some evidence suggests that low-income and minority populations experience elevated risk of contracting foodborne disease. The reasons are multifaceted and underexplored, but they are believed to be related to food consumption patterns, food-handling behaviors, and knowledge gaps around safe food-handling at home, and different patterns of access to supermarkets and restaurants.[14] For the purposes of this case study, we chose to focus on the latter.

In many low-socioeconomic-status neighborhoods, fast food and take-out restaurants are more readily available, while limited access to supermarkets (food deserts) leaves residents with fewer options.

Eating at restaurants is a risk factor for contracting a foodborne disease.[7] Minority populations may also disproportionately rely on independent ethnic restaurants. Research conducted on independent ethnic, chain ethnic, independent non-ethnic, and chain non-ethnic restaurants in Kansas showed that independent ethnic restaurants had more critical and noncritical violations than the other three restaurant types.[15] Although inspection results do not track perfectly to outbreak risk, these results reveal a potential risk factor. Quinlan[14] noted the absence of investigation into the relative safety of food services in food deserts compared with food environments characteristic of higher income populations. Given that eating at restaurants is a risk factor for contracting foodborne disease, and that those living in food deserts rely more heavily on food-service restaurants, this area clearly calls for further exploration.

Foodborne illness risk may also affect low-income and minority populations in more subtle ways. Lund and O'Brien[16] state that between 15 and 20 percent the general population are more susceptible to foodborne illness. Health conditions that can make people more susceptible include diabetes, liver, and kidney disease, excess iron in the blood, immune conditions, malnutrition, and pregnancy. Behavioral risk factors such as tobacco use and heavy alcohol consumption are also known to adversely affect immune system function. Those undergoing cancer treatment with immune-suppressing drugs or radiation, as well as the very old and the very young, are also more likely to contract a foodborne disease. Furthermore, some minority populations are at greater risk for immune-suppressing chronic diseases such as diabetes; people of low SES are more likely to die from diabetes,[17] and there is a disproportionate burden associated with behavioral risk factors within lower-socioeconomic-status populations. As a result, these interconnected risk factors contribute to the disproportionate effect of foodborne illness on minority and low-income groups. Differences in health care-seeking behaviors may also have an impact on rates of foodborne illness in specific populations.

Foodborne illness, and its differential effects on low SES and minority populations, could be more thoroughly investigated using electronically sourced data and agent-based models. Mobile technologies—which now enjoy widespread and heavy use among people of low SES—could be used to collect data on factors related to foodborne illness risk, including, for example, occurrences of gastrointestinal illness, location data that pinpoints when and where people visit food service outlets, and point-of-sale data. These technologies could also allow researchers to investigate relationships between behaviors and eating patterns related to smoking, shift work, stress, exercise, and more. We believe these technologies could be invaluable for identifying new relationships and risk factors related to foodborne disease, many of which could yield insights into the likely disproportionate effect of foodborne illness on minority and low-income populations.

Methods

The purpose of the agent-based model[1] that we describe here is to explore the possibilities for using Big Data mobile technologies to control foodborne illness. We investigated the possible outcomes of equipping a small proportion of the population, referred to as sentinels, with a mobile technology that allows them to collect data on restaurants that they visit, report subclinical signs of foodborne illness, and transmit this information to public health inspectors in the event of an outbreak. The outcomes that we investigated were health impacts on individuals and the length of public health investigations.

The model contains three entities: consumers, restaurants, and an inspector. The consumers have two important state variables: (1) whether or not they are ill, and if they are, whether they are experiencing either mild-to-moderate or severe symptoms; and (2) whether or not they are sentinels. Consumers also have parameters that govern how frequently they eat in restaurants and whether or not they practice good food-handling habits when cooking at home. Restaurants may either be in a contaminated or uncontaminated state; one restaurant is contaminated at the model's initialization. The inspector begins in the routine inspection state, and if an outbreak occurs, changes its inspection strategy to focus on the restaurants most frequently reported as having been visited by ill consumers.

---

1   View this model in the CoMSES Model Library: https://www.openabm.org/model/4325/version/1/view

The model was implemented in AnyLogic (version 6.9.0). Model time is continuous and measured in days, and there is no fixed stop time; the model stops when the inspector finds the contaminated restaurant. The model is does not depend on spatial relationships, but the implementation in AnyLogic used some spatial elements to improve understanding and allow for easier communication and debugging. The following processes occur continuously, not sequentially.

Inspections: The inspector conducts routine inspections by first forming a collection of all restaurants, ordered randomly. The inspector goes through the list in a round-robin fashion, inspecting one restaurant per day. The inspector has a 50 percent chance of correctly identifying a contaminated restaurant; this estimate is meant to reflect the fact that inspectors may inspect a restaurant when it is less busy and sloppy errors in food handling may be less likely to occur; or when staff members who are more safety conscious may be working and violations do not happen to be visible. A contaminated restaurant will comply with routine inspection 50 percent of the time. If the inspector correctly identifies the affected restaurant during a routine inspection, and if the restaurant complies with the inspector, the model realization ends. No empirical data was available in this area; these estimates were informed through discussion with an expert in the field and are used for illustration purposes.

Consumer behavior: Consumers eat once per day either at home or at a restaurant. The likelihood of a consumer becoming ill depends on where they are eating; if they are eating at home, their likelihood of becoming ill depends on whether they practice safe food-handling behaviors, and if they are eating at a restaurant it depends on whether they have been to the contaminated restaurant in the model. The risks associated with food-handling practices were derived from empirical data; for further details, please see the calculations summarized in the appendix.

Illnesses: Once a consumer has been exposed to a pathogen, either in the home or in a restaurant, the consumer will transition from the healthy state to the illness exposure state, where they remain for one day in model time. Next, the consumer either experiences mild-to-moderate or severe symptoms. Symptoms severe enough to warrant a visit to the doctor and subsequent reporting to public health authorities were assumed to occur in about 0.5 percent of cases and last for five days. Mild to moderate cases, which were not reported to a physician and hence were unrecognized by public health authorities, were assumed to last for two days.

Outbreaks: Two severe cases trigger an outbreak investigation. If an outbreak is declared, the severely ill consumers update a list of visited restaurants. Recollection is treated as imperfect, as consumers have a certain chance per day of forgetting restaurant locations that they have visited, and they are more likely to forget restaurant visits, which occurred more distantly in the past. The consumers then pass their list of visited restaurants to the inspector, who maintains a count of reports originating in each restaurant. Once an outbreak has been triggered, and on an ongoing basis until the contaminated restaurant is identified, the inspector will seek to visit the restaurant with the highest cumulative count of reports that has not yet been visited as part of the outbreak investigation. This process continues until the inspector correctly identifies the contaminated restaurant, which ends the model realization. During an outbreak investigation, the model treats the inspector as capable of recognizing the contaminated restaurant with perfect sensitivity and specificity; the elements of uncertainty in identification and compliance that are present in routine inspections are not used in outbreak investigations, because inspectors have more information to guide their investigation and could shut down the affected restaurant.

Sentinels: Sentinel consumers behave in accordance with all of the above consumer processes, with minor changes depending on the scenario. The first scenario involves sentinels whose mobile devices track which restaurants have been visited, allowing them to report with greater accuracy than consumers who must remember where they have been, and sentinels report mild-to-moderate symptoms of foodborne disease. In the second scenario, sentinels report mild-to-moderate symptoms and report which restaurants they have visited with the same imperfect memory as non-sentinel consumers once an outbreak has been triggered. In both of these scenarios, four sentinels reporting any symptoms, or two severe cases, will trigger an outbreak. In the third scenario, sentinels do not report symptoms; however, if they experience mild-to-moderate illness, they provide visited restaurant data to the inspector once two severe cases have been reported.

Outbreak indicators: An output file is created that keeps track of the time of the first severe case, the time between the first severe case and the inspector beginning an outbreak investigation, the length of the investigation, the count of severe illnesses, the count of mild-to-moderate illnesses, the number of sentinel consumers who experienced mild-to-moderate illness, the number of consumers who become sick eating at home, the number of consumers who become sick from eating at restaurants, the total time length of the simulation, and the number of routine inspections.

Model initialization: The model is initialized with 5,000 consumers and 100 restaurants, one of which is contaminated. There is one inspector in the model. Upon model initialization, consumers are placed in categories based on frequency of eating in restaurants: 6.7 percent of consumers eat out daily, 30.9 percent three times a week, 23 percent once a week,[18] and the remaining 39.4 percent of consumers visit a restaurant once every two weeks. Although this survey data did not explicitly consider the reasons why consumers were accessing restaurants at that frequency, given that low-income populations with less access to supermarkets eat at food service facilities more frequently, this parameter likely reflects income disparity. Each consumer selects a subset of 10 restaurants with uniform probability to form their list of possible restaurants to visit. Consumers are also randomly assigned to either practice good or poor hygiene while cooking at home: 20 percent practice good food-handling habits, and 80 percent do not. Studies observing food safety practices while preparing meals in the home[19,20] were used to inform this aspect of the model; however, the data reported by these studies is quite nuanced, so the 80-to-20 percent figure is an abstraction. The per-day hazard of illness from eating a home meal prepared with good food safety practices, which is based on empirical data, is approximately 0.00015.[2] We conducted 1,000 realizations with no sentinels (baseline), and then 1 percent, 2 percent, and 4 percent sentinels for each of the three scenarios.

Analysis: The results from the model were analyzed in R (version 2.15.1). The Kruskal-Wallis rank sum test was used to compare the results within each scenario with 1 percent of the population acting as sentinels, 2 percent, and 4 percent, to the baseline (tables 1–3), as well as the results between scenarios with the same percentages of the population as sentinels (table 4). Next, post-hoc analysis using pairwise Mann-Whitney-Wilcoxon tests was completed, using the Holm correction to account for multiple comparisons. Unless otherwise stated, the pairwise analysis results are statistically significant ($p < 0.001$).

---

2   See the Appendix for details.

Table 1

Statistical Results for Scenario One, for Baseline, 1%, 2% and 4% Sentinels

| | Scenario 1: Sentinels Report Subclinical Symptoms and Restaurant Visits | | | | | | | | |
| | Baseline | | 1% Sentinels | | 2% Sentinels | | 4% Sentinels | | KW Test |
	Mean	SD	Mean	SD	Mean	SD	Mean	SD	P Value
Length of investigation	18.59	51.91	10.21	34.37	10.85	28.35	6.42	15.77	<0.001
Count clinical illnesses	1.26	1.02	0.97	0.92	0.78	0.86	0.49	0.70	<0.001
Count subclinical illnesses	249.20	205.38	199.01	138.78	155.42	100.40	92.67	53.21	<0.001
Count sentinel subclinical	0	0	1.97	1.62	2.92	1.70	3.61	1.51	<0.001
Number of Routine Inspections	211.90	177.05	174.07	119.21	133.29	84.35	79.98	45.2	<0.001

Findings

Scenario one: Where sentinels report both mild or moderate symptoms and visited restaurants, the total number of sick consumers declines as the percentage of sentinels increases. The length of time required to identify the affected restaurant in an outbreak investigation also decreases as sentinels are added, and the variability is substantially reduced. However, the Mann-Whitney-Wilcoxon test showed no effect on length of increasing the amount of sentinels from 2 percent to 4 percent ($p = 0.34$) (table 1).

A related measure, the overall length of time that passes until the model run ends, also declines; because clinical cases are rare, relying on a second clinical case in order to trigger an outbreak results in longer model run times, which also means that there is more time for a greater number of consumers to become ill. When sentinels can report mild or moderate symptoms, the outbreak investigation occurs earlier and is completed more quickly because inspectors have access to additional information on visited restaurants (figure 1).

Scenario two: In scenario two, where sentinels report mild or moderate symptoms, the total number of sick consumers decreases as sentinels are added although the decrease is not as substantial as in scenario one. The difference between the baseline and having 1 percent sentinels was significant for the number of consumers who became ill from home cooking ($p = 0.023$), ill from eating at restaurants ($p = 0.031$), and the overall length of time of the model ($p = 0.02$). The most interesting result from this scenario was that the length of outbreak investigation for all sentinel percentages was greater than for the baseline ($p < 0.001$).

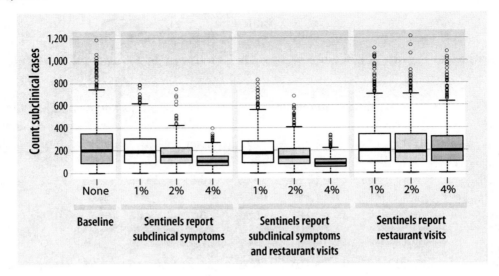

Figure 1. Subclinical cases, all scenarios

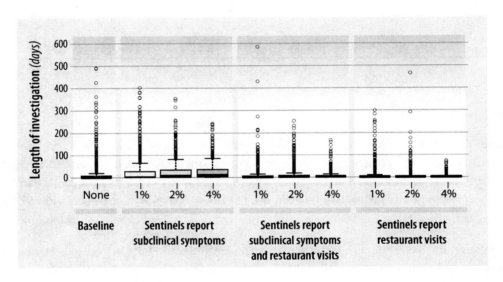

Figure 2. Length of investigation, all scenarios

Scenario three: In scenario three, where sentinels only report restaurant visits, the number of cases of foodborne illness was not substantially reduced (table 2). Generally, there were few statistically significant differences between the baseline and sentinels. The difference between the baseline and 1 percent sentinels for the length of investigation was significant ($p = 0.0013$), but the difference between 2 percent and 4 percent sentinels was not statistically significant ($p = 0.079$). Overall, the outbreak investigations in this scenario were the shortest of all three scenarios (figure 2). The difference between the baseline and 1 percent sentinels was statistically significant ($p = 0.02$) for the length of time from the beginning of the model when a pathogen first appears until the outbreak investigation completes.

Table 2

Statistical Results for Scenario Two, for Baseline, 1%, 2% and 4% Sentinels

	Scenario 2: Sentinels Report Subclinical Symptoms								
	Baseline		1% Sentinels		2% Sentinels		4% Sentinels		KW Test
	Mean	SD	Mean	SD	Mean	SD	Mean	SD	P Value
Length of investigation	18.59	51.91	27.79	57.62	26.85	45.70	25.16	36.91	< 0.001
Count clinical illnesses	1.26	1.02	10.02	1.01	0.84	0.93	0.56	0.77	< 0.001
Count subclinical illnesses	249.20	205.38	214.38	153.19	164.8	102.74	112.55	63.91	< 0.001
Count sentinel subclinical	0	0	2.17	1.82	3.30	2.07	4.40	2.31	< 0.001
Number of routine inspections	211.90	177.05	170.48	119.59	126.47	77.87	80.11	45.12	< 0.001

Table 3

Statistical Results for Scenario Three, for Baseline, 1%, 2% and 4% Sentinels

	Scenario 3: Sentinels Report Restaurant Visits								
	Baseline		1% Sentinels		2% Sentinels		4% Sentinels		KW Test
	Mean	SD	Mean	SD	Mean	SD	Mean	SD	P Value
Length of investigation	18.59	51.91	9.06	30.08	5.70	24.04	1.97	6.90	< 0.001
Count clinical illnesses	1.26	1.022	1.17	0.97	1.17	0.93	1.15	0.91	0.16
Count subclinical illnesses	249.20	205.38	245.56	196.80	236.41	188.72	234.57	185.80	0.66
Count sentinel subclinical	0	0	2.49	2.54	4.75	4.56	9.27	8.03	< 0.001
Number of routine inspections	211.90	177.05	217.70	178.63	212.6	171.88	214.44	169.70	0.74

The results from scenario one show the greatest reductions in the number of sick consumers in both severe and mild cases (figure 1). However, this scenario only performs marginally better than scenario two; the difference between these two scenarios for the number of mild illnesses was not statistically significant, with 1 percent sentinels ($p = 0.046$), but was significant with 2 percent sentinels ($p = 0.021$) and 4 percent sentinels ($p < 0.001$). Overall, these two scenarios performed comparably (table 4).

Table 4

Kruskal–Wallis Test Results for all Scenarios

	1% Sentinels		2% Sentinels		4% Sentinels	
	Kruskal–Wallis test		Kruskal–Wallis test		Kruskal–Wallis test	
	Chi-sq (2DF)	P Value	Chi-sq (2DF)	P Value	Chi-sq (2 DF)	P Value
Length of investigation (days)	78.31	<0.001	305.1	<0.001	715.29	<0.001
Count clinical illnesses	26.08	<0.001	111.08	<0.001	345.27	<0.001
Count subclinical illnesses	15.42	<0.001	85.13	<0.001	427.56	<0.001
Count sentinel subclinical	6.13	<0.05	60.44	<0.001	412.97	<0.001
Number of routine inspections	23.64	<0.001	132.63	<0.001	601.43	<0.001

Implications

This chapter has provided a glimpse of the complex and multifaceted relationship between simulation modeling and Big Data. These approaches support each other and support decision-making and learning more quickly, deeply and reliably from evidence. We have introduced a model that is used to evaluate the possible health benefits from using Big Data in the area of foodborne illness.

This case study model provides a proof of concept for using mobile technology to enhance foodborne illness surveillance. We have shown that even a small proportion of the population serving as sentinels can substantially reduce the number of illnesses present in the population, pointing to the technology's feasibility.

The model has generated three important insights. First, having sentinels report visited restaurants, without reporting subclinical symptoms to trigger the identification of an outbreak, does not substantially reduce the number of illnesses. We can infer that it is not helpful for the inspector to only receive restaurant reports from sentinels; early reports of milder symptoms of foodborne illness that can trigger an outbreak are needed for the intervention to have an effect.

Second, the model illuminates Peter Drucker's quote, "What gets measured, gets managed," as it applies to public health policy. Because the model assumes perfect reporting of subclinical cases, the length of investigation is longer when sentinels only report subclinical symptoms, but fewer people are ill overall. However, if a health department was to deploy this technology and authorities were unaware or unconvinced of the reduction in illnesses—in part because many of these subclinical cases are unknown to begin with—they may think that the technology is actually making things worse because of the apparent adverse effect on the duration of outbreak investigations.

Third, the model shows that adding sentinels can result in more stable and predictable levels of illness within the population, which is likely to be more easily managed by the public health system. Wide and unpredictable swings in outcomes can be taxing on resources and contribute to negative perceptions of public health and food safety.

Crowdsourcing offers interesting possibilities for public involvement in public health.[1,10,11,21] Crowdsourcing using mobile technology may be particularly fruitful for studying populations, and individual habits and experiences, such as the relationship between low SES and foodborne illness.

There some limitations to this work, plus two key assumptions for future research. In the model, we have assumed that sentinel consumers carry the device and use it consistently all of the time, and that there is always one contaminated restaurant in the model. While past studies with similar technology have shown less-than-perfect compliance,[1] it is possible that the true number of sentinels required to show an effect in a pilot study might need to be slightly higher, to account for less than perfect compliance and a fuzzier definition of a contaminated restaurant.[3] However, our own work (not presented here) has demonstrated exceptional degrees of participant reporting of illness and eating with financial compensation. Implementation of this work would need to be conducted in close collaboration with local health departments to ensure that their needs are met and that the incoming data does not overburden staff. Future research should take SES and the type of restaurant into account, to reflect food consumption patterns by populations of interest.

The main advantage of the model presented here is that it provides a starting point for study design. To fully synthesize simulation with novel mobile technology, we would use the data resulting from a pilot study deploying mobile technology to collect reports of foodborne illness symptoms to further refine and restructure the model's assumptions. This is especially relevant for foodborne illness because data is uncertain, in part due to under-reporting, and many argue that interventions can prevent some cases of foodborne disease.[4-6] Mobile technologies also provide a new way of focusing research on foodborne illness related to restaurant and other food vendor use in low socioeconomic areas as compared to high socioeconomic areas, something which has not been extensively researched to date, but where there are reasons to believe that the burden is significantly higher. Mobile technologies offer a fruitful, effective and efficient way to collect more information about populations of interest and their different experiences with foodborne illness and restaurant use. The techniques described offer new ways of using data models to cover gaps in other research methods. By linking mobile technologies and models in a fundamental way, we can provide better evidence to inform decision-making in public health.

---

3   The percentage of sentinels used in the model could be taken as indicating the fraction of reliably compliant individuals; however, the model does not provide assistance with determining how many sentinels would need to be recruited in order to achieve this percentage.

References

1. Hashemian M, Knowles D, Calver J, et al. iEpi: an end-to-end solution for collecting, conditioning and utilizing epidemiologically relevant data. In: *Proceedings of the 2nd ACM International Workshop on Pervasive Wireless Healthcare*. Hilton Head, South Carolina; 2012:3–8.

2. Hashemian M, Qian W, Stanley KG, Osgood ND. Temporal aggregation impacts on epidemiological simulations employing microcontact data. *BMC Med Inform Decis Mak.* 2012;12:132.

3. Hashemian M, Stanley K, Osgood N. Leveraging H1N1 infection transmission modeling with proximity micro-data. *BMC Med Inform Decis Mak.* 2012;12:36.

4. Buzby JC, Roberts T. The economics of enteric infections: human foodborne disease costs. *Gastroenterology.* 2009;136:1851–1862.

5. Schlundt J. New directions in foodborne disease prevention. *Int J Food Microbiol.* 2002;78:3–17.

6. Batz MB, Doyle MP, Morris JG, et al. Attributing illness to food. *Emerg Infect Dis.* 2005;11(7):993–999.

7. Jones TF, Angulo FJ. Eating in restaurants: a risk factor for foodborne disease? *Clin Infect Dis.* 2006;43(10):1324–1328.

8. Centers for Disease Control and Prevention (CDC). 2011 Estimates: Findings. CDC Estimates of Foodborne Illness in the United States. http://www.cdc.gov/foodborneburden/2011-foodborne-estimates.html. Updated January 8, 2014. Accessed June 2, 2014.

9. Public Health Agency of Canada. Estimates of Food-borne Illness in Canada. http://www.phac-aspc.gc.ca/efwd-emoha/efbi-emoa-eng.php. Published May 9, 2013. Accessed May 17, 2013.

10. Sadilek A, Brennan S, Kautz H, Silenzio V. nEmesis: Which restaurants should you avoid today? In: *Proceedings of the First AAAI Conference on Human Computation and Crowdsourcing*. Palm Springs, CA: 2013:138–146.

11. Harrison C, Jorder M, Stern H, et al. Using Online Reviews by Restaurant Patrons to *Identify Unreported Cases of Foodborne Illness - New York City, 2012–2013*. Centers for Disease Control and Prevention; 2014:441–445.

12. IBM. IBM Research Breakthrough Helps Public Health Officials Improve Food Safety. IBM News Releases. https://www-03.ibm.com/press/us/en/pressrelease/44295.wss. Published July 3, 2014. Accessed July 8, 2014.

13. Jones GT. Agent-based modeling: use with necessary caution. *Am J Public Health.* 2007;97(5):780–781.

14. Quinlan J. Foodborne illness incidence rates and food safety risks for populations of low socioeconomic status and minority race/ethnicity: a review of the literature. *Int J Environ Res Public Health.* 2013;10(8):3634–3652.

15. Roberts K, Kwon J, Shanklin C, Liu P, Yen W. Food safety practices lacking in independent ethnic restaurants. *J Cul Sci Tech.* 2011;9:1–16.

16. Lund BM, O'Brien SJ. The occurrence and prevention of foodborne disease in vulnerable people. *Foodborne Pathog Dis.* 2011;8(9):961–973.

17. Saydah S, Lochner K. Socioeconomic status and risk of diabetes-related mortality in the U.S. *Public Health Rep.* 2010;125(3):377–388.

18. Canadian Restaurant and Foodservices Association. *Canada's Restaurant Industry: Putting Jobs and Economic Growth on the Menu.* 2010. http://www.crfa.ca/pdf/ipsos_report.pdf.

19. Redmond EC, Griffith CJ, Slader J, Humphrey TJ. Microbiological and observational analysis of cross contamination risks during domestic food preparation. *Br Food J.* 2004;106(8):581–592.

20. Anderson JB, Shuster TA, Hansen KE, Levy AS, Volk A. A camera's view of consumers food-handling behaviors. *J Am Diet Assoc.* 2004;104(2):186–191.

21. Paul MJ, Dredze M. You are what you tweet: analyzing Twitter for public health. In: *Proceedings of the Fifth International AAAI Conference on Weblogs and Social Media.* Barcelona, Spain: AAAI Press; 2011:265–272.

22. Smith DeWaal C, Glassman M. *Outbreak Alert! 2014: A Review of Foodborne Illness in America from 2002–2011.* Washington, DC: Center for Science in the Public Interest; 2014:1–15. http://cspinet.org/reports/outbreak-alert2014.pdf.

APPENDIX: SUPPLEMENTAL MATERIAL

The following formula introduces forgetfulness over time regarding the location of a meal occurring at time t_{meal}, where U(a,b) denotes a uniform continuous distribution sampling from the interval (a, b], and t denotes the current time, and both t and t_{meal} are measured in days. By using a uniform distribution, there is a hazard rate between 0.05 and 0.20 probability per day of the consumer forgetting to recall the location of a meal:

$$\exp(-U(0.05, 0.2)^*(t - t_{meal})$$

To determine the probability of a consumer becoming sick per meal, the following stylized facts were used:

- Approximately 1 in 8 Canadians become ill each year from foodborne illness.[9]
- Consumers have been divided into categories based on how frequently they eat in restaurants: 6.7 percent of consumers eat out daily, 30.9 percent three times per week, and 23 percent eat out once per week;[18] the remaining 39.4 percent visit a restaurant once every two weeks.
- Restaurants are responsible for twice as many outbreaks as private homes.[22]
- Most consumers use poor food-handling practices while cooking at home;[19,20] in the model, 80 percent of the consumers use poor food-handling practices and 20 percent use safe practices when cooking at home. We assume that consumers who use poor practices are twice as likely to contract an illness as those who use safe practices.
- We also know that in the model 1 out of 100 restaurants is contaminated.
- Finally, a key assumption is that agents eat one meal per day; this means the per meal and per day chance of becoming ill are equivalent.

p refers to the probability of becoming ill from eating a meal prepared safely at home.

First, we derive the chance of becoming ill from an average home meal, based on the above.

$(2 * 0.8 + 1 * 0.2)p$ = the chance of becoming ill from an average home meal

Next, we derive the average chance of becoming ill from a restaurant meal, which is twice the likelihood of becoming ill from the average home meal.

$2(2 * 0.8 + 1 * 0.2)p$ = the average chance of becoming ill from a restaurant meal

Next, we determine the weighted average of becoming ill from any restaurant, which should equal twice the likelihood of becoming sick from a home-cooked meal. We assume that there is no risk of becoming ill from a non-contaminated restaurant.

$$p(GettingSickInRestaurant)$$
$$= Fcontaminated * p\left(\frac{sick}{contaminated}\right)$$
$$+ (1 - Fcontaminated)p(\frac{sick}{non-contaminated})$$

Which becomes:

$$2(2 * 0.8 + 1 * 0.2)p = \frac{1}{100} * p\left(\frac{sick}{contaminated}\right) + 0$$
$$360p = p(\frac{sick}{contaminated})$$

Now, we know that certain segments of the population eat at restaurants more or less frequently and can use that to determine the overall fraction of meals at restaurants:

Frestaurantmeals

$$= (0.067 * \frac{7}{7} + 0.309 * \frac{3}{7} + 0.23 * \frac{1}{7} + 0.394 * \frac{1}{14})$$
$$Frestaurantmeals = 0.2604$$

This means that our overall chance per day of contracting foodborne illness, or α, is as follows:

$\alpha = (Fhomemeals * $ *chance of becoming ill from home meals* $+ Frestaurantmeals$ $*$ *chance of becoming ill from restaurant meals*$)$

We also know that approximately 1 in 8 Canadians become sick each year, so we must use this in determining our per day chance of illness:

$e^{-\alpha t}$, where t refers to 365.25 days.
The fraction getting sick over a year would be $1 - e^{-\alpha * 365.25}$

$$\ln\left(1 - \frac{1}{8}\right) = -\alpha * 365.25$$
$$\alpha = -\frac{\ln\left(1 - \frac{1}{8}\right)}{365.25}$$
$$\alpha = 2.2688p$$

We then use α to solve for p, the chance of becoming sick per day from a safely prepared home meal: $p = 0.000161138588$

CHAPTER 14

USING COMPLEX SYSTEMS APPROACHES IN THE STUDY OF POPULATION HEALTH AND HEALTH DISPARITIES: SEVEN OBSERVATIONS

Sandro Galea, MD, DrPH
Robert A Knox Professor and Dean
School of Public Health
Boston University

Ana V. Diez Roux, MD, PhD, MPH
Distinguished University Professor and Dean
Dornsife School of Public Health
Drexel University

Carl P. Simon, PhD
Professor of Mathematics, Complex Systems and Public Policy
University of Michigan

George A. Kaplan, PhD
Thomas Francis Collegiate Professor Emeritus of Public Health
University of Michigan

The contributors to this book present a number of illustrations of how complex systems approaches can be used to address questions of interest to the study of two disciplines—systems science and population health. In particular, the chapters attest to the potential of interdisciplinary groups of investigators to come together to advance understanding of the causes and consequences of health disparities, bringing to bear approaches from multiple disciplines to tackle challenging, complex questions.

These projects, most arising from the work of the Network on Inequalities, Complex Systems, and Health (NICH), are the result of several years of work. The group of investigators developed a common vocabulary for bridging disciplinary differences, built suitable models, and tested hypothesis, which resulted in the analyses presented here. As we noted in the introductory chapter, NICH was explicitly designed to bring together scientists from across diverse disciplines to catalyze a synthesis of thinking in complex systems and population health science, with a focus on health disparities.

In this concluding chapter, we highlight seven core observations that stayed with us after the work of the network concluded, which represent both challenges and opportunities. We present them here to surface the tensions that arise in this work. We draw on the work documented in the preceding chapters, to show how the members of the NICH network grappled with challenges and point the way to opportunities may move fruitfully the field forward.

1. Insight from Complex Systems Approaches Depends on Asking the Right Questions

This book is animated by the promise of complex systems approaches for population health, with health disparities as an overriding concern. However, as the preceding chapters amply illustrate, these computational approaches to population health are not straightforward, nor are they quick to implement. This raises the bar for when we should be engaging these approaches; when are they suitable and necessary for a particular question, and when will a simpler, noncomplex, systems approach do? This question urges us to clarify our thinking about which questions that we can (and should) be tackling with complex systems approaches. Our experience with the network and in our own work suggests that honing in on the particular question that is suitably tackled using these approaches may indeed most difficult part of this exercise.

In chapter 5, for example, Stange and colleagues were interested in the primary health care systems, an extraordinarily complex system and one that would defeat any attempt at comprehensive modeling. However, through the use of agent-based modeling focused on a specific representation of the system, Stange and colleagues show that access to primary care actually increased the effectiveness of specialty care in treating individual diseases. Further, their model was able to show that this somewhat surprising finding emerged because primary care physicians refer patients selectively to the right specialist, improving specialist performance over cases where self-referring patients approach specialists whose skills may not be as well suited to their health problems.

Honing in on the right question is particularly critical in emerging transdisciplinary fields, which have not yet built a body of work to educate a generation of scholars in articulating questions that build on was learned previously. In complex systems science, some of the most promising alternative scenarios respond to changing contexts, helping us to understand what might happen if we changed the structural drivers of population health. This is well illustrated in chapter 3, which aims to understand the dynamic foundational factors that produce black-white gaps in obesity; Orr, Galea, and Kaplan show that improvements in school quality take longer, but have a longer-lasting effect on narrowing black-white gaps in obesity than improvements in neighborhood infrastructure for physical activity. This could galvanize a line of work in the field that considers the outcomes of policy manipulations, identifying the time-steps of particular policies and clarifying areas of action to maximize the public health returns on investments. As the field matures other prominent question sets will emerge, furthering our understanding of how these approaches can be used to study health disparities.

2. The Utility of Complex Systems Approaches Depends on the Development of a Shared Language of Scholarship

The contributions of the NICH arose from its explicit efforts to bring together a group of scholars from different disciplines—including epidemiology, sociology, economics, demography, political science, computer science, mathematics, and systems science—to promote a transdisciplinary synthesis that could productively tackle difficult population health and health disparities questions. Fortunately, the network had the gift of time on it side. Thanks to generous sponsorship by the OBSSR at the National Institutes of Health, the network brought together these scholars over an extended time period, giving them the opportunity to get to know each other and understand different approaches to population health and health disparities, develop synergies based on mutual interest, and identify shared questions that would benefit from complementary areas of expertise.

The network's successes, however, also reveal a core challenge to this work. Although solutions for population health challenges—including persistent and intractable health disparities—rest at the interstices of disciplines, science continues to train scholars primarily in disciplinary siloes, such as epidemiologists, computer scientists, political scientists, and biostatisticians. However, the adoption of complex systems approaches to population health rests on bringing these disciplines (and more) to the table.

Trained and socialized within our own disciplines, we frequently share little common scientific vocabulary or explanatory tools with colleagues in other disciplines. Without specific reasons to come together—as was the case with NICH—we seldom meet long enough to generate collaborative work with suitable motivations, shared goals, mutual interests, and time. Our academic systems discourage dedicating time to develop shared languages of scholarship. The path for young scholars on the way to promotion remains quickest within her discipline, applying the tools she knows well from her training to questions that are rewarded by the relevant disciplinary journals and promotion committees. The rewards of cross-disciplinary work are more distant, albeit just, if not more, worthwhile.

The NICH network demonstrated that computer scientists, population health scientists, and others could find common ground to tackle questions that neither could separately. The challenge of how to bridge these disciplinary divides without the luxury of a subsidized network remains. OBSSR has pioneered several educational efforts to help bridge this gap, aiming to create a generation of scientists who are comfortable with multiple approaches and can forge ahead with this transdisciplinarity in their own work; this book contributes to that effort. Chapter 2 (Hammond, Osgood, and Wolfson) presents a synthesis of systems modeling steeped in social epidemiology, and chapter 13 (McPhee-Knowles and Osgood) demonstrates the intersection of systems modeling and the emergence of big data technologies. These chapters can serve as a first step for readers who wish to further their training and apply these methods to their own work.

3. Data Suitability Limits Complex Systems Approaches

The application of complex systems approaches to population health questions rests on the adoption of computational methods that simulate the real and complex world. Most early work in the field relied on simulated data experiments with only scant attention to connecting models to real life. For example, prominent early work in the field illustrated the dynamics behind spatial residential segregation, building on observed norms of behavior but not tied to specific cities, spaces or actual data on individual preferences. This approach gave way to modeling that was grounded in empirically observed data across a range of disciplines. Grounding models in real data allows inferences in situations that more closely mimic the range of conditions observed in the real world, and it may make the modeling effort more useful for identifying the effects of specific policies, a key goal of population health. Perhaps more fundamentally, the modeling exercise itself often identifies the need for data that is not currently available and must be collected in order to improve the model's validity.

Researchers whose work is presented in this book parameterize their models using data from a range of sources, including publically available data and data collected for other purposes. Yet these data are always imperfect for the task. This is well illustrated by the authors of chapter 9, who aim to test the theory that correlations between income inequality and health are contingent on country-specific factors. Their model provides important insights but is limited, as the authors note, by the lack of comparable neighborhood-level data for Canadian and U.S. cities that can be compared to higher quality international data on educational effects on income.

Data collected for particular studies reflect the circumstances of those studies. For example, data may come from a city that is characterized by factors not measured in the data, are from a specific population, were collected cross-sectionally or prospectively, and may or may not adjust or not for confounding or mediating factors. Therefore, the modeler must make decisions: are the available data good enough to parameterize models in a way that can provide generalizable, real-world inferences? Complicating the issue further is that the data needed to parameterize a model to answer a particular question typically come from different studies, often with different populations and measures. The central question then emerges: to what extent can data from different studies be usefully combined, and to what extent are inferences from these data combinations useful beyond the particular modeling exercise? The answer to this question must rest on a careful reading of a particular study and on sensitivity analyses that aim to articulate the boundaries of certainty around particular findings.

4. Useful Models Should be as Simple as Possible, but not Simpler

Albert Einstein's aphorism, "Everything should be made as simple as possible, but not simpler," has found currency in the growing scholarly discourse around complex systems approaches to population health. Like all aphorisms it is undoubtedly wrong, but nonetheless useful. While previously discussed challenges pertain to finding suitable data to parameterize models, the challenge of simplicity rests on an ancillary question: how much data, and how much complexity, do we really need to answer important questions? Computational approaches to population health provide tremendous opportunities to model the nonlinearities, discontinuities, feedback, dynamics, and emergent properties that characterize populations and population health. But to what extent do all these rich characteristics of the systems of interest need to be taken into account to address a particular question? This question bedevils population health modelers, and it is amplified when using complex systems approaches, with their ability to incorporate multiple characteristics. Certainly, everything about a population may matter. But what matters most, and what needs to be taken into account in a particular modeling exercise? For example, if we are interested in modeling a policy environment that might influence physical activity, do we also need to take into account the full set of transportation policies that affect gasoline prices and road construction as determinants of car congestion and likelihood of population preferences for walking? Perhaps. But just as likely we may not need to model this full range of complexity, accepting that some informed and well-articulated assumptions about car availability will do.

This point is illustrated well in chapter 6. Yang and colleagues built two agent-based models to understand how walking behavior within a hypothetical city is affected by interactions with the environment and between people. Several important insights emerge from these relatively parsimonious models. For example, the investigators show that for low-socioeconomic-status populations, improved attitudes toward walking may have a short-term effect, which does not last long unless the environment is modified to be safer. This has real implications for large-scale national efforts such as the Let's Move! initiative, which are broadly based on motivational approaches. In a nice example of how different models provide validation of a concept and build evidence to influence policy, the authors of chapter 7 used an agent-based model to assess the potential determinants of leisure-time physical activity in black men and women. That model also found that improving exercise infrastructure and neighborhood safety are both needed to encourage outdoor activity.

On a different topic, in chapter 11, Kreuger, Flint MacBride and Osgood explore interventions aimed at encouraging preventive care as a way of reducing inter-group disparities in oral health. They show that for persons with lower SES, the rate-limiting step to accessing preventive care is limited material ability, while for individuals of moderate SES, the rate-limiting step appears to be their relationship with care clinics, centering around trust. This provides an example of a "one size does not fit all" set of solutions that can only be understood through the use of models that take into account all the dynamic and complex interactions.

Adding more dynamic interactions to models like this one does not come without costs. In addition to real and substantial costs in human effort, added complexity embeds within it new parameter assumptions and the need for sensitivity testing, which may further shake our confidence in the model's findings, or at the least dramatically enlarge the magnitude of the effort. In the end, these decisions about model parsimony or comprehensiveness must be made on a project-by-project basis, informed by an understanding of the core issues and an understanding of which factors are sufficiently distal from the health indicators of interest. Setting boundaries is always a key challenge in complex systems models. But by being explicit about what is included and what is not, these approaches allow a richer scientific discussion about what may matter to answer particular research questions. In some cases sensitivity analyses can be used to determine the impact of including or excluding factors under different conditions.

The core motivation behind adopting complex, dynamic modeling approaches is the imperative not to oversimplify, and to grapple with the full set of dynamic interactions that contribute to the health of populations. At the same time, adding too much complexity may make models difficult to evaluate, require many assumptions, and shake confidence in model results. The challenge is to find the right balance, and indeed, the modeler's art is to make things as simple as possible, but not simpler.

5. Complex Systems Approaches can Usefully Present "What Happens if" Scenarios

Populations are complex systems and, as such, complex systems approaches lend themselves to better characterizations of these systems than simpler analytic approaches. While recognizing the technical challenges in parameterizing complex models, and the conceptual challenges in focusing on the key questions of interest to which these approaches should be applied, one clearly emerging utility of these modeling approaches to population health is their capacity to help us answer "what if" questions. Population health science is informed by the exigencies of public health, by the pragmatic need to improve health in populations. The tools of public health have, in some respects, served it well over the past century, helping to improve the health of populations worldwide. However, as we enter an era marked by more complex drivers of population health and by diseases with multifactorial roots (e.g., non-communicable diseases such as cardiovascular disease), it will be more useful to have in our population health science armamentarium the capacity to model the potential impacts of different manipulations of the multiple factors that produce health.

In the era dominated by infectious disease, the improvement of population health rested on efforts to eradicate the infectious agent, minimize its transmission, and to treat related pathologies. In an era dominated by complex health concerns such as obesity, hypertension, and diabetes, it is far less clear where the best return on investment for public health action lies. Is it in improving walkable environments, restricting trans fats in food, or changing dietary guidelines? Complex systems approaches allow alternate *in silico* environments to be considered where these different manipulations can be considered as complements or substitutes, under scenarios of resource constraints. We now have an opportunity to ask, "What happens if we change dietary guidelines?" or, "Would changing dietary guidelines have a greater impact than efforts to restrict trans fats?" Clearly our capacity to usefully address these "what if" questions is circumscribed by the accuracy of our complex systems approaches themselves. But even here, identifying data to fully parameterize our models can become a virtue. Sensitivity analyses provide the clarity to pursue "what happens if...within a range of assumptions" questions, which both (1) allow the articulation of the potential outcomes of interventions, and (2) allow us to understand those outcomes while testing the robustness of the assumptions informing our scenario-planning. In pushing us to highlight the assumptions that inform our thinking, complex systems approaches bring clarity to our quantitative scholarship. In particular, these approaches help us find answers to questions that simply cannot be answered in other ways.

This is illustrated elegantly in chapter 4, in which Boyce and colleagues pursue questions around classroom hierarchy and its role in well-being and depression, using an agent-based model. They aptly note that such models are an *in silico* laboratory, which can provide a "plausible and useful alternative" to conducting national randomized experiments that may be too costly to be feasible, and perhaps unethical. This point is further made, on an entirely different topic in chapter 12. Wolfson and Rowe simulate what a measure of population health—the Health Adjusted Life Expectancy (HALE)—would be in the counter factual world. Their results are provocative and surprising, including, for example, that a world where everyone is always somewhat overweight, with a body mass index of 27, was protective for overall health, in sharp contrast to our current understanding of the role of weight in health. The authors prudently note that "considerable work remains to corroborate or contradict our conclusions." However, in employing models to simulate "what if" scenarios, Wolfson and Rowe succeed in pushing us towards a critical re-examination of observations that have become canonical, and which may benefit from a re-thinking that is grounded in the full complexity of the factors influencing population health.

6. Modeling Can Help Clarify What We Need to Know

Building computational models to describe and analyze population health questions challenges our store of available data, pushing us to adapt available data to the model's purpose while being acutely aware of the limitations of the data available for that purpose. While this is clearly a challenge, it is also an opportunity. Complex systems approaches require an explicitly articulated conceptual model (e.g., a logic model) that describes the how the factors shaping health indicators of interest interact. This leads us to a search for data that can adequately represent the links between and among these factors, in order to parameterize the computational model. It also, however, can lead to greater clarity about the data we do not have, which are needed to build a denser and richer understanding of the drivers of population health and the interconnections between risk factors traditionally considered to act independently of one another. By focusing on conceptual clarity, we can clarify what we need to know and the studies needed to provide data to illuminate causal pathways in population health.

For example, in chapter 8 Kassman and Klassik use agent-based models to assess the mechanisms that lead to racial and socioeconomic disparities in secondary and college enrollment. Their illuminating modeling showed that, for example, even extreme versions of affirmative action based on SES would not replicate the racial diversity that can be achieved in colleges that use race-based affirmative action. These models raise many important new questions for research; they did not address cost or financial aid, and it remains unclear these factors would affect the observed model results. This model provides many answers, but importantly suggests additional policy-relevant questions.

7. Complex Systems Approaches can Help Move the Health Conversation Forward

As currently practiced, population health methods predominantly rest on assessing relative risk, quantifying the likelihood of particular outcomes given particular exposures. While these methods have clear utility and have served the field well, our findings can be difficult to explain to non-scientific audiences. Insofar as the goal of public health is to improve the conditions that make people healthier, its advocates must be able to consistently and persistently translate their knowledge to policymakers who can shape those conditions. The capacity to present simulated environments and alternate scenarios for different policy actions can help to bridge the gap between scientist and policymaker. Complex systems approaches can provide us with common language to inform and perhaps influence action, presenting a tremendous opportunity to translate our scholarship into public health successes. Any such utility is mitigated by models that are inaccurate or misrepresent the world, or that do not have adequate humility to articulate the full set of assumptions that inform their conclusions. However, if properly wielded, the modeling of complex systems has tremendous potential to shape public health. In chapter 10, Simon and colleagues show that agent-based models can be fruitfully applied to help us understand the dynamics of crime within complex social systems. Their model presents a new approach that considers the best types of interventions to reduce long-run disparities in the school-to-prison pipeline, and bolsters hope that the country can tackle an intractable social problem in a new way.

8. Conclusion

It has been a privilege to be part of NICH for the past five years. As our work evolved during the arc of this network's life, the field of complex systems modeling has also blossomed; articles bringing complex systems approaches to population health questions have been published in mainstream journals, and have been presented at high-profile plenaries at professional meetings. Best of all, a new generation of scholars is beginning to grapple with how to make these methods another tool to help reduce health disparities and improve population health. As these scholars make their mark, it will be exciting to see where the field goes in the next decade.

ABOUT THE AUTHORS

EDITORS

George A. Kaplan, PhD, is the Thomas Francis Collegiate Professor Emeritus of Public Health; a Research Professor Emeritus at the Institute for Social Research; founder and former Director of the Center for Social Epidemiology and Population Health; and a former Chair of the Department of Epidemiology, all at the University of Michigan, He was a member of the Canadian Institute for Advanced Research Population Health Group, and is an Institute for Integrative Health Scholar Emeritus. Among his honors are elected membership in the National Academy of Medicine (formerly the Institute of Medicine), the National Academy of Social Insurance, and the Academy of Behavioral Medicine Research; election to the Presidency of the Society for Epidemiologic Research; and winner of the American Public Health Association's Abraham Lilienfeld Award and the Patricia Barchas Award from the American Psychosomatic Society. Professor Kaplan was also the first public-health scientist to be invited to address the Nobel Forum at the Karolinska Institute in Sweden. Professor Kaplan has published extensively on the links between "social divides" and "health divides," and his work has been cited more than 45,000 times. Since 2005, Kaplan has been leading a major interdisciplinary effort to build bridges between researchers in population health and complexity and systems science, to more fully capture the dynamic, multilevel and multiscale, nonlinear complex processes that produce patterns of population health and health disparities. In that role, he was Chair of the National Institutes of Health–funded Network on Inequality, Complexity, and Health.

Ana V. Diez Roux, MD, PhD, MPH, is a Distinguished University Professor of Epidemiology and Dean of the Drexel University School of Public Health. Before joining Drexel University, she served on the faculties of Columbia University and the University of Michigan, where she was Chair of the Department of Epidemiology and Director of the Center for Social Epidemiology and Population Health at the School of Public Health.

Dr. Diez Roux is internationally known for her research on the social determinants of population health and the study of how neighborhoods affect health. Her research areas include social epidemiology and health disparities, environmental health effects, urban health, psychosocial factors in health, cardiovascular disease epidemiology, and the use of multilevel methods. Recent areas of work include social environment–gene interactions and the use of complex systems approaches in population health. She has been a member of the MacArthur Network on Socioeconomic Factors and Health and was Co-Director of the Network on Inequality, Complexity, and Health. Dr. Diez Roux has served on numerous editorial boards, review panels, and advisory committees. She was awarded the Wade Hampton Frost Award for her contributions to public health by the American Public Health Association.

GROWING INEQUALITY

Sandro Galea, MD, MPH, DrPH, a physician and epidemiologist, is Dean and Robert A Knox Professor at the Boston University School of Public Health. Prior to his appointment at Boston University, Dr. Galea served as the Anna Cheskis Gelman and Murray Charles Gelman Professor and Chair of the Department of Epidemiology at the Columbia University Mailman School of Public Health. He previously held academic and leadership positions at the University of Michigan and at the New York Academy of Medicine. He was named one of TIME magazine's epidemiology innovators in 2006. He is past-president of the Society for Epidemiologic Research and an elected member of the National Academy of Medicine and the American Epidemiological Society.

Dr. Galea is centrally interested in the social production of health of urban populations, with a focus on the causes of brain disorders, particularly common mood-anxiety disorders and substance abuse. He has long had a particular interest in the consequences of mass trauma and conflict worldwide, including as a result of the September 11 attacks, Hurricane Katrina, conflicts in sub-Saharan Africa, and the American wars in Iraq and Afghanistan. He has published over 500 scientific journal articles, 50 chapters and commentaries, and 9 books, and his research has been featured extensively in current periodicals and newspapers. He was a Co-Director of the Network on Inequality, Complexity, and Health.

Carl P. Simon, PhD, is a Professor of Mathematics, Economics, Complex Systems and Public Policy at the University of Michigan. He was the founding Director of the University of Michigan Center for the Study of Complex Systems (1999-2009). He has served as the Associate Director for Social Science and Policy of the Michigan Energy Institute and as Director of the University of Michigan Science and Technology Policy Program. His research interests center around the theory and applications of dynamic systems. He has applied dynamic modeling to the spread of AIDS (in particular the role of primary infection), staph infection, malaria, and gonorrhea; the spread of crime; and to the evolution of ecological and economic systems.

His research team won the 1995 Howard M. Temin Award in Epidemiology for Scientific Excellence in the Fight against HIV/AIDS and the 2005 Kenneth Rothman Epidemiology Prize for paper of the year in Epidemiology. He was named the University of Michigan LS&A (Literature, Science and the Arts) Distinguished Senior Lecturer for 2007 and received the University of Michigan Distinguished Faculty Achievement Award in 2012. Simon was also a Co-Director of the Network on Inequality, Complexity, and Health.

CONTRIBUTORS

Reed F. Beall is a Vanier Scholar and PhD Candidate in Population Health at the University of Ottawa, Canada. He investigates the nonmedical (social) determinants of health, how these health outcomes pattern according to socioeconomic factors, and which policy interventions make the biggest difference for the populations who need them most. He is a mixed-methods, interdisciplinary researcher interested in collaborative projects on intersectoral topics that have implications for population health and health inequities. He is affiliated with the Faculties of Medicine and of Law. Beall discovered agent-based, micro-simulation modelling as an emerging methodology within theoretical social epidemiology during his first year of doctoral studies. He is a research and teaching assistant with Professor Michael Wolfson's research group, which is developing the Theoretical Health Inequalities Model (THIM) discussed in this book.

W. Thomas Boyce, MD, is the Lisa and John Pritzker Distinguished Professor of Developmental and Behavioral Health in the Departments of Pediatrics and Psychiatry, University of California, San Francisco; and head of the Division of Developmental Medicine within the Department of Pediatrics. Previously, he was Professor of Pediatrics and the Sunny Hill Health Centre–BC Leadership Chair in Child Development at the University of British Columbia; a member of the Human Early Learning Partnership; and with the Child and Family Research Institute of BC Children's Hospital. Dr. Boyce has served as a member of Harvard University's National Scientific Council on the Developing Child and UC Berkeley's Institute of Human Development, as well as a founding co-Director of the Robert Wood Johnson Foundation Health & Society Scholars Program at UC Berkeley and UCSF. He co-directs the Child and Brain Development Program for the Canadian Institute for Advanced Research; serves on the Board on Children, Youth and Families of the National Academies and was elected in 2011 to the National Academy of Medicine.

Dr. Boyce's research addresses individual differences in children's biological sensitivity to social contexts, such as the family, classroom, and community. His work, which has generated nearly 200 scientific publications, demonstrates that a subset of children ("orchid children") show exceptional biological susceptibility to their social conditions and bear higher risks of illness and developmental disorders in settings of adversity and stress. Taken together, findings from his research suggest that the supportiveness of early environments have important effects on children's health and well-being.

Jeanne Brooks-Gunn, PhD, is the Virginia and Leonard Marx Professor of Child Development at Teachers College and the College of Physicians and Surgeons at Columbia University. She is also the co-director of the National Center for Children and Families (www.policyforchildren.org). Dr. Brooks-Gunn is a developmental psychologist who studies children, youth, and families over time. She is interested in the family and neighborhood conditions that influence how children and youth thrive or do not and how conditions at different ages influence development. She also does policy work as well as designing and evaluating interventions for children and families (home visiting clinic-based programs, early childhood education programs, and after-school programs).

Daniel G. Brown, PhD, is a Professor in the School of Natural Resources and Environment at the University of Michigan. His work—published in over 150 refereed articles, chapters, and proceedings papers—has aimed at understanding human–environment interactions through a focus on land-use and land-cover changes, modeling these changes, and spatial analysis and remote sensing methods for characterizing landscape patterns. Recent work has used agent-based and other spatial simulation models to understand and forecast landscape changes that have impacts on carbon storage and other ecosystem services, and human health and well-being. He has conducted fieldwork on three different continents: North America, Asia, and Africa. He has chaired the Land Use Steering Group and Carbon Cycle Steering Group and was a lead coordinating author for the third National Climate Assessment, all under the auspices of the U.S. Climate Change Science Program. In 2009, he was elected fellow of the American Association for the Advancement of Science.

Sarah T. Cherng, MPH, is a PhD candidate at the University of Michigan School of Public Health in the Department of Epidemiology and at the Center for Social Epidemiology and Population Health. She has a broad background in health policy and health care operations research, and focuses primarily on machine learning, agent-based modeling, and other complex adaptive systems research methods.

Amanda M. Dettmer-Erard, PhD, is a Senior Postdoctoral Fellow at the Laboratory of Comparative Ethology at the Eunice Kennedy Shriver National Institute of Child Health and Human Development at the National Institutes of Health. She is a primate behavioral neuroscientist studying the early life organization of brain and behavioral development in rhesus monkeys. Her particular focus is on early life determinants of chronic stress susceptibility and resiliency, and how that chronic stress further shapes social and cognitive functioning across development. Dr. Dettmer earned her PhD at the University of Massachusetts, Amherst, in 2009 and has been working with nonhuman primate models of child development since she was an undergraduate at the University of Washington (BS, Zoology), where she graduated in 2001.

Margo Gardner, PhD, is a Senior Research Scientist at the National Center for Children and Families at Teachers College, Columbia University. She earned her PhD in developmental psychology at Temple University, and her BA in psychology at Duquesne University. Dr. Gardner's work is aimed at exploring child and youth development in low-income and otherwise at-risk populations. Her past research has focused on adolescent risk-taking, the development of juvenile offending, and the consequences of youth exposure to neighborhood and family violence. Currently, Dr. Gardner is working on projects related to young adult development, postsecondary access and credentialing, and postsecondary gains among low-income mothers of young children.

Ross A. Hammond, PhD, is a Senior Fellow in Economic Studies at the Brookings Institution, where he is also Director of the Center on Social Dynamics and Policy. His primary area of expertise is modeling complex dynamics in economic, social, and public health systems using methods from complexity science. His current research topics include obesity etiology and prevention, food systems, tobacco control, behavioral epidemiology, health disparities, childhood literacy, crime, corruption, segregation, and decision-making. He has authored numerous scientific articles in prominent journals such as *Lancet*, *JAMA Pediatrics*, *American Journal of Public Health*, *PNAS*, *Evolution*, and *Journal of Conflict Resolution*, and his work has been featured in *The Atlantic Monthly*, *New Scientist*, *Salon*, *Scientific American*, and major news media.

Hammond is a member of the advisory council for the National Institute of Minority Health and Health Disparities. He has served on committees at the National Academy of Medicine of the National Academies of Science, including one assembled for a recent report on the food system, and he serves as a Public Health Advisor at the National Cancer Institute and as an advisory Special Government Employee at the FDA Center for Tobacco Products. Hammond is also an appointed member of the newly formed Lancet Commission on Obesity. He has been a member of four research networks funded by the National Institutes of Health using complex systems approaches: MIDAS (Models of Infectious Disease Agent Study), ENVISION (part of the National Collaborative on Childhood Obesity Research), NICH (Network on Inequality, Complexity, and Health), and SCTC (State and Community Tobacco Control). Hammond currently holds academic appointments at the Harvard School of Public Health, the Santa Fe Institute, and Washington University in St. Louis. He has taught computational modeling at Harvard, the University of Michigan, the National Cancer Institute, and the NIH/CDC Institute on Systems Science and Health.

Laura Homa, PhD, is a Research Associate in the Department of Family Medicine at Case Western Reserve University. She received her PhD in applied mathematics from CWRU in 2013. Her research interests include mathematical modeling of complex systems, and her current work is in developing a mathematical model of the natural history of colorectal cancer recurrence.

Peter S. Hovmand, PhD, MSW, is an Associate Professor of Practice and the founding director of the Brown School's Social System Design Lab at Washington University in St. Louis. His research and practice focus on advancing participatory group model building methods to involve communities and other stakeholders in the process of understanding system behavior and finding high-leverage solutions using system dynamics computer modeling and simulation. His most recent work focuses on the social determinants of health, from a feedback perspective with applications in energetics and cancer, sexual assault prevention, child and maternal health, and obesity prevention.

Matt Kasman, PhD, is a research associate at the Brookings Institution Center on Social Dynamics and Policy. He received his doctorate in Educational Policy at Stanford University in 2014. Through both his doctoral research and work at Brookings he has gained extensive experience in applying complex systems approaches to educational policy analysis, public health topics, and biological systems. His current research interests include school choice, affirmative action in higher education, teacher labor markets, educational equity, tobacco regulatory policy, and childhood obesity prevention efforts.

Daniel Klasik, PhD, is an Assistant Professor of Higher Education Administration at the George Washington University Graduate School of Education and Human Development. He has professional experience working both in selective college admissions and doing education policy research. He received his doctorate in Education Policy from Stanford University. In his research, he investigates inequality in college opportunity, access, and choice. This agenda includes looking at how individuals make college enrollment decisions, and how federal, state, and institutional policies influence students' college enrollment and success.

Alison Kraus, MSW, received a Bachelor of Arts in psychology and political science from Washington University in St. Louis. She received a Master of Social Work with a clinical mental health concentration, also from Washington University in St. Louis. Kraus's practice focuses on engaging communities and stakeholders in understanding systems and designing systemic solutions to community-level challenges. She has applied group methods in clinical settings and participatory processes, such as group model building. During her tenure at the Social System Design Lab, Alison facilitated projects in application areas including maternal and child health, mental health, cancer, obesity, educational equity, and designing for sustainability and scale-up. Kraus currently works for a behavioral health collective impact organization in the St. Louis, Missouri, region.

Kurt Kreuger, MSc, is a PhD student in the Computer Science department of the University of Saskatchewan. His background is in engineering (BEng) and physics (MSc). He has worked as an electrical engineer and as a university lecturer. His current work involves using various dynamic modeling techniques, including agent-based system dynamics and discrete event approaches, to study issues of health inequalities and human behavior. This transition to the computational field was motivated by his desire to use his STEM training in the public health discourse. Currently, Kreuger's interests are in human behavior modeling for tobacco addiction, where he is collaborating with National Institutes of Health researchers on building behavioral simulations of human addiction patterns. Much of his work has used iEpi, a smartphone-based tool that gathers micro-level person data and allows the interpreting of participant location, activity, and day-night cycles, alongside more traditional ecological momentary assessment surveys, all correlated in time. Kreuger is interested in how this powerful microdata can be more meaningfully integrated with dynamic simulation models, and he is currently undertaking studies of this type in the area of cigarette and e-cigarette use.

Shiriki Kumanyika, PhD, MPH, is a Professor Emerita at the University of Pennsylvania and Research Professor in Community Health and Prevention at the Drexel University Dornsife School of Public Health. During her 15-year tenure at Penn, Dr. Kumanyika was Professor of Epidemiology in Biostatistics and Epidemiology, with a secondary appointment in Pediatrics, and Associate Dean for Health Promotion and Disease Prevention in the School of Medicine. She was also the founding director of Penn's university-wide,

Master of Public Health program. Dr. Kumanyika's research over more than three decades has focused on the primary and secondary prevention of chronic diseases related to nutrition and obesity, with a particular focus on improving the health profiles of black Americans in these areas. At Drexel, she leads the African American Collaborative Obesity Research Network (AACORN), which she founded in 2002 and continues to chair. AACORN is a national affinity group and collaboration platform for academic and community-based researchers and research partners with a commitment to addressing nutrition, physical activity, and weight issues in black American communities.

Dr. Kumanyika is a member of the National Academy of Medicine (formerly the Institute of Medicine [IOM]) and chaired the IOM standing committee on obesity prevention from 2008 to 2013. She was Vice-Chair of the U.S. Department of Health and Human Services Secretary's Advisory Committee on National Health Promotion and Disease Prevention Objectives for 2020; is immediate past President of the American Public Health Association; and is a member of the Centers for Disease Control and Prevention Task Force on Community Preventive Services. In the international sphere, Dr. Kumanyika co-chairs the Policy and Prevention Section of the World Obesity Federation and is a nutrition advisor to the World Health Organization, the World Cancer Research Fund, and the Access to Nutrition Foundation. She has pursued her interest in systems-science approaches to addressing critical public health issues through membership in the Network on Inequality, Complexity, and Health and the Johns Hopkins Global Center on Obesity Prevention.

Bobbi S. Low, PhD, is a Professor of Resource Ecology in the School of Natural Resources and Environment, University of Michigan. Her research focuses on the use of evolutionary theory to understand human activities, particularly patterns of resource use and conservation. Her studies include resources and reproductive variance, and reproductive and resource trade-offs for modern women. She has authored or co-authored over 120 reviewed papers and six books, including *Why Sex Matters: A Darwinian Look at Human Behavior*. 2nd ed. (Princeton University Press).

She was co-founder and President of the Human Behavior and Evolution Society and the Director of the Evolution and Human Adaptation Program at the University of Michigan. In 2007 she was awarded the University of Michigan's Outstanding Graduate Mentor Award.

Robin Flint MacBride, MPH, is doctoral candidate (DrPH) in Health Policy and Management at the UCLA Fielding School of Public Health, and she holds a lecturer appointment in the UCLA Section of Pediatric Dentistry. She has over 20 years of experience directing and managing state and federal grants related to improving access to quality care for children. Her research interests include systems of care and quality improvement, health behaviors, population health and health disparities, policy issues, and the use of complex systems approaches. Her dissertation applies complex systems and dynamic modeling to examine the relationship between dental clinical practices, caries, and population oral health; its ultimate goal is to understand current system drivers, determine health optimization strategies, and reduce expenditures and health disparities.

Austen Mack-Crane is a research assistant at the Brookings Institution Center on Social Dynamics and Policy. He has experience designing and implementing agent-based and microeconomic models of social systems with diverse applications including game theory, social-ecological interactions, public health, network analysis, and community dynamics.

David B. McMillon is a doctoral student at the University of Chicago's Harris School of Public Policy. He was a Marjorie Lee Brown Fellow at the University of Michigan, where he earned two Master's degrees, in Applied Mathematics and Operations Research. He was awarded the National Science Foundation's Graduate Research Fellowship Honorable Mention and the Ford Fellowship in 2014. His research interests lie in the application of cutting-edge quantitative techniques and complex systems theory to contemporary issues in social policy that affect low-income groups. He constructs mathematical and agent-based models of the spread of crime, mass incarceration, and the school-to-prison pipeline. These interests emerge from the combination of his mathematical training, upbringing in inner city Saginaw, Michigan, and conviction that systems thinking is the key to generating sustainable improvements in social and urban policy.

Sara McPhee-Knowles, PhD, is a policy analyst with the Government of Yukon. Prior to entering the public service, she completed her PhD in public policy at the Johnson-Shoyama Graduate School of Public Policy at the University of Saskatchewan. Her research interests include the application of agent-based models to the policy cycle, specifically focusing on modeling food safety inspection systems and consumer choices.

Jeffrey Morenoff, PhD, is a Professor in the Department of Sociology at the Gerald R. Ford School of Public Policy, and at the Institute for Social Research, University of Michigan. He is also the Director of the Population Studies Center at the University of Michigan. He conducts research on neighborhood environments and their influence on health and well-being, the causes and consequences of crime, and the influence of the criminal justice system on population dynamics and the health and well-being of people with criminal records. In 2014, he was recognized in the Thomson Reuters list of Highly Cited Researchers 2014, ranking him among the top 1 percent most cited for his subject field in that year.

Mark G. Orr, PhD, is a Research Associate Professor, Social and Decision Analytics Laboratory, Biocomplexity Institute of Virginia Tech. He was originally trained as a cognitive psychologist at the University of Illinois at Chicago and had postdoctoral fellowships in computational modeling (Carnegie Mellon), neuroscience (Albert Einstein College of Medicine), and epidemiology/complex systems (Columbia University). Over the past decade, his work has focused on understanding dynamic processes and drivers of risky behavior and decision-making, primarily in a public health context, at the scale of the individual and populations.

Nathaniel D. Osgood, PhD, is an Associate Professor in the Department of Computer Science and Associate Faculty in the Department of Community Health and Epidemiology at the University of Saskatchewan. His research is focused on providing cross-linked simulation, ubiquitous sensing, and inference tools to inform understanding of population health trends and health policy trade-offs. His applications work has addressed challenges in the communicable, zoonotic, environmental, and chronic disease areas. Dr. Osgood is the co-creator of two novel, wireless, sensor-based epidemiological monitoring systems, most recently the Google Android-based "iEpi" smartphone system. He has contributed innovations to improve dynamic modeling quality and efficiency, introducing novel techniques that hybridize multiple simulation approaches and simulation models with decision analysis tools, and which leverage such models using data gathered from wireless epidemiological monitoring systems. Dr. Osgood has led many international courses in simulation modeling and health around the world, and his online videos on the subject attract thousands of views per month. Prior to joining the University of Saskatchewan faculty, he served as a Senior Lecturer at the Massachusetts Institute of Technology and worked for a number of years in a variety of academic, consulting, and industry positions.

William Rand, PhD, is an Assistant Professor of Business Management at the Poole College of Management at North Carolina State University. He examines the use of computational modeling techniques—such as agent-based modeling, geographic information systems, social network analysis, and machine learning—to help understand and analyze complex systems, such as the diffusion of innovation, organizational learning, and economic markets. He received his doctorate in Computer Science from the University of Michigan in 2005, where he worked on the application of evolutionary computation techniques to dynamic environments; and was a regular member of the Center for the Study of Complex Systems, where he built a large-scale, agent-based model of suburban sprawl. He previously was awarded a postdoctoral research fellowship at Northwestern University in the Northwestern Institute on Complex Systems (NICO), where he worked with the NetLogo development team studying agent-based modeling, evolutionary computation, and network science.

Over the course of his research experience, he has used computer models to help understand a large variety of complex systems, such as the evolution of cooperation, suburban sprawl, traffic patterns, financial systems, land-use and land-change in urban systems, and other phenomena.

Rick L. Riolo, PhD, is a Research Professor Emeritus in the Center for the Study of Complex Systems (CSCS) at the University of Michigan. He was the founding director of the Center's Computing Lab and played an instrumental role in the founding of CSCS and curriculum development for the graduate certificate in complex systems. Recent projects involve applying agent-based models as part of a wide range of interdisciplinary research projects, including modeling: urban sprawl and its ecological impacts; the co-evolution of cooperation, competition, and other interaction patterns in the context of niche formation; the relationship between phenotype plasticity and the structure and dynamics of food webs; the ecological effects of logging in central Africa; processes that generate inequalities in population health; the spread of antibiotic resistance in nursing homes; and the effect of mandates on HPV vaccination attitudes and use. Dr. Riolo was also a member of the Swarm Board of Directors (SDG) and the Repast Organization for Architecture and Development (ROAD), the two groups responsible for the development and distribution of Swarm (see http://swarm.org) and Repast (http://repast.sourceforge.net) software packages for creating agent-based models.

Daniel A. Rodríguez, PhD, is a Distinguished Professor of Sustainable Community Design in the Department of City and Regional Planning; directs the Center for Sustainable Community Design, a unit within the Institute for the Environment; and is Adjunct Professor of Epidemiology, all at the University of North Carolina, Chapel Hill. His research focuses on the reciprocal relationship between the built environment and transportation, and its effects on the environment and health. He has a distinguished publication record, include co-authoring the book *Urban Land Use Planning* (University of Illinois Press). He serves in the editorial board of the *Journal of the American Planning Association*, *International Journal of Sustainable Transportation*, *Journal of Architectural Planning and Research*, *Journal of Transportation and Health*, and the *Journal of Transport and Land Use*.

Johnie Rose, MD, PhD, is a preventive medicine physician and health services researcher specializing in the development of simulation models of systems involving populations. He serves as Assistant Professor in the Department of Family Medicine and as Preventive Medicine Residency Program Director at Case Western Reserve University School of Medicine. His research and methodological work have involved modeling the population impact of vaccination programs in the developing world, developing methods for stakeholder participation in the development of agent-based models, and modeling recurrence and post-treatment surveillance in colorectal cancer.

Jacob Rosen, MS, is a Co-Founder & CTO of Deftr, a company that uses data visualization and artificial intelligence techniques to clarify and simplify tax law. Previously, he developed quantitative methodologies to detect tax evasion and Medicare fraud for The MITRE Corporation, and also was a complex systems researcher who focused on linguistic evolution and data visualization for agent-based models.

Geoff Rowe, PhD, is a demographer with University of Alberta, and is now retired after 30 years working at Statistics Canada. For much of his career, he worked on the design, content development, and implementation of a range of microsimulation models focused on labor market, taxation, demographic, and health issues.

Kurt C. Stange, MD, PhD, is a family and public health physician practicing at Neighborhood Family Practice, a federally qualified community health center in Cleveland, Ohio. At Case Western Reserve University, he is a Distinguished University Professor, and is the Gertrude Donnelly Hess, MD Professor of Oncology Research, and Professor of Family Medicine and Community Health, Epidemiology and Biostatistics, Oncology and Sociology. He is an American Cancer Society Clinical Research Professor, and serves as editor for the *Annals of Family Medicine* (www.AnnFamMed.org). He is working on Promoting Health Across Boundaries (www.PHAB.us), and is active in practice-based, multimethod, participatory research and development that aims to understand and improve primary health care and community health. He is a member of the National Academy of Medicine.

Stephen J. Suomi, PhD, is Chief of the Laboratory of Comparative Ethology at the Eunice Kennedy Shriver National Institute of Child Health and Human Development (NICHD), National Institutes of Health in Bethesda, Maryland. Dr. Suomi was a Professor at the University of Wisconsin-Madison before moving to the NICHD in 1983. Dr. Suomi's present research at the NICHD focuses on the general issues: the interaction between genetic and environmental factors in shaping individual developmental trajectories; the issue of continuity versus change and the relative stability of individual differences at multiple level of analysis throughout development; and the degree to which findings from monkeys studied in captivity generalize not only to monkeys living in the wild but also to humans living in different cultures. He has been the recipient of numerous awards and honors, including the Donald O. Hebb Award and a Presidential Citation from the American Psychological Association, the Distinguished Primatologist Award from the American Society of Primatologists, and the Arnold Pfeffer Prize from the International Society of Neuropsychoanalysis. To date, he has authored or co-authored over 450 articles published in scientific journals and chapters in edited volumes.

Melicia C. Whitt-Glover, PhD, is President and CEO of Gramercy Research Group, an independent research firm in Winston-Salem, North Carolina. She is also Director of Community Outreach and Engagement in the Maya Angelou Center for Health Equity at Wake Forest School of Medicine, and a Charter Member of the African American Collaborative Obesity Research Network. Dr. Whitt-Glover is currently involved in community-based/community-engaged research studies designed to identify effective strategies to increase weight loss and weight gain prevention, and to promote adherence to national recommendations for diet and physical activity in high-risk populations. Dr. Whitt-Glover served on the faculties at the University of Pennsylvania School of Medicine and Wake Forest University School of Medicine before starting Gramercy Research Group in 2009.

Michael C. Wolfson, PhD, is Canada Research Chair in Population Health Modeling/Populomics in the Faculty of Medicine at the University of Ottawa. With training in mathematics, computer science, and economics, he was formerly Assistant Chief Statistician, Analysis and Development (which included the Health Statistics program and the central R&D function) at Statistics Canada in 2009. Prior to joining Statistics Canada, he held increasingly senior positions in the Treasury Board Secretariat, the Department of Finance, the Privy Council Office, the House of Commons, and the Deputy Prime Minister's Office. While a senior public servant, he was also a founding Fellow of the Canadian Institute for Advanced Research Program in Population Health.

Yong Yang, PhD, is an Assistant Professor in the School of Public Health at the University of Memphis. He holds degrees in geography and health geography. His research examines how human health-related behaviors including physical activities are influenced by the built and social environments, how to estimate the corresponding impacts on humans' health, and to provide implications for policy interventions. As an interdisciplinary researcher, his research is based on the integration of methodologies from Epidemiology, Systems Science, and Geography. He has served as a reviewer for more than 30 academic journals and grant agencies including the European Research Council, Medical Research Council (UK), Economic and Social Research Council (UK), and Swiss National Science Foundation.

CPSIA information can be obtained
at www.ICGtesting.com
Printed in the USA
LVOW09s1501010617
536600LV00004B/59/P